A Textbook of
Community Nursing

Edited by
SUE CHILTON, HEATHER BAIN,
ANN CLARRIDGE and KAREN MELLING

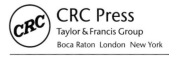
CRC Press
Taylor & Francis Group
Boca Raton London New York

CRC Press is an imprint of the
Taylor & Francis Group, an **informa** business

CRC Press
Taylor & Francis Group
6000 Broken Sound Parkway NW, Suite 300
Boca Raton, FL 33487-2742

© 2012 by Taylor & Francis Group, LLC
CRC Press is an imprint of Taylor & Francis Group, an Informa business

Visit the Taylor & Francis Web site at
http://www.taylorandfrancis.com

and the CRC Press Web site at
http://www.crcpress.com

CONTENTS

CONTRIBUTORS

Fiona Baguley MSc
Lecturer in Public Health/Community
School of Nursing and Midwifery
Robert Gordon University
Aberdeen

Heather Bain
Lecturer/Course Leader BN (Hons) Community Health
School of Nursing and Midwifery
Robert Gordon University
Aberdeen
Chair of the Association of District Nurse Educators

Donna Baker Dip HE Nursing Cert Ed BSc (Hons) RN SCPHN (HV)
Learning Environment Lead
NHS Isle of Wight

Sue Chilton
Senior Lecturer in Health
University of Gloucestershire
Staff Nurse
District Nursing Service
Gloucestershire Care Services

Reverend Ann Clarridge MSc BSc (Hons) Dip Th PCCEA RN DN
Assistant Priest
Holy Trinity Church
Northwood, Diocese of London
formerly Principal Lecturer
London South Bank University

Caroline A W Dickson MSc PG Cert Prof Ed BA RN Dip DN RNT
Lecturer in Nursing/Programme Leader for Community Health Nursing: SPQ Community Nursing
in the Home/District Nursing, Division of Nursing
Occupational Therapy and Arts Therapies, School of Health Sciences
Queen Margaret University
Edinburgh

Dee Drew (Dr) PhD MSc DN RN
Award Leader Doctorate in Health and Wellbeing
School of Health and Wellbeing
University of Wolverhampton
West Midlands

Margaret Fergus SRN RHV PGCE(A)
Lecturer in Nursing Studies
University of Southampton

Helen Gough RGN RM DN BSc Health Studies PgC RNT MEd
Programme Leader MSc Healthcare Education
Programme Leader BSc/BSc Hons Health Studies
School of Health and Life Sciences
Glasgow Caledonian University

Jill Y Gould RGN DN BSc (Hons) CSPPgD Primary Care Studies
Msc Healthcare Education
SPQ/Teacher/Nurse Prescriber NMC
Treasurer ADNE Programme Leader
MSc/BSc Hons Community Specialist Primary Care Nursing
Sheffield Hallam University

Sue Harness PGCE Bsc (Hons)
Community Specialist Practice RGN
Senior Lecturer in Community and Public Health
Programme Lead Community Specialist Practice
University of Cumbria

Kirsten Jack RN BA (Hons) MSc PhD
    Senior Lecturer, Adult Nursing
    Department of Nursing
    Manchester Metropolitan University

Gina King RN DN Dip BSc
    Clinical Facilitator for End of Life Care
    NHS Gloucestershire(Hons)
    Chair of the EoLC Facilitators Regional Network (South West)

Helen R McVeigh MA BSc (Hons) RNT RGN
    Senior Lecturer in Primary Care
    School of Nursing and Midwifery
    De Montfort University
    Leicester

Karen Melling TD MA PGCEA RDNT PWT DN RN SEN
    Formerly Course Leader Specialist
    Practitioner Community Nursing Programme

Sue Miller RGN RSCN, DN, Cert Ed, BSc (Hons), MSc

Virginia Radcliffe MA BSc (Hons) SPDN N Prescriber RNT RN
    Senior Lecturer in Nursing and Prescribing
    Centre for Primary Health & Social Care
    London Metropolitan University

Mark Rawlinson RGN DNCert/Dip BA (Hons) PCED CPT
    Pathway Leader
    District Nursing Faculty of Health Sciences
    University of Southampton

Jo Skinner
    Director of the Centre for Health and Social Care
    London Metropolitan University

Anne Smith MSc BSc (Hons) (Dist Nurs) PGCHE QN RN
    Honorary Fellow
    University of Reading
    Berkshire

Debra Smith MA BSc (Hons) DN RN
    Senior Lecturer in Primary Care
    School of Health and Wellbeing
    University of Wolverhampton
    West Midlands

Sally Sprung MA BSc (Hons) SPDN RNT QN
    Programme leader for Specialist Community Practitioner Programmes
    Liverpool John Moores University
    Member of the Association of District Nurse Educators

Rose Stark BSc (Hons) MA PGCE
    Senior Lecturer, Primary Care
    Faculty of Health & Social Care
    London South Bank University
    London

Linda Watson PgCert HELT MSN-FNP BSN BScPodM DipPodM
    Clinical Tutor
    Aberdeen Medical School
    Aberdeen

Patricia M Wilson PhD MSc BEd (Hons) RN NDN
    Research Lead Patient Experience & Public Involvement
    Centre for Research in Primary & Community Care
    University of Hertfordshire
    Hatfield

FOREWORD

Community nursing is a specialism whose time has come. It is the lifeboat to the health services' Titanic. After decades of lip service to the movement of healthcare out of hospitals and into people's homes and community settings, there is now real recognition that this must and will happen.

Community-based care is the future. It is no longer a matter of policy or political ideology. It is a matter of demography, technology and economics. The UK has a rapidly growing population of older people, and a continuing rise in the number of people living with long-term conditions. No government can afford to continue to use hospitals as the default option for healthcare delivery. Instead, they must develop, resource and improve community-based services, if people are to receive the care they need and the national health systems – in their different forms across the UK – are to remain solvent and successful.

This is not a new idea. Florence Nightingale called hospitals 'an intermediate stage of civilization' and held the view that 'the ultimate object is to nurse all sick at home'. Similarly, the man who invented organized district nursing in Liverpool in the 1870s, William Rathbone, wrote in his 1890 history of the movement of the reasons why patients should be cared for at home: it would be their choice, rather than to go into hospital; the hospitals lacked capacity to deal with the demand, and anyway were unsuitable for people with chronic conditions; and home-based care was cheaper than institutional care.

It took 100 years for healthcare policy to begin to catch up. Now we can add three more reasons for the move to community-based health care. First, technology has made highly complex care possible outside of acute settings, and freed patients with serious, even life-threatening conditions from the misery of months or years in hospital. Second, the increasing professional freedom of community nurses, and their allied health professional colleagues, has expanded their scope to care. They can assess, diagnose, prescribe, follow up and discharge, completing the healthcare journey with the patient or client. And lastly, but importantly, we are now much more aware of the causes of disease and ill health than the Victorians Rathbone and Nightingale were. We know that the public health, health promotion and safe-guarding roles of nurses in the community are vital to reduce the burdens of disease, injury, social isolation and the health consequences of deprivation.

So community nursing today is more important than ever before. And without a doubt, the demands on its practitioners, so well described in this book, make it a specialist area of practice, for which specialist preparation is needed. How that specialist preparation is delivered has been the subject of intense debate across the four countries of the UK for decades. There have been many changes of approach, and there is now great diversity in opportunity for the aspiring community nurse.

Any nurse in the community, or contemplating a move into community-based nursing, would be well advised to study this book. It maps the territory, explores the professional requirements, and shares the wisdom and learning of expert practitioners. It shows just how different community nursing is from hospital nursing, and introduces the new and different skills a nurse will need. It will help the community novice to chart a safe course across some of the most exciting, challenging and rewarding waters in a nursing career.

Rosemary Cook CBE
Director, Queen's Nursing Institute

INTRODUCTION

Sue Chilton, Heather Bain, Ann Clarridge and Karen Melling

This book has been designed to support staff who may be new to working in a community setting and is an essential guide to practice. We envisage that it will be useful for pre-registration students on community placement, community staff nurses and nurses moving from an acute work environment to take up a community post. The aim of the book is to develop and support nurses to work safely and effectively in a range of community locations.

Community nurses work in a great diversity of roles and a variety of settings – including schools, the workplace, health clinics and the home (Naidoo and Wills, 2009). They empower individuals, families and communities to have control over their health and to improve their wellbeing. They also work across the lifespan, and with a range of social groups that includes those who are vulnerable, experience inequalities and are socially excluded. Not only do community nurses work autonomously in leading, managing and providing acute and long-term health and social care, anticipatory care and palliative care, but they also have a public health remit. They have a pivotal role in health protection, ill-health prevention and health improvement.

Community practice is dynamic, forever changing and in a constant state of flux. Baguley *et al.* (2010) have conceptualized community nursing in Fig. 1, which illustrates that, in the promotion of optimum health and wellbeing, community practitioners work in a range of locations – with individuals, families and communities. The overlapping spheres demonstrate the intricacies and relationships between individuals, families and communities.

Community nursing is complex but essentially falls within the following four continuums, which are all addressed within this book:

- **Birth to death**: they work with all ages across the lifespan.
- **Vulnerability and resilience**: individuals, families and communities fluctuate in and out of vulnerability and resilience throughout their life.
- **Assessment and intervention**: community practitioners work within a cycle of assessment of needs and interventions to address the needs and support individuals, families and communities.
- **Leadership and autonomy**: community practitioners work in varying degrees of autonomy and leadership in advancing practice, evidencing practice and providing the best practice.

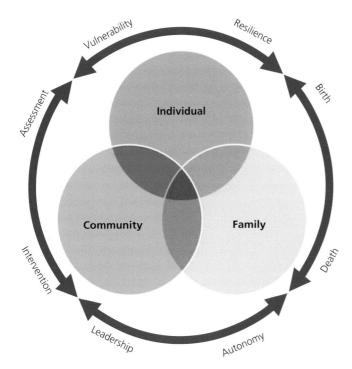

Figure 1 Promotion of optimum health and wellbeing (Baguley *et al.*, 2010).

A range of topics relating to professional issues in community nursing is addressed within the book. The text reflects recent and current government health and social care policy reforms and the effect of these on the roles and responsibilities of community nurses. It is acknowledged that the devolution of political power to the four countries within the UK has influenced health policies. There is now a much greater degree of freedom in relation to the health policies they produce. All recognize the shifting balance of care from the acute sector to the community, with an increasing focus on the management of long-term conditions to reduce hospital admissions. There are, however, various political stances providing differing opinions on how to develop their own health services that take the demographics of each of the four countries into consideration (Jervis, 2008).

Community nursing is seen in the context of not only political but also social and environmental influences. The authors take an inclusive approach, working from a health and social care perspective to meet the needs of service users. Interpersonal and practical skills, as well as the knowledge base required by community nurses, are critically analyzed and linked to relevant theory. The use of activities, examples and case studies/scenarios relating to the range of community nursing disciplines are included throughout the book to stimulate the reader's creative thinking. Themes running through the text are evidence-based practice, reflection, vulnerability and current government policy drivers across the four UK countries. Each chapter has been written by a contributor(s) with in-depth knowledge and experience of the specific subject area, resulting in a range of writing styles.

Topics covered within this text inform key aspects of the community nurse's role. A brief summary of each chapter is detailed below:

Chapter 1 – Nursing in a community environment – explores definitions of 'community' and acknowledges its complex nature. A range of factors influencing the delivery of community healthcare services and the expertise required of community nurses is discussed.

Chapter 2 – Public health and the promotion of wellbeing – analyzes the role of Public Health in community nursing and ways of determining health need. Opportunities for positively influencing care delivery are explored.

Chapter 3 – Professional approaches to care – discusses the concept of 'professionalism', comparing and contrasting the traditional, hierarchical and individualistic model of professional practice with a more inclusive partnership model.

Chapter 4 – Managing risk – explores health and safety considerations in relation to community nursing with particular emphasis upon vulnerable groups – people with mental health issues, older people and children.

Chapter 5 – Therapeutic relationships – discusses the challenges and issues involved in establishing therapeutic relationships between service users and community nurses.

Chapter 6 – Care across the lifespan – considers how an understanding of the lifespan can enhance the quality of care provision by exploring different theories of growth and development.

Chapter 7 – Community nursing assessment – explores the notion of 'assessment' and the concept of need. Assessment frameworks and decision-making processes are discussed.

Chapter 8 – Carers – the keystone of communities and families – discusses the role of carers identifying some of the inherent challenges and rewards. Carer assessment tools and carer support networks are considered.

Chapter 9 – Spirituality: a neglected aspect of care – highlights the importance of developing self awareness and using appropriate tools to assess and address a person's spiritual needs.

Chapter 10 – Collaborative working: benefits and barriers – examines the importance of collaborative working including some of the opportunities and constraints.

Chapter 11 – Approaches to acute care in the community – defines acute care in the community setting and identifies the knowledge and skills required by community nurses to manage it.

Chapter 12 – Emerging issues in long-term conditions – describes contributing factors and the potential impact of a long-term condition on individuals, families and communities.

Chapter 13 – Providing quality in end-of-life care – highlights the importance of a holistic and timely assessment in order to effectively manage the end-of-life care needs.

Chapter 14 – Organization and management of care – critically analyzes work organization and care delivery in the community setting with particular reference to prioritization, delegation and skill mix.

Chapter 15 – Clinical leadership and quality care – explores the role of leadership and clinical governance at practice level within community nursing.

Chapter 16 – Learning and teaching in the community – discusses the importance of identifying learning needs and exploiting clinical learning opportunities.

Chapter 17 – eHealth – defines the terminology used in telehealth and telecare and appraises its potential use in community nursing practice.

Chapter 18 – Development of community nursing in the context of changing times – identifies contemporary political influences and discusses new ways of working and responding as community nurses.

Within each chapter further reading and resources are suggested. You may also find it useful to access the NHS Education for Scotland (2012) toolkit to support Modernising Nursing in the Community, at **www.mnic.nes.scot.nhs.uk**. This is a developing resource which is presented in three platforms: adults and older people; children and young people; and work and well being. Within each platform there are elements to support safe and effective person-centred care. Although the resource focuses on Scottish policy there are useful sections on supporting evidence and examples from practice which can be applied equally across the four countries of the UK, and will complement many of the theories and concepts considered within this book.

We hope you find this book informative and inspirational in developing your professional practice.

The editors would like to thank colleagues from the Association of District Nurse Educators (ADNE), many of whom have contributed to the book. The ADNE (www.adne.co.uk) is committed to raising the profile of district nursing and its purpose is the educational preparation and support of district nurses and other health professionals working in primary and community care across the UK. At various stages along the way, members of this professional group have offered guidance and support.

REFERENCES

Baguley F, Bain H and Cowie, J (2010) *Concept of Community Nursing,* Aberdeen: Robert Gordon University

Jervis P (2008) *Devolution and Health.* London: Nuffield Trust

Naidoo J and Wills J (2009) *Health Promotion,* 3rd edn. Edinburgh: Elsevier

FURTHER RESOURCES

www.mnic.nes.scot.nhs.uk – NHS Education for Scotland toolkit to support Modernising Nursing in the Community

Nursing in a community environment

Sue Chilton

LEARNING OUTCOMES

- Compare and contrast definitions of 'community', exploring the contexts in which the term is used and, specifically, how it is interpreted within community nursing
- Explore the environmental, social, economic, professional and political factors influencing the delivery of community healthcare services and critically appraise ways in which local services aim to be responsive to the specific needs of their population
- Develop insight into the complex nature of the environment of community healthcare
- Identify the skills and qualities required of nurses working in the community and describe a range of community nursing roles, including the key responsibilities of the eight community specialist practitioner nursing disciplines

---

INTRODUCTION

This chapter considers the complex environment within which community nurses practise and offers some definitions of 'community' and ways in which the term is used. It explores the wide range of factors impacting upon the services community nurses provide for patients and discusses ways of tailoring care to respond to local needs. Key skills and qualities required by community nurses are identified and a variety of roles is described, including the eight community specialist practice disciplines.

DEFINITIONS OF 'COMMUNITY'

Changes in terms of the location and nature of community nursing care provision have occurred over the years in response to a variety of influencing factors. More recently, we have seen a distinct shift of services from the hospital setting to primary care and community locations (McGarry, 2003). Current health and social care policy directives indicate that still more services will be provided within the community context in the future (Scottish Government, 2007; Welsh Assembly, 2009; Scottish Government, 2010; DHSSPS, 2010; DH, 2010a). In order to provide the required administrative and managerial infrastructure to accommodate these changes, several major organizational reconfigurations have taken place across the UK in recent years. In England, for example, GP Fundholding was replaced by Primary Care Groups, which then developed into Primary Care Trusts (DH, 1997). Currently, we are witnessing the largest structural reorganization of the NHS since its inception in 1948, involving the development of GP consortia (DH, 2010a), which will have wide-ranging responsibilities for commissioning services and managing 80% of the NHS budget.

Although, from an academic perspective, the notion of 'community' has been discussed widely across a range of disciplines, including sociology and anthropology (Cohen, 1985), clarity with regard to a definitive definition eludes us.

ACTIVITY 1.1

Reflection point
Compile a list of words that helps to define 'community' for you. Identify any recurring themes that emerge when considering different types of community or different contexts within which the term is used.

Laverack (2009) offers four key characteristics of a 'community' which help to summarize many of the definitions found in the literature. These are:

- spatial dimension – referring to a place or location
- interests, issues or identities that heterogeneous groups of people share
- social interactions that are often powerful in nature and tie people into relationships or strong bonds with each other
- shared needs and concerns that can be addressed by collective and collaborative actions.

Although the essence of 'community' is difficult to capture within a definition, the word itself largely conveys a positive impression conjuring up feelings of harmony and cooperation. It is unsurprising to find that it is a word used frequently by politicians within government documents to create just that effect.

The uncertainty with regard to the true meaning of the word 'community' also applies within community nursing (Hickey and Hardyman, 2000). It is pivotal (Carr, 2001) that the context within which care takes place, including physical and social aspects among many others, is considered alongside the geographical location of care. By attempting to include the wide array of elements involved, the true complexity of nursing within the community begins to emerge. Although some of the challenges, such as interacting with patients and families in their own homes, are acknowledged within the literature (Luker *et al.*, 2000), the meaning of community within community nursing is often assumed and taken for granted (St John, 1998).

St John (1998: 63) interviewed community nurses who explained the nature of the communities they worked within in terms of 'geography; provision of resources; a network and target groups'. Some nurses described their communities as a 'client' or an entity, particularly where members of the community were connected. If a population was not connected, nurses defined community as the next largest connected element such as a group or family.

It would appear that definitions of community often include the dimensions of people, geography or space; shared elements, relationships or interests; and incorporate some form of interaction. Many of these common themes are captured in the following definition of 'community' as:

> ... a social group determined by geographical boundaries and/or common values and interests. Its members know and interact with each other. It functions within a particular social structure and exhibits and creates certain norms, values and social institutions.
>
> *(WHO, 1974)*

Awareness of the networks that exist within a community helps in identifying opportunities or strategies to engage 'hidden' members of the population. 'Social capital' is a term used to explain networks and shared norms that form an essential component of effective community development (Wills, 2009). It is proposed that poor health is linked to low social capital and social exclusion where poverty or discrimination exist (Wilkinson, 2005). According to the National Occupational Standards in Community Development Work, the main aim of community development work is

> collectively to bring about social change and justice by working with communities to identify their needs, opportunities, rights and responsibilities; plan, organise and take action and evaluate the effectiveness and impact of the action all in ways which challenge oppressions and tackle inequalities.
>
> *(Lifelong Learning UK, 2009)*

Community development work is inclusive, empowering and collaborative in nature and is underpinned by the principles of equality and anti-discrimination, social justice, collective action, community empowerment, and working and learning together.

A study by McGarry (2003) identifies the central position of the home and relationships that take place within it in defining the community nurse's role. Four key themes emerging from her research are 'being a guest' within the home, the maintenance of personal–professional boundaries, notions of holistic care and professional definitions of community. The findings highlight the tensions for nurses in embracing their personal perceptions of community nursing while trying to work effectively within the constraints of organizational and professional boundaries.

Kelly and Symonds (2003), in their exploration of the social construction of community nursing, discuss three key perspectives of the community nurse as carer, the community nurse as an agent of social control and community nursing as a unified discipline. The authors discuss the proposition that community nurses are still reliant on others to present the public image of community nursing that is portrayed. They argue, interestingly, that community nurses may not possess enough autonomy to define their own constructs and articulate these to others.

FACTORS INFLUENCING THE DELIVERY OF COMMUNITY HEALTHCARE SERVICES

Community nurses face many challenges within their evolving roles. The transition from working in an institutional setting to working in the community can be somewhat daunting at first (Drennan *et al.*, 2005). As a student on community placement or a newly employed staff nurse, it soon becomes apparent that there is a wide range of factors influencing the planning and delivery of community healthcare services. Within the home/community context, those issues that impact upon an individual's health are more apparent. People are encountered in their natural habitats rather than being isolated within the hospital setting. Assessment is so much more complex in the community, as the nurse must consider the interconnections between the various elements of a person's lifestyle. Chapter 7 explores the concept of assessment in more detail. In addition, community nurses are often working independently, making complex clinical decisions without the immediate support of the wider multidisciplinary team or access to a range of equipment and resources as would be the case in a hospital or other institutional healthcare environment. It is recognized, for example, that district nurses are frequently challenged with managing very complex care situations which require advanced clinical skills, sophisticated decision-making and expert care planning (Baid *et al.*, 2009). Barret *et al.* (2007) also acknowledge the need for specialist district nurse practitioners to have expert knowledge and advanced clinical skills as well as highly developed interpersonal skills and a clear understanding of a whole systems approach.

Defining health is complex as it involves multiple factors. According to Blaxter (1990), health can be defined from four different perspectives: an absence of disease, fitness, ability to function and general wellbeing. The concept of health has many dimensions such as physical, mental, emotional, social, spiritual and societal. All aspects of health are interdependent in a holistic approach. It is prudent to view an individual within the context of their wider socioeconomic situation when considering issues relating to their health (Fig. 1.1).

There are acknowledged inequalities in health status between different people within society and major determinants include social class, culture, occupation, income, gender and geographical location. Several reports have been published since the 1980s, across the countries making up the UK, providing comprehensive reviews of the literature/research available on inequalities in health (DHSS, 1980; Acheson Report, 1998; Welsh Assembly, 2005; DHSSPS, 2007; Scottish Government, 2008; Marmot Review, 2010). Although these documents have sought to inform the national public health agenda of the day, the reality is that unacceptable inequalities remain.

In England, *Fair Society, Healthy Lives* is the title of the most recent of these reports by Marmot (2010). The main recommendations are:

- giving every child the best start in life
- enabling all children, young people and adults to maximize their capabilities and have control over their lives
- creating fair employment and good work for all

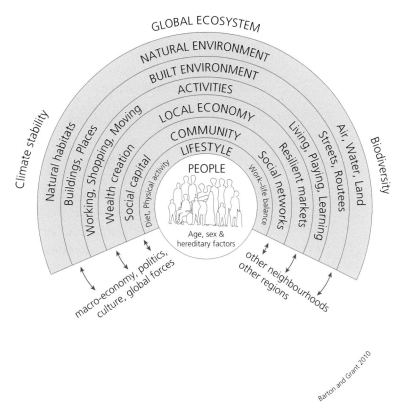

Figure 1.1 The health map (Barton and Grant, 2010). The determinants of health and wellbeing in our neighbourhoods.

- ensuring a healthy standard of living for all
- creating and developing healthy and sustainable places and communities
- strengthening the role and impact of ill-health prevention.

The report states that people living in more disadvantaged communities die 7 years earlier on average than people living in more prosperous communities. Those in the poorest neighbourhoods will also experience more of their lives with a disability – an average difference of 17 years.

In order to improve health inequalities, Marmot (2010) suggests that health professionals, including community nurses, can contribute in three ways. First, they can help to remove any social and ethnic barriers to receiving healthcare. Second, they should act as advocates for their service users and work in collaboration with other health and social care providers. Finally, they should base health improvement initiatives/best practice on rigorous evidence and research so that strategies used are effective and replicable. In response to this, the DH (2010b) recognizes that disadvantaged areas face the toughest challenges and are set to receive greater rewards for any health improvements made.

The increased emphasis lately on the development of a primary care-led NHS has come about in response to demographic, technological, political and financial influences, among others. An increasing population of older people, shorter hospital stays, improvements in technology and patient preference have all contributed to the movement of resources from the acute to the primary care sector.

The development of new competencies to provide services away from hospital settings means that an increasing number of people with both acute and long-term conditions will eventually receive care at home or in a range of other locations within the community. It is envisaged that hospitals will mainly provide diagnostic and specialist services in the future (DH, 2010a).

MEETING THE NEEDS OF THE LOCAL POPULATION

Community nurses can identify the needs of their given population by conducting a health needs assessment, which is a process of gathering information from a variety of sources in order to assist the planning and development of services. As society is constantly changing, health needs assessment is not a static exercise. According to the King's Fund (1994), data are required regarding disease patterns (epidemiology) and public health in a particular area (locality/community/neighbourhood) as well as information regarding local environmental factors/resources (knowledge base/ experience of community service providers). In other words, a combination of 'hard' (statistical/research-based/quantitative) data and 'soft' (experiential/anecdotal/ qualitative) data.

Qualitative information may include newspapers; meetings of agencies; diaries, meeting notes of local workers; projects undertaken by students on programmes of study; photographs and videos. Quantitative data will be obtained from a variety of sources but will consist mainly of statistical evidence and research-based studies (Hawtin and Percy-Smith, 2007).

Three key approaches to health needs assessment described by Coles and Porter (2008) are epidemiological, comparative and corporate. A comprehensive assessment would normally incorporate more than one of these approaches.

ACTIVITY 1.2

Reflection point
Consider the area/team within which you are working at present. What sources of information would help to inform you regarding the specific needs of your client group/population? Make a list and try to divide the information into either 'hard' or 'soft' data.

Explore the different sources of data available to inform a health and social needs assessment of your local community. Much information can be obtained from the local council, libraries and Internet sources (see list at the end of the References list).

In capturing the 'essence' of a locality, the term 'community profile' is frequently used to describe an area in relation to its amenities, demography (characteristics of the population), public services, employment, transport and environment. Traditionally, health visitors, in particular, have been required to produce community profiles as a form of assessment during their training.

'Community profiling' can be defined as:

> a comprehensive description of the needs of a population that is defined, or defines itself, as a community and the resources that exist within that community, carried out with the active involvement of the community itself, for the purpose of developing an action plan or other means of improving the quality of life of the community.
>
> *(Hawtin and Percy-Smith, 2007: 10)*

There are three interacting levels identified within profiling, which are:

- community – assessment of need within a locality/neighbourhood
- practice – assessment of need within a GP practice
- caseload – assessment of need within a health professional's caseload.

Any attempt to analyze the series of complex processes that makes up a living community without the participation of local residents/consumers is a fairly fruitless exercise. In gathering information from a large community population, a variety of methods may prove useful. An approach entitled Participatory Rapid Appraisal has been described elsewhere (Coles and Porter, 2008) and involves community members in the collection of information and related decision-making. Originally used in developing countries to assess need within poor rural populations, it has been employed in deprived urban areas. A wide variety of data-collection methods is used and Participatory Rapid Appraisal involves local agencies and organizations working together. By working in partnership with local residents, action is taken by community members who have identified issues of local concern/interest and discussed potential solutions. Clearly, Participatory Rapid Appraisal could be used to help tackle specific issues as well as large-scale assessments.

Current government policy (DH, 2010a,b) stresses the importance of a localized approach to community healthcare service provision. Each locality is different in terms of its characteristics, which might include its demography, geographical location, environment, amenities, transport systems, unemployment levels, deprivation scores, work opportunities and access to services, for example. As a result of these potential variations, it is important to interpret national guidelines according to local needs. Each locality will have its own individualized local targets for public health tailored to the specific requirements of the local population. Such targets are usually chosen following an examination of local information sources, such as epidemiological data collected by the Public Health department, general practice profiles and caseload analysis data obtained from local healthcare practitioners, for example.

By systematically reviewing local information sources and working within government/professional guidelines, community nurses have an opportunity to develop practice and more collaborative ways of working.

Example 1.1

From general practice profile information, one locality identified a significantly high percentage of the older population with dementia. As a result, the community psychiatric nurse team working with older people in the locality liaised with the district nurses and practice nurses across the identified GP practices with a view to discussing the provision of support for the carers involved.

DH (2010a) highlights the importance of frontline staff taking responsibility for implementing changes in the NHS. This will involve community nurses becoming more actively involved in health needs assessment. It has been recognized that there are populations whose healthcare needs are unmet (Coles and Porter, 2008), which presents community nurses with the challenge of redefining their services to more accurately respond to the needs of their particular patient group. Responding more appropriately is not an easy task as many of these unmet needs often require seeking out and might exist within the more disadvantaged sectors of society. It is not unreasonable to assume that many community nurses will require a greater understanding of different cultural issues and social value systems before they are able to identify specific unmet needs. The inverse care law means that, ironically, the more advantaged people in society tend to receive better healthcare services (Acheson, 1998). Current NHS policy is attempting to rectify this anomaly and end the so-called 'postcode lottery', which suggests you are able to determine your health status from the place where you live.

Although National Service Frameworks (NSFs) are national guidelines produced to encourage the dissemination of best practice in relation to particular conditions or client groups, it is the responsibility of frontline staff to implement them locally and interpret them according to local conditions.

ACTIVITY 1.3

Action point
In relation to the locality in which you are based within the community, find out about ways in which the NSFs are being implemented at a local level. Gather information regarding local initiatives and examples of any community nurses working in collaboration with other individuals/organizations/agencies in addressing the NSF guidelines.

THE COMPLEX NATURE OF THE ENVIRONMENT OF COMMUNITY HEALTHCARE

Kelly and Symonds (2003) discuss how community nurses have been obliged to conform to current views and power structures since the beginning of the nineteenth century. Even the caring nature of their role has been often overlooked as a result of influence from more powerful groups to conform to more stereotypical female roles and medical models of care. Recent shifts into community and primary healthcare have prompted community nurses to re-examine their position, which has involved empowering the more disadvantaged groups within society in the form of 'social support'. However, the development of the caring aspect of community nursing has been compromised by models of primary healthcare delivery in favour of activity that is more medically rather than socially focused.

A new understanding of community care as 'process' rather than 'context' is proposed by Clarke (1999) to enable us to value community nursing as advanced specialist practice in its own right rather than as institutional or acute care nursing in another setting. Appreciation of the true complexity of meeting the health and social care needs of service users in the community only really becomes evident with experience. Eng *et al.* (1992) encourage an 'understanding that a community is a "living" organism with interactive webs of ties among organisations, neighbourhoods, families and friends'.

ACTIVITY 1.4

Reflection point

Reflect on a health problem/issue that you or a family member or friend may have experienced. Consider the effects of this experience on everybody involved and the health and social care needs that resulted.

- Make a list of the identified health and social care needs of all those people involved.
- Were all of the needs addressed or met? If not, why not?
- Who was involved in meeting these needs?
- Consider the different sources of support, information, care, treatment and advice offered and given. Was the overall package of care well coordinated?
- Were there other potential sources of help that were untapped at the time?
- Were sources of care and support readily available or did they need seeking out?
- Were self-care strategies employed in any way?
- With hindsight, how would you rate the quality of care and support received/obtained?
- What do you consider to be the most important elements of high-quality care provision?

On reflecting on the above activity, you may have identified service providers from statutory, voluntary or charitable agencies and organizations. Individuals responsible for assessing, planning, delivering and evaluating care based on apparent needs may have been professionally qualified or not. Sources of support may have come from recognized services or consisted of more informal networks. Information to help you make sense of the experience could be accessed in a variety of ways. Frustrations, concerns and reassurance at the time will probably have linked to a range of factors – such as interpersonal communication, transport, accessibility of services, effectiveness of treatment, information available and financial issues, for example.

The National Nursing Research Unit (NNRU) (2011) has conducted research measuring patient experience in the primary care sector that included patients with different illnesses/conditions. Generic themes that were important to patients included being treated as a person; staff who listen and spend time; individualized treatment and no labelling; feeling informed, receiving information and given options; patient involvement in care-efficient processes; and emotional and psychological support. The authors highlight the need for policy-makers to start to consider the relational aspects of a patient's experience more – such as compassion, empathy and emotional support – as well as the functional aspects of service provision – such as access, waiting and food. Such information can only be collected from patients and carers themselves.

The community environment is a fascinating yet complicated matrix of elements. There are myriad individuals, groups, agencies and organizations involved in the delivery of health and social care. Potential barriers to effective coordination of services and support include different management systems and ways of working between organizations, conflicting ideologies or philosophies of care of service providers, a variety of communication networks and channels, and power differentials and stereotyping between different groups in society.

COMMUNITY NURSES: KEEPING THE FOCUS ON PERSON-CENTRED CARE

Clearly, there are differences between communities in terms of the locations in which community healthcare services are offered to service users. Provision will vary considerably between a very rural community as opposed to an urban one. For example, in a rural location, there might tend to be more community hospitals, providing more accessible local services that are not of a specialist nature whereas walk-in centres, for example, tend to be located in more densely populated areas such as city centres and airports.

Community nursing takes place in a wide variety of settings.

ACTIVITY 1.5

Action point
From personal or professional experience, list as many different locations as you can where community nurses provide care. This might help you to identify a wide range of community nursing roles.

In the early 1990s, the United Kingdom Central Council for Nursing, Midwifery and Health Visiting (UKCC) conducted the PREP project to clarify the future training requirements for post-registration nurses in terms of education and practice. At the time, eight community specialist practice disciplines were identified and included occupational health nursing, community children's nursing, community nursing learning disability, community mental health nursing, general practice nursing, school nursing, health visiting and district nursing. The UKCC (1994) proposed a common core-centred course for all specialities, which was to be at first degree level at least and 1 year in length. According to the UKCC (1994), the remit of community specialist practice embraces 'clinical nursing care, risk identification, disease prevention, health promotion, needs assessment and a contribution to the development of public health services and policy'. Clearly, a higher level of decision-making is involved in specialist community nursing practice.

A brief synopsis of each of the eight community specialist practice nursing roles is offered below. For a more detailed discussion of the roles of these community nurses, please refer to Sines *et al.* (2009).

Occupational health nursing

Occupational health nursing is a relatively new nursing discipline that has developed from its origins in 'industrial nursing' in the mid-nineteenth century when the role was mainly curative rather than preventative (Chorley, 2001). Occupational health nurses (OHNs) work within the wider occupational health services and engage in preventative activities to advise employers, employees and their representatives on health and safety issues in the working environment and the adaptation of the working environment to the capabilities of the employees (RCN, 2005).

Key skills of the OHN include risk assessment, health surveillance and health promotion and health protection. Attendance management and the use of strategies to enable a successful return to work following an accident or serious illness are seen as important elements of the role of the OHN (Harriss, 2009).

OHNs holding an appropriate qualification are eligible for registration on the third part of the NMC register for Specialist Community Public Health Nursing (SCPHN), which was established in 2004.

Community children's nursing

Over the past decade, there has been a rapid expansion of community children's nursing (CCN) services with a current total of 243 CCN services throughout the UK (RCN, 2008). This development has been supported by a number of pertinent government reports.

There are three key elements within the delivery of CCN services, which are (1) first contact/acute assessment, diagnosis, treatment and referral of children; (2) continuing care, chronic disease management and meeting the imperatives of the Children's National Service Framework; and (3) public health/health protection and promotion programmes – working with children and families to improve health and reduce the impact of illness and disability (DH/DfES, 2004).

It has been acknowledged that if they are to meet the wide-ranging needs of local child populations in the future, 'CCNs will need to change and adapt to new models of service delivery, taking on novel and emerging roles in order to ensure that all children with nursing are managed closer to home' (Whiting *et al.*, 2009: 159).

Community nursing learning disability

According to Barr (2009), there was recognition of the need for more community-based services to be provided for people with learning disabilities living at home and their families in the mid-1970s. Around this time, different models of service were developing around the notion of 'normalization', which is the underlying philosophy of many of the services provided for people with learning disabilities. Normalization may be defined as 'a complex system which sets out to value positively devalued individuals and groups' (Race, 1999).

Service principles for learning disability services should place people with learning disabilities at the centre of care; provide care in an attractive environment; have clear arrangements for safeguarding; provide access to independent advocacy services; be open to internal and external scrutiny; and have comprehensive training in place for staff (HCC, 2007).

The role of community nursing learning disability nurses (CNLDs) has changed markedly over the past few years. It is becoming more health focused and a particular emphasis in the future will be with people who have increasingly complex physical and mental health needs. CNLDs must 'take seriously their role to support people with learning disabilities and their families through the provision of high-quality, person focused and coordinated services' (Barr, 2009: 231).

Community mental health nursing

The community mental health nursing (CMHN) service has been well documented since its inception in the mid-1950s. The expertise of the CMHN lies in assessing the mental health of an individual within a family and social context. CMHNs may be located in health centres, GP practices, voluntary organizations and accident and emergency departments. They represent people with mental health needs and provide high-quality therapeutic care. Five elements underpin the professional practice of CMHNs (McLaughlin and Long, 2009). First, a guiding paradigm, which within CMHN involves respecting, valuing and facilitating the growth unique within each individual (Rogers, 1990). Second, therapeutic presence is needed to restore clients' dignity and worth as healthy, unique human beings. Third, the therapeutic encounter, which is essential for healing and growth. Fourth, the principles of CMHN, which include the search for recognized and unrecognized mental health needs; the prevention of a disequilibrium in mental health; the facilitation of mental health-enhancing activities; therapeutic approaches to mental healthcare and influences on policies affecting mental health, and, finally, the National Service Framework (DH, 1999).

Although several models are emerging in the organization, delivery and evaluation of community mental health services, the guiding principles remain the same. Collaboration between government, local authorities, the voluntary and statutory services, and community groups both nationally and locally is pivotal in improving the nation's mental health (McLaughlin and Long, 2009).

General practice nursing

Nurses have been working in general practice for almost 100 years (Selvey and Saunders, 2009). Since the early 1990s, the number of practice nurses has grown considerably in response to the demands of general practice. The full-time equivalent workforce has expanded by 23% since 1996 (Drennan and Davis, 2008).

Practice nurses frequently fulfil the role of 'gatekeeper' and are relatively easily accessible and acceptable to patients as they are located within GP surgeries. The role of the practice nurse is wide ranging and covers all age groups within the practice population. Three key aspects of the role are first contact, public health and long-term condition management (Selvey and Saunders, 2009). Practice nurses have become involved in the implementation of National Service Framework guidelines at a local level and often play a key role in establishing nurse-led clinics to tackle public health targets.

In order to develop innovative ways of delivering services with a changing skill mix within general practice, practice nurses will require well-developed leadership and management skills in the future (Selvey and Saunders, 2009).

School nursing

School nurses have been employed within the school health service for more than 100 years and are seen as central to child-focused public health practice (Jameson and Thurtle, 2009).

Key aspects of the school nurse's role include the assessment of health needs of children and school communities, agreement of individual and school plans and delivery of these through multidisciplinary partnerships; playing a key role in immunization and vaccination programmes; contributing to personal and health and social education and to citizenship training; working with parents to promote positive parenting; offering support and counselling, promoting positive mental health in young people and advising and coordinating healthcare to children with medical needs.

School nurses holding an appropriate qualification are eligible for registration on the third part of the NMC register for SCPHN:

> With the development of children's trusts and the provision of statutory guidance on interagency working and cooperation to improve the well-being of children and young people, school nurses need to work hard to build links with education and social care teams.
>
> *(Jameson and Thurtle, 2009)*

Health visiting

The health visiting service has been in existence for more than 100 years and has its roots in public health and concern about poor health. The overall aim of the service is the promotion of health and the prevention of ill health. According to the CETHV (1977) the four main elements of the health visitor's (HV) role include the search for health needs; stimulation of awareness of health needs; influence on policies affecting health; and facilitation of health-enhancing activities.

HVs holding an appropriate qualification are eligible for registration on the third part of the NMC register for SCPHN.

HVs need to engage actively in public health work, with individuals, families, groups and communities working collaboratively with the full range of community services (Frost and Horner, 2009). Recent government directives (DH, 2010a) have highlighted the need for HVs to maintain a focus on children and families. At the same time, the profession is keen to develop their future roles in consultation with the public they serve.

District nursing

District nurses can trace their roots back to the mid-1800s at least, and the historical development of the service is well recorded. They used to work in relative isolation but are more likely nowadays to work within a team. The role of the district nurse has evolved over time in response to political influences and the changing needs of the populations served. Although it is acknowledged that the role of the district nursing service is not clearly defined, it involves the assessment, organization and delivery of care to support people living in their own homes (Audit Commission, 1999). The current work of the district nurse includes responsibility for providing pathways of nursing care during acute, long-term and terminal illness (Boran, 2009). The majority of people on the district nurse's caseload tend to be from the older generation – an often vulnerable and marginalized group of people within society.

The Queen's Nursing Institute (2010) is currently lobbying to maintain and develop the role of the district nurse, and Smith (2010) and Cook *et al.* (2011) highlight the need for clear policy, professional standards and funding to support district nurse education in the future.

In addition to the community specialist practitioner nursing roles identified above, there are, of course, many other community nursing roles. Numerous specialist nurses work within the community environment and these include roles that link specifically to a particular condition or illness (such as the specialist nurse for diabetes) or to a group of conditions, such as long-term conditions (Community Matron). Other community nurses work with specific client groups, such as homeless or older people. A range of different titles exists for various roles and often the terms 'specialist' or 'advanced' practitioner are applied. Such a plethora of titles can cause confusion and forms part of the wider ongoing specialist–generalist debate within community nursing circles (McKenna and Bradley, 2003).

THE FUTURE VISION

In order to provide high-quality care to patients, community nurses need the necessary skills, knowledge and expertise, and it is the responsibility of individual practitioners and their employing authority to ensure that appropriate preparatory education and training are organized. Workforce planning assists employing authorities in predicting future demand in terms of recruitment and education of new staff and the continuing professional development of existing staff. In addition, employers develop and update policies and procedures in relation to the clinical responsibilities of community nurses, and these should relate to the latest benchmarking criteria and government/professional guidelines. The views of service users and carers should influence the preparation of health and social care service providers (NNRU, 2011) and evidence will be required that this is the case in the future (DH, 2010a).

Recent government reforms in terms of the structures and systems that form the NHS (DH, 2010a) have led to an acknowledgement by community nurses that their roles and responsibilities need to be examined and redefined in preparation for the new challenges ahead. Leadership, practice development and partnership working are key elements within the roles of all community nurses (QNI, 2010).

Hyde (1995) states that applying the concept 'community nurse' across all the different community nursing disciplines is unhelpful and confusing and that the concept has become popular as a result of the following myths:

- Community nursing is the same as hospital nursing: skills are simply transferred to a different setting.
- Community nursing is peripheral to the centrality of hospital nursing.
- Community nursing is primarily about visiting the sick.
- All community nurses share a unified vision of the nature of care.

(Hyde, 1995: 2)

Kelly and Symonds (2003) suggest it is important for community nurses to critically examine the concept of 'community nurse' and how it has evolved over time if they are to influence their future professional development and emphasize their caring role.

At present, the future educational preparation of many community nursing disciplines is under review by the government, relevant professional bodies and community nurses themselves as current professional standards are no longer relevant and require updating (Cook *et al.*, 2011). At a time of qualified staff reductions due to the economic climate, increasing demand for health services is leading to an emphasis on improving productivity by changing the skill mix within community nursing teams and working in different ways. Many community nurses are fearful that care will be compromised if person-centred approaches are replaced by task allocation models of care. Concerns revolve around the potential loss of a holistic approach, which would lead to fragmentation of care, lack of continuity and poorer quality services.

A recent report by the Parliamentary and Health Service Ombudsman (2011) on the treatment of older people by institutions within the NHS concluded that it too often failed to treat them with 'care, compassion and respect'. Many community nurses are concerned that these findings will be replicated in the community if nurses are not adequately prepared for their demanding and challenging roles. Interestingly, Community Links (2011) has produced a literature review of the role of effective relationships in public services entitled *Deep Value*. This review describes the value created when relationships in public services are effective, including both improved service outcomes and wider benefits for service users. It concludes that improving the effectiveness of relationships is therefore an important strategy for improving quality and performance.

DH (2008: 1) proposes that:

Community services are in a central position ... and of critical importance in delivering our vision for the future of primary and community care ...

increased influence for community staff in service transformation, through a commitment to multi-professional engagement in practice based commissioning and the piloting of more integrated clinical collaborations.

In rising to such challenges and embracing these opportunities, Sines *et al.* (2009) stress the importance for community nurses of developing effective leadership and innovative approaches to practice. They state that nurses must continue to act as advocates for their service users, families and communities and influence local and government policy agendas. In addition, they should maintain confidence and competence in performing risk assessment and delivering safe practice.

REFERENCES

Acheson D (1998) *Independent Inquiry into Inequalities in Health Report.* London: The Stationery Office.

Audit Commission (1999) *First Assessment: a Review of District Nursing Services in England and Wales.* London: Audit Commission.

Baid H, Bartlett C, Gilhooly S, Illingworth A and Winder S (2009) Advanced physical assessment: the role of the district nurse. *Nursing Standard* 23:41–6.

Barr, O (2009) Community Nursing Learning Disability. In: Sines D, Saunders M and Forbes-Burford J (eds) *Community Health Care Nursing,* 4th edn. Chichester: Wiley-Blackwell.

Barret, A, Latham, D and Levermore, J (2007) Defining the unique role of the specialist district nurse practitioner. *British Journal of Community Nursing* 12:442–8.

Barton H and Grant M (2006) A health map for the local human habitat. *The Journal of the Royal Society for the Promotion of Health* 126:252–3.

Blaxter M (1990) *Health and Lifestyles.* London: Routledge.

Boran S (2009) Contemporary issues in district nursing. In Sines D, Saunders M and Forbes-Burford J (eds) *Community Health Care Nursing,* 4th edn. Chichester: Wiley-Blackwell.

Carr S (2001) Nursing in the community – impact of context on the practice agenda. *Journal of Clinical Nursing* 10: 330–6.

Chorley A (2001) Occupational health nursing. In Sines D, Appleby F and Raymond E (eds) *Community Health Care Nursing,* 2nd edn. Oxford: Blackwell Science.

Clarke J (1999) Revisiting the concepts of community care and community health care nursing. *Nursing Standard* 14:34–6.

Cohen AP (1985) *The Symbolic Construction of Community.* London: Routledge.

Coles L and Porter E (eds) (2008) *Public Health Skills: a Practical Guide for Nurses and Public Health Practitioners.* Oxford: Blackwell Publishing.

Community Links (2011) *Deep Value. A Literature Review of the Role of Effective Relationships in Public Services.* London: Community Links.

Cook R, Bain H and Smith A (2011) Educating community nurses. *Nursing Times* 107:20–2.

Council for the Education and Training of Health Visitors (CETHV) (1977) *An Investigation into the Principles of Health Visiting.* London: CETHV.

Department of Health (DH) (1997) *The New NHS: Modern, Dependable.* London: HMSO.

DH (1999) *National Service Framework for Mental Health: Modern Standards and Service Models.* London: Department of Health.

DH (2008) *NHS Next Stage Review: Our Vision for Primary and Community Care: What It Means for Nurses, Midwives, Health Visitors and AHPs.* London: The Stationery Office.

DH (2010a) *Equity and Excellence: Liberating the NHS.* London: HMSO.

DH (2010b) *Healthy Lives, Healthy People.* London: HMSO.

Department of Health/Department for Education and Skills (DH/DfES) (2004) *National Service Framework for Children, Young People and Maternity Services: Core Standards.* London: The Stationery Office.

Department of Health and Social Security (DHSS) (1980) *Inequalities in Health (The Black Report).* London: HMSO.

Department of Health, Social Services and Public Safety (DHSSPS) (2007) *Health Inequalities Report: Second Update Bulletin.* Belfast: DHSSPSNI.

DHSSPS (2010) *Healthy Futures 2010–2015: The Contribution of Health Visitors and School Nurses in Northern Ireland.* Belfast: DHSSPSNI.

Drennan V and Davis K (2008) *Trends Over 10 Years in the Primary Care and Community Nurse Workforce in England.* London: DH.

Drennan V, Goodman C and Leyshon S (2005) *Supporting People with Long Term Conditions: Supporting Experienced Hospital Nurses to Move into Community Matron Roles.* London: DH.

Eng E, Salmon ME and Mullan F (1992) Community empowerment: the critical base for primary health care. *Family and Community Health* 15:1–12.

Frost M and Horner S (2009) Health visiting. In Sines D, Saunders M and Forbes-Burford J (2009) (eds) *Community Health Care Nursing*, 4th edn. Chichester: Wiley-Blackwell.

Harriss A (2009) Occupational health nursing. In Sines, D, Saunders M and Forbes-Burford J (2009) (eds) *Community Health Care Nursing*, 4th edn. Chichester: Wiley-Blackwell.

Hawtin M and Percy-Smith J (2007) *Community Profiling: A Practical Guide.* Milton Keynes: Open University Press.

Healthcare Commission (HCC) (2007) *A Life Like No Other: A National Audit of Specialist Inpatient Healthcare Services for People with Learning Difficulties in England.* London: Healthcare Commission.

Hickey G and Hardyman R (2000) Using questionnaires to ask nurses about working in the community: problems of definition. *Health and Social Care in the Community* 8:70–8.

Hyde V (1995) Community nursing: a unified discipline? In Cain P, Hyde V and Howkins E (eds) *Community Nursing: Dimensions and Dilemmas.* London: Arnold.

Jameson M and Thurtle V (2009) School nursing. In Sines D, Saunders M and Forbes-Burford J (eds) *Community Health Care Nursing*, 4th edn. Chichester: Wiley-Blackwell.

Kelly A and Symonds A (2003) *The Social Construction of Community Nursing.* Basingstoke: Palgrave Macmillan.

King's Fund (1994) *Community-oriented Primary Care.* London: King's Fund.

Laverack G (2009) *Public Health. Power, Empowerment and Professional Practice.* Basingstoke: Palgrave Macmillan.

Lifelong Learning UK (2009) *National Occupational Standards for Community Development.* London: Lifelong Learning UK.

Luker K, Austin L, Caress A and Hallett C (2000) The importance of 'knowing the patient': community nurses' constructions of quality in providing palliative care. *Journal of Advanced Nursing* 31:775–82.

Marmot Review (2010) *Fair Society, Healthy Lives: Strategic Review of Health Inequalities in England post-2010*. London: The Marmot Review.

McGarry J (2003) The essence of 'community' within community nursing: a district nursing perspective. *Health and Social Care in the Community* 11:423–30.

McKenna H and Bradley M (2003) Generic and specialist nursing roles in the community: an investigation of professional and lay views. *Health and Social Care in the Community* 11:537–45.

McLaughlin D and Long A (2009) Community mental health nursing. In Sines D, Saunders M and Forbes-Burford J (eds) *Community Health Care Nursing*, 4th edn. Chichester: Wiley-Blackwell.

National Nursing Research Unit (NNRU) (2011) *Measuring Patient Experience in the Primary Care Sector: Does a Patient's Condition Influence What Matters?* London: NNRU.

Parliamentary and Health Service Ombudsman (2011) *Care and Compassion? Report of the Health Service Ombudsman on Ten Investigations into NHS Care of Older People*. London: The Stationery Office.

Queen's Nursing Institute (QNI) (2010) *Position Statement March 2010. Nursing People in their Own Homes – Key Issues for the Future of Care*. London: QNI.

Race DG (1999) *Social Role Valorisation and the English Experience*. London: Whiting and Birch.

Rogers CR (1990) *Client Centred Therapy*. London: Constable.

Royal College of Nursing (RCN) (2005) *Competencies: An Integrated Career and Competency Framework for Occupational Health Nursing*. London: Royal College of Nursing.

RCN (2008) *Directory of Community Children's Nursing Services*. www.rcn.org.uk.

Scottish Government (2007) *Better Health, Better Care: Action Plan*. www.scotland.gov.uk/Publications/2007/12/11103453/0.

Scottish Government (2008) *Equally Well: Report of the Ministerial Task Force on Health Inequalities*. Edinburgh: Scottish Government.

Scottish Government (2010) *The Healthcare Quality Strategy for NHS Scotland*. Edinburgh: Scottish Government.

Selvey K and Saunders M (2009) General practice nursing. In Sines D, Saunders M and Forbes-Burford J (eds) *Community Health Care Nursing*, 4th edn. Chichester: Wiley-Blackwell.

Sines D, Saunders M and Forbes-Burford J (2009) (eds) *Community Health Care Nursing*, 4th edn. Chichester: Wiley-Blackwell.

Smith A (2010) District nursing: an endangered species? *Journal of Community Nursing* 24:44.

St John W (1998) Just what do we mean by community? Conceptualisations from the field. *Health and Social Care in the Community* 6:63–70.

UKCC (1994) *Standards for Specialist Education and Practice*. London: UKCC.

Welsh Assembly (2005) *Inequalities in Health: The Welsh Dimension 2002–5*. Cardiff: Welsh Assembly Government.

Welsh Assembly (2009) *Setting the Direction: Primary and Community Services Strategic Delivery Programme*. Cardiff: Welsh Assembly Government.

Whiting M, Myers J and Widdas D (2009) Community children's nursing. In Sines D, Saunders M and Forbes-Burford J (eds) *Community Health Care Nursing*, 4th edn. Chichester: Wiley-Blackwell.

Wilkinson R (2005) *The Impact of Inequality. How to Make Sick Societies Healthier*. London: Routledge.

Wills J (2009) Community development. In Sines D, Saunders M and Forbes-Burford J (eds) *Community Health Care Nursing*, 4th edn. Chichester: Wiley-Blackwell.

World Health Organization (WHO) Expert Committee on Community Health Nursing (1974) *Community Health Nursing, Report of a WHO Expert Committee* (Technical Report Series no. 558). Geneva: World Health Organization.

FURTHER RESOURCES

www.ons.gov.uk – Independent information to improve our understanding of the UK's economy and society

www.neighbourhood.statistics.gov.uk – Detailed statistics within specific geographical areas

www.imd.communities.gov.uk

www.census.gov.uk – Index of Multiple Deprivation – statistics available at ward level

www.poverty.org.uk – UK site for statistics on poverty and social exclusion

www.direct.gov.uk – Public services all in one place – according to postcode

www.ic.nhs.uk – NHS Information Centre for health and social care

www.qof.ic.nhs.uk – Quality and Outcomes Framework – GP practice results database

www.marmotreview.org – Baseline figures for some key indicators of the social determinants of health, health outcomes and social inequalities for specific geographical areas

2

Public health and the promotion of wellbeing

Mark Rawlinson, Donna Baker and Margaret Fergus

LEARNING OUTCOMES

- Critically analyze why public health is an everyday part of community nursing
- Critically analyze the concept of health and ways of determining health need
- Explore opportunities to positively influence care delivery in order to improve health and wellbeing

INTRODUCTION

Public health is everyone' business according to Cowley (2007). The aim of this chapter is to encourage all nurses (including pre-registration nurses) to reflect upon the relevance of this statement, and to explore their understanding of and identify their current involvement in public health. The intention is to reaffirm the importance and highlight the opportunities you have as a community nurse or any practitioner experiencing community nursing to positively influence the health of the public and promote wellbeing. This could be at an individual level through opportunistic health promotion, which is the main focus of discussion in the second half of the chapter, or at a community (population) level identified through needs analysis and delivered and evaluated through planned interventions. Throughout the chapter reference to the four underpinning tenets of public health (health protection, health promotion, illness prevention and reducing inequalities (Skills for Health, 2008)) will also be made.

The chapter will initially discuss 'what' public health might be (then and now) by presenting a very brief history about its development, highlighting current government policy. It will go on to explore 'why' public health is important and to whom by considering the determinants of health and the need for the community nurse to be politically aware of such influences, for example how lifestyle choices and living conditions can combine to affect health and illness. Finally the chapter will address (through the presentation of a case study) the challenge of 'how' you can be involved in public health as a community nurse by promoting health and wellbeing.

The activities presented throughout the chapter are there to act as stimuli for personal learning and development; they are also intended to act as catalysts to foster a deeper understanding of public health through reflection and informed discussion.

PUBLIC HEALTH: THEN AND NOW

The concept of health and, conversely, illness has been the subject of much debate in society, both before and after the inception of the NHS in 1948. A major criticism of contemporary healthcare provision was made by Lord Darzi, who observed that the NHS has been overwhelmingly concerned with treatment of the sick, and that it should move from a 'sickness service to a wellbeing service' (Darzi, 2007: 37). This inclusion of wellbeing in policy acts to encourage services to be organized in such a way as to place greater emphasis on social health.

According to Raymond (2005), health has been conceptualized from the perspectives shown in Box 2.1.

Box 2.1 Concepts of health (Raymond 2005)

- A biomedical point of view, which emphasizes medical interventions to treat disease, and is mainly concerned with functional capacity.
- A behavioural point of view, which emphasizes individual responsibility for health-influencing behaviour.
- A social point of view, which focuses on social and political determinants of health and emphasizes social justice.
- A postmodernist point of view, which according to Naidoo and Wills (1998, cited in Raymond, 2005) challenges the adequacy of the preceding perspectives and suggests that no single theory sufficiently explains health experience.

Although this typology does not define what health actually is, it does indicate the differing views from which health can be examined. The World Health Organization (WHO) however did define health in 1946 in its constitution document; its definition came into effect in 1948 and remains unchanged:

> Health is a state of complete physical, mental and social well-being and not merely the absence of disease or infirmity.

> *(WHO 1946: 2)*

Even though the deconstruction of health as a concept is not the focus of this chapter, it is however a relevant point to be cognisant of. The WHO definition reflects a somewhat idealistic view of health, although it does acknowledge that it is a multidimensional issue. Subsequent WHO publications have contextualized this definition and presented it in light of the importance of recognizing the underpinning determinants of health (WHO, 2006). This is particularly relevant when it comes to discussing public health: that being, that health is determined by the wider social milieu within which populations live (Reading, 2008).

In modern times the association between health and social determinants can be traced back in policy to some of the work of the early social reformers. Edwin Chadwick, one of the more well known, produced a report in 1842 entitled *Report of the Sanitary Conditions of the Labouring Population of Great Britain,* (Chadwick, 1965) in which the relevance of social conditions of the poor and their ability to influence their plight were made explicit in relationship to individuals' health. This report to the poor law commissioners resulted in the first Public Health Act in 1884.

Since then public health has been part of (although not always at the centre of) this country's healthcare provision. The UK has seen many different approaches (emphases) to public health over the past 150 years, each reflecting a more detailed/broader understanding of health and illness in society. Activities have included interventions to address inequalities on a population level, through the provision of state education and increased employment opportunities, to programmes of illness prevention through mass vaccination of children. More recently there has been increased recognition of the need to engage in more active health protection, resulting in the establishment of the Health Protection Agency in 2003. Although it would seem that the state has adopted the position of being responsible for the health of the nation, this has obvious limitations, one being that you cannot legislate for all eventualities, especially when it comes down to individual choice! It would therefore seem that if society is to become 'healthier' the state and individuals need to work together to achieve the long-term aim of reducing inequalities and improving life opportunities for all.

ACTIVITY 2.1

The development of public health
The table below identifies key developments in public health over the last century. Consider these developments in relation to the facets of health as purported by Raymond 2005. How has the focus of public health developed over the years?

Nineteenth Century	Twentieth Century	Twenty-first Century
John Snow, Edwin Chadwick (The Sanitary Movement 1842)	First BCG vaccine for TB (1921)	Acheson Report (1998)
First Public Health Act (1848)	Beveridge Report (1942)	Health Protection Agency (2003)
	Founding of the NHS (1948)	Choosing Health (2004)
	Vaccines for Children Programme (1960s)	Healthy lives, Healthy people (2010)

Acheson (1988) defined public health as 'the science and art of preventing disease, prolonging life and promoting health through the organised efforts of society'. This conceptualization became a major influence in the development of what became known as new public health, and ultimately was a main building block of New Labour's health reforms (1997–2010). This vision of the collective efforts of society empowering individuals and groups was clearly expressed in the White Paper *Saving Lives: Our Healthier Nation* (DH, 1999: 3), in which the strategic intent of the government was set out as that being to improve the health of the population as a whole by increasing the length of life and the number of years people spend free from illness; to improve the health of the worst off in society and to narrow the health gap.

This intent was further enhanced by Wanless (2004: 27), who went on to define public health as

the science and art of preventing disease, prolonging life and promoting health through the organised efforts and informed choices of society, organisation, public and private communities and individuals.

Wanless's definition builds upon Acheson's ideas by expanding the definition to include the idea that choice is a critical component when discussing health and the public. This emphasis on personal responsibility signifies the importance of the role of the individual and not the healthcare practitioner when it comes to making lifestyle decisions. However, the role of the healthcare practitioner (in this case the community nurse) is crucial to achieving health-related goals, as community nurses are often in a position to assist individuals to either access services or support individuals in making informed decisions about their health and wellbeing.

In 2010 the coalition government clearly stated its commitment to developing a public health service by producing its vision in the form of a White Paper (DH, 2010a) in which it set out a strategy for improving the nation's health by preventing illness. Central to this guidance is the idea that promoting health and wellbeing through prevention of illness is achievable through the collective efforts of society. Furthermore, it emphasizes that everyone (not just a select articulate few) should have services tailored for them at the right times in their life from the professionals closest to them.

On a global level public health is an omnipresent issue, with the WHO in 2006 reaffirming its commitment to improve the health of all by setting out a framework to achieve the millennium development goals in its eleventh programme of work entitled *Engaging for Health: A Global Health Agenda 2006–2015*. This document, as well as stating an understanding of the determinants of health and the measures required to improve health, recognizes health as a shared resource and a shared responsibility.

PUBLIC HEALTH

Simply put, public health strategies exist to improve and protect health and wellbeing in a population. To apply a degree of depth to this statement, the UK's Public Health Skills and Career Framework broadens this intention through expressing that

the purpose of public health should improve health and wellbeing in the population, prevent disease and minimise its consequences, thus prolonging valued life and reducing inequalities in health.

(Skills for Health, 2008)

Furthermore they consider that this is achieved through a culture which 'mobilises the organised efforts of society' (Skills for Health, 2008) by empowering individuals and by tackling the wider social, economic, environmental and biological determinants of health and wellbeing.

Determinants of health

There is growing recognition of the impact of the wider determinants of health and health inequalities, in addition to the acknowledgement that addressing these root causes of ill health requires public health to be everyone's business and responsibility (Wilkinson and Marmot, 2003).

The social determinants of health have been described as 'the causes of the causes' (LGID, 2010). They are the social, economic and environmental conditions that influence the health of individuals and populations. They include the conditions of daily life and the influences upon them, and determine the extent to which a person has the resources to meet needs and deal with changes to their circumstances (LGID, 2010).

Dahlgren and Whitehead (1991) developed a model demonstrating how health is influenced, either positively or negatively, by a variety of factors (Fig. 2.1).

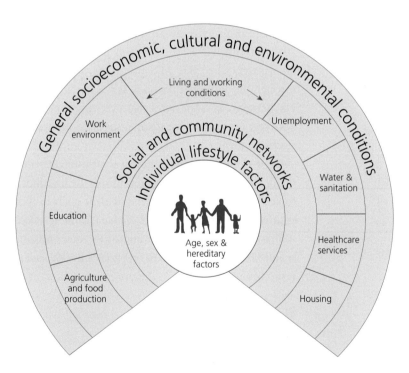

Figure 2.1 Social determinants of health (Dahlgren and Whitehead, 1991).

The centre of the model represents age, sex and hereditary factors, which are genetic or biological in nature. These are by and large fixed entities; however, they lie within the wider determinants of health arising from social, environmental, economic and cultural conditions. Such factors can directly influence our health, or have a bearing on the lifestyle decisions we make and our ability to make such choices. The existence in the UK of inequity in health (unfair differences in health between different sectors of the population) has been well documented in successive surveys of the nation's health, such as the Black Report (1980), the Acheson Report (1998), the Wanless Report (2004) and the Marmot Review (2010). All these reports indicated that socioeconomic factors were strong indicators for health. The negative impact from these determinants leads to disadvantage which can take on many forms. It may be absolute or relative, affecting individuals and communities, for example a single parent living in isolated, low-quality housing, a teenager having a poor education, or communities and populations whose economy is compromised from insecure employment opportunities.

The social gradient, in which social and economic circumstances impact upon health, is viewed as a highly significant measurement of health inequality (Wilkinson and Marmot, 2003). There is a substantial body of evidence which indicates that individuals further down the social ladder have more disease and die earlier (Donkin *et al.*, 2002). This trend within the social gradient and its relation to health is evident among the most affluent countries where measurable differences exist not just in health. These differences are inextricably linked to income and power distribution (Wilkinson and Pickett, 2009).

ACTIVITY 2.2

The spirit level
Visit the website www.equalitytrust.org.uk/resource/the-spirit-level. Watch the short film, summarizing the findings of a book entitled *The Spirit Level* (Wilkinson and Pickett, 2009). This book has been described as 'profoundly important' (Richard Layard, London School of Economics), with the potential to change political thinking on both sides of the Atlantic. Initially the book united the political classes; however, more recently this position has begun to be challenged.

Closer to home the pattern is similar, drawing attention to the evidence that most people in the UK are not living as long as the best off in society and spend longer in ill health. Tackling these persistent health inequalities has traditionally seen government policy funnel resources towards specific individuals or groups within society through targeted services. Public health requires services to focus upon the underlying social and contextual causes of the problems, suggesting that to improve health for all of us action is needed across the social gradient (Marmot, 2010). The previous Labour administration, through key social policies, sought to promote and protect health. The Health Act (1999) saw specific 'partnership arrangements' designed to develop multi-agency services to address the wider determinants of health. However, subsequent health policy (DH, 2000) focused less on public health and health promotion. Recognition of wide and increasing health inequalities (DH, 2003) led to the development of a plethora of policies to address them. The recommendation that public, private and voluntary sectors work together to adopt a 'public health mindset' (DH, 2004, 2006) enabled greater collaboration through the creation of local strategic partnerships in England.

There is evidence that the coalition government's Secretary of State for Health is placing tackling health inequalities high on the political agenda. The White Paper *Equity and Excellence: Liberating the NHS* (DH, 2010b) with its ambitious objectives certainly places public health at the centre of this particular government's agenda for reforming the NHS through plans to devolve greater responsibility to Local Authorities for improving public health.

Complementing this vision, the White Paper *Healthy Lives, Healthy People* (DH, 2010a) claims to be the life course framework for tackling the wider social determinants of health. Underpinned by an empowerment approach, it sets out to harness a population resilient to the determinants affecting health. The principles behind the idea of their 'Big Society', which propose that private and voluntary sectors mobilize to provide a network of effective and sustainable support, will be imperative towards achieving this aim.

Assessing community health needs

As previously discussed, many people, through the influence of social determinants, have measurable differences in their health status. All too often this is compounded by inequitable access to healthcare. Disadvantaged individuals and groups, despite having the greatest overall need, are the least likely to access services (Tudor-Hart, 1971).

It is generally viewed that a need, if met, will result in an improvement in people's health (Haughey, 2008); however, what constitutes need is widely contested. Needs are variable; they can be objective and measurable, obvious or hidden. Conversely, they too are subjective, personal and interchangeable according to context (Cowley, 2008). Taxonomies exist (Bradshaw, 1972, cited in Haughey, 2008) that capture the wider dimensions of need, thus compounding the complexity of it as a concept. Despite this, undertaking an assessment of needs and priorities within populations is essential to improve and protect health and wellbeing as a result of meeting the public health agenda.

Cowley (2008) implies that the contested concept of health, coupled with the added dimensions of what constitutes need, lends a significant degree of complexity to this task. In recent years there has been an increased fusion between health and social care services, a pattern set to increase with local authorities being given lead responsibility for public health and for the first time a ring-fenced budget. However, not all services involved in the delivery of public health will be under the control of local authorities. Community nurses and specialist community practice public health nurses, e.g. health visitors and occupational health nurses, are likely to remain outside the control of local authorities. This fragmentation of service provision, combined with the differing underpinning values, may well pose a particular challenge to conducting needs assessments, in particular when it comes to developing a consensus of what the need is and how to respond to it. The health needs assessment (HNA) has been described as 'a systematic method of identifying the health and healthcare needs of a population and making recommendations for changes to meet these needs' (Wright, 2001). The evolution of the HNA as a tool has provided public health practitioners with a framework for undertaking this complex and important task in an evidence-based way.

Approaches to assessing need

Stevens and Raftery (1994) depict three main approaches to needs assessment characterized as epidemiological, comparative and corporate.

An epidemiological approach to needs assessment, proposed by Williams and Wright (1998), combines the three elements of identifying health status through incidence/prevalence data, effectiveness and cost-effectiveness of interventions, and the current level of service provision. The benefit of this approach is that its systematic and objective method quickly identifies specific problems; however, it can assume uniform prevalence and focus upon medical rather than social need (Haughey, 2008). A comparative approach can be used cross-nationally and locally and compares levels of service provision between these localities, for example the service provision in one town compared with another of similar demography. Thus it is often used to provide a timely and inexpensive assessment. An approach which considers making the needs assessment responsive to local concerns is characterized as corporate. This approach collects the knowledge and views of the stakeholders of the issues being addressed in the needs assessment. The stakeholders can be a collective of practitioners, in both primary and secondary care settings, health and social care service managers, commissioners of services, experts in the field and service users.

Stevens and Raftery (1994), recognizing the limitations of each of the three approaches above, developed the pragmatic approach to needs assessment. This process combines all of the above approaches, drawing upon evidence from a variety of sources, thus offering a more realistic assessment, which, they argue, is needed to support interventions that focus upon the wide-ranging needs of specific communities (Stevens and Raftery, 1994).

Identifying individual and public health needs through the use of assessment affords nurses the opportunity to promote health and wellbeing in the communities within which they work. This can be on an individual level – for example while undertaking a routine wound dressing an assessment of need may identify the opportunity for health promotion in relation to healthy eating. This could then lead the community nurse to investigate the individual's circumstances pertaining to their lifestyle choices surrounding diet and nutrition and in addition give them the opportunity to discuss with the individual how this may impact upon their wound healing. Additionally there are numerous examples of nurse-led projects (www.qni .org.uk/project-funding/funded-projects.html) that illustrate the positive impact nurses can have on improving the public's health at a community and population level, thus demonstrating that when equipped with the appropriate knowledge and skills nurses have the capacity and the capability to influence behaviour change within a health-promoting milieu.

PROMOTING HEALTH AND WELLBEING

Community nurses are involved in public health activity through their day-to-day contact with patients, clients, families and carers; delivering health promotion activity, planned or unplanned.

By its very nature health and the associated term wellbeing are both very difficult to define. Health (as previously discussed) comprises both objective and subjective components and is informed by theories from biological sciences, psychology, sociology, epidemiology and health sciences which all contribute to the understanding of health and the barriers to achieving it for individuals, populations and societies (Seedhouse, 2001).

The term wellbeing was analyzed by the Sustainable Development Research Network (SDRN, 2005), finding that the term encompassed the concepts of life satisfaction (happiness, quality of life), physical health, income and wealth, relationships, work and leisure, personal stability and lack of depression. The idea of health and wellbeing has been embedded in government policy, for example the DfES (2004) document *Every Child Matters*, which set goals in the following areas: for children to be healthy, stay safe, enjoy and achieve, make a positive contribution and achieve economic wellbeing. Additionally health and wellbeing were identified in the Key Stage Skills Framework (2004) as a key skill area for all nurses to achieve and the DH (2010b) document *Equity and Excellence* directed local authorities to set up Health and Wellbeing Boards to commission and to ensure delivery of appropriate services for local public health.

Contribution of community nurses in promoting health and wellbeing

Community nurses are in a strong position to promote health and wellbeing. Their knowledge of the local community and access to clients and their families in their own homes enables community nurses to develop a deep understanding of the factors that influence the health of individuals, families and communities. Their ability to influence the care received by individuals and to influence local health policy development is high. However, the extent of the contribution of community nurses to the public health agenda has been the subject of much debate in relation to its role (WHO, 2001; Clarke, 2004; Carr, 2005), and its contribution (Poulton *et al.*, 2000; Turner *et al.*, 2003; Poulton, 2008).

Poulton *et al.*'s (2000) study explored the contribution of community nurses to the public health agenda and found that activity relating to primary prevention techniques fell more to nurses undertaking health visiting and school nursing roles in contrast to GP practice nurses and district nurses, whose activity was focused more within secondary and tertiary prevention techniques and chronic disease management. While this may be as expected as health visitors and school nurses fall under the umbrella term of the Specialist Community Public Health Nurse (SCPHN), what became apparent in a later study by Poulton (2008) was the contribution of more community-focused public health nursing practice among district nurses. Public health nursing practice should address the needs of populations as well as individuals; however, evidence suggests that a trend exists towards more individual-focused as opposed to community-focused activity (Turner *et al.*, 2003; Poulton, 2008), thus indicating a gap between the rhetoric and the reality of community public health nursing.

For community nurses (at every level) the challenge will be to articulate their contribution to promoting health and wellbeing, not just to commissioners but to other health and social care professionals, through effective leadership and use of evidenced-based practice.

Health promotion

The WHO (1984) succinctly defined health promotion as 'the process of enabling people to increase control over and to improve their health'. This definition is still relevant today, underpinning current government policy, actively placing the patient/client at the centre of care and encouraging patient involvement in the decision processes in order to take control of health decisions: 'No decision about me without me' (DH, 2010b). Therefore, it can be concluded that health promoters (such as community nurses) should aim to enhance participation, equity and fairness to improve the health of individuals, families and communities.

However, a complex theoretical picture of health promotion has emerged from a wide variety of academic disciplines. The following models represent a small selection of those available – most seek to describe health promotion activity at individual, group and population levels. Ewles and Simnett (2003) proposed a model that described five approaches to health promotion: medical, behaviour change, educational, client centred and societal change. The values which underpinned the approaches were represented in a corresponding gradient from professional-led to client-led activity. Tonnes and Tilford (2001) identified educational, preventative, empowerment and radical approaches but viewed empowerment as central to health promotion. Tannahill (1985) identified prevention, health education and health protection in overlapping spheres to describe the services and activities that constituted health promotion practice. Beatie (1991, cited in Katz *et al.*, 2000) developed an analytical model that highlighted the interplay of intervention (authoritative or negotiated which equates to professional or client led) and the focus of intervention (individual or society). Other theories that contribute towards the understanding of the effect of health promotion interventions on the client and why people seek help are the psychological theories of behaviour change which aim to explain why and how people can change their behaviour. Examples are Becker's Health Belief Model (cited in Wills and Earle, 2007), Ajzen and Fishbein's Theory of Reasoned and Planned Action (cited in Wills and Earle, 2007), and Prochaska and DiClemente's (1983) Transtheoretical Stages of Change Theory.

ACTIVITY 2.3

Promoting health
Think of a patient/client or family you have been regularly involved with recently. Make a list of the needs identified in partnership with the individual(s). What opportunities were there to promote health and wellbeing?

In order for community nurses to have a positive impact on the health of individuals it is necessary to have the underpinning knowledge and skills associated with promoting health and wellbeing; central to this is having a developed understanding of the importance of effective communication.

Communication theory underpins the delivery of health promotion; communication between the professional and the client is the main determinant of success.

Most of the above theories describe or analyze health promotion practice, but the skill of health promotion practice requires a deep understanding of communication and partnership working theory to achieve the goal, which is to enable people to increase control over and to improve their health. Rollnick *et al.* (1999) proposed a client-centred model of partnership working (Motivational Interviewing) to complement Prochaska and DeClemente's (1983) Transtheoretical (stages of change) Theory. The aim was to facilitate individuals to move through the stages of precontemplation – contemplation – making changes – maintaining changes. Rollnick *et al.* suggested that a practitioner could reduce resistance to change by relationship building using a therapeutic approach based on trust and information exchange to negotiate the agenda and to set achievable goals based on the individual's vision of importance and their confidence to make the change. Gallant *et al.* (2002) conducted a very informative concept analysis of partnership working which identified three phases to the partnership working relationship: the initiating phase, the working phase and an evaluation phase. To work in partnership one needs to build a professional therapeutic relationship based on trust. The professional must be competent and honest and display professional integrity (to work in the best interests of the client/ patient) at all times and the client must be a willing partner (Pilgrim *et al.*, 2011).

APPLYING THEORY TO PRACTICE

The framework in Figure 2.2 has been heavily influenced by the work of Rollnick, Gallant, Prochaska and DiClemente, Ewles and Simnett, Becker and Tonnes and Telford, and as such is an eclectic representation of existing theoretical approaches.

Community nurses usually either work in the client's own home or a location nearby. They develop very complex relationships with the client and often other family members. For clients who rely on their family for care the nurse must assess and work with the client, being respectful of the needs of both client and carer/ family. Many clients may also have other professionals involved in their care. Community nurses as the principal care providers in the client's home need to work in partnership with other professionals who may work for health, other statutory agencies, the voluntary or independent sectors, although this can be difficult to achieve at times. When working with other professionals in partnership the same principles of trust, which include honesty, competence and integrity, apply. Communication between professionals that is respectful, open and honest is essential to achieve the best outcomes for clients and their families. Although health promotion is often defined in terms of work with populations and work with individuals is defined as health education, all interventions that aim to enable people to take control over their own health on an individual or population basis are considered to be health-promoting interventions (Whitehead and Irvine, 2010).

In order to assist established community nurses or those experiencing community nursing, the case study, and subsequent analysis and action planning, have been developed around the framework for promoting health and wellbeing (Fig. 2.2). It is anticipated that this simple practical example will assist community nurses in the delivery of client-led health-promoting activity, which may also improve an individual sense of wellbeing.

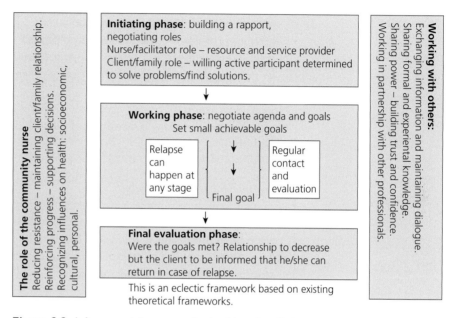

Figure 2.2 A framework for promoting health and wellbeing.

CASE STUDY

Mr John Smith is an 82-year-old gentleman who lives with his wife Mary (72 years old) in a semi-detached house. The house has one bathroom situated upstairs and no toilet downstairs. Mr Smith is a retired dockyard worker who smokes 20 cigarettes per day and used to enjoy an active social life centred on the local social club. An extended family comprising a son and his wife also lives nearby.

Mr Smith's mobility has gradually declined over the last 5 years and he is presently housebound because of chronic obstructive pulmonary disease (COPD). He is able to walk around the house but becomes very breathless when walking upstairs. He is reliant on Mary as his main carer. Mr Smith has a history of chronic bronchitis for 20 years and two episodes of pneumonia in the last 5 years; he is not oxygen dependent but maintained on inhaled steroids and bronchodilators; he has smoked since he was a child; he is partially deaf and wears hearing aids.

Mr Smith had recently suffered a bout of pneumonia, which was treated in hospital, where he was advised to seek support with stopping smoking. He has also developed a leg ulcer that requires weekly dressings.

After a comprehensive assessment the nurse in partnership with Mr Smith may decide that it would be beneficial for him to consider changing his health behaviour to improve his quality of life.

During the '**initiating phase**' one would attempt to build a relationship with Mr Smith and his wife using the assessment documentation as a focus for discussion, asking about their life present and past.

Examples of open questions that may help in the **initiating phase**

> **Nurse:** I see that you were advised to seek support with giving up smoking while in hospital. How do you feel about this?
>
> **Client:** It's probably too late to make any difference now.
>
> **Nurse:** In my experience if a person in your situation can stop or cut down on smoking this does improve their quality of life (Include his wife in the conversation)
>
> **Nurse:** How you tried to give up smoking before?
>
> **Nurse:** Stopping smoking is a really hard thing to do but there is support available.

Moving into the **working phase:**

> **Nurse:** There are lots of support services available today, for example there are trained professionals who could help you by phone.
>
> **Nurse:** Would you like to take one of these cards which has the local NHS stop smoking helpline numbers on it?

Next visit: **working phase continued:**

> **Nurse:** How did you get on with the helpline?
>
> **Client:** It was really helpful. The counsellor and I have made an action plan. He said that I should ask you to prescribe Nicorette patches and to try to cut down gradually by one per day for a week and then another one.
>
> **Nurse:** Yes, I am a nurse prescriber and will be delighted to do this for you. This would entail us working together with your counsellor to ensure that the treatment is effective. How do you feel about that?

As can be seen from the communication above the nurse is allowing the client to take control, to make the decisions, and is being open and honest about her involvement with other professionals. This way power can be shared. The client shared his experiences of trying to give up smoking in the past and the nurse shared her formal knowledge in a working partnership and the roles of both client and professional were being established.

As part of the weekly intervention (for his leg ulcer treatment) there will be an evaluation of success and support to achieve the small realistic goals which will build the client's confidence, and as Mr Smith starts to see positive results in his health this will hopefully be a driver to continue.

At the end the success of the intervention will be evaluated with the client. The nurse may need to discuss the possibility of relapse with Mr Smith while reassuring him that support is always available to him should this occur.

CONCLUSION

As services are redesigned to deliver care closer to home, there is an increased emphasis upon the next generation of nurses to experience the delivery of nursing care in community environments. It is widely acknowledged that community environments are where there is an emphasis on health promotion and prevention of ill health and a recognition of how 'external influences and social factors can impact upon nursing assessment, interventions and activities' (NMC, 2010: 38). It is therefore incumbent on the current nursing workforce to develop an approach to community nursing that goes beyond the idea that nursing is just about assessing, planning and implementing/evaluating the delivery of care associated with a set of clinical tasks. Effective community nursing must identify and engage in public health activity, in order to promote health and wellbeing in society.

Through the presentation of relevant underpinning theory/policy and the use of the case study this chapter has demonstrated that public health is everyone's business and that community nurses are in a position to enable and empower individuals and communities across all levels, from some of the hard-to-reach groups in the population, such as the housebound, to those eagerly involved with promoting their own health and improving their own sense of wellbeing.

It is hoped that this exposure will embed a public health mindset into all nurses and future graduate nurses, who will in turn rise to the challenge of improving the health and wellbeing of the population.

REFERENCES

Acheson D (1988) *Public Health in England.* London: HMSO.

Acheson D (1998) *Independent Inquiry into Inequalities in Health.* London: HMSO.

Black Report (1980) *Inequalities in Health – Report of the Research Working Group.* London: DHSS.

Carr SM (2005) Refocusing health visiting: sharpening the vision and facilitating the process. *Journal of Nursing Management* 13(3):249–56.

Chadwick E (1965 [1842]) *Report of the Sanitary Conditions of the Labouring Population of Great Britain.* Edinburgh: Edinburgh University Press.

Clarke J (2004) Public health nursing in Ireland: a critical Overview … developed from a presentation made at the Annual Conference of the Institute of Community Health Nursing, Ireland, 29 September 2001. *Public Health Nursing* 21(2):191–8.

Cowley S. (2007) Foreword. In Coles L and Porter E (eds) (2008) *Public Health Skills: A Practical Guide for Nurses and Public Health Practitioners.* Oxford: Blackwell, p. vii.

Cowley, S. (2008) *Community Public Health in Policy and Practice: A Sourcebook,* 2nd edn. London: Bailliere Tindall.

Dahlgren G and Whitehead M (1991) In Acheson D (1998) *Part 1 Independent Inquiry into Inequalities in Health.* London: HMSO.

Darzi A (2007) *Our NHS Our Future: The Next Stage Review Interim Report.* London: NHS COI for the Department of Health.

Department for Education and Skills (DfES) (2004) *Every Child Matters: Change for Children.* Nottingham: DfES Publications.

Department of Health (DH) (1999) *Saving Lives: Our Healthier Nation.* London: Department of Health.

DH (2000) *The NHS Plan. A Plan for Investment. A Plan for Reform.* Cm 4818-I. London: The Stationery Office.

DH (2003) *Tackling Health Inequalities.* London: Department of Health.

DH (2004) *Choosing Health: Making Healthier Choices Easier.* London: The Stationery Office.

DH (2006) *Our Health, Our Care, Our Say: A New Direction for Community Services.* London: The Stationery Office.

DH (2010a) *Healthy Lives, Healthy People.* London: The Stationery Office.

DH (2010b) *Equity and Excellence: Liberating the NHS.* London: The Stationery Office.

Donkin A, Goldblatt P and Lynch K (2002) Inequalities in life expectancy by social class 1972–1999. *Health Statistics Quarterly* 15:5–15.

Ewles L and Simnett I (2003) *Promoting Health: A Practical Guide,* 5th edn. Edinburgh: Bailliere Tindall.

Gallant H, Marcia C and Carnevale F (2002) Partnership: an analysis of the concept within the nurse–client relationship. *Journal of Advanced Nursing* 40:149–57.

Haughey R (2008) *Assessing and Identifying Health Needs.* In Coles L and Porter E (eds) *Public Health Skills: A Practical Guide for Nurses and Public Health Practitioners.* Oxford: Blackwell.

HM Government (2010) *Healthy Lives, Healthy People. Our Strategy for Public Health in England.* (Accessed 14 December 2010) www.dh.gov.uk/prod_consum_dh/groups/dh_ digitalassets/@dh/@en/@ps/documents/digitalasset/dh_122347.pdf.

Katz J, Peberdy A and Douglas J (2000) *Promoting Health: Knowledge and Practice,* 2nd edn. Milton Keynes: Open University Press.

Local Government Improvement and Development (LGID) (2010) *Understanding and Tackling the Wider Social Determinants of Health.* (Accessed 12 October 2010) www.idea. gov.uk/idk/core/page.do?pageId=14114189.

Marmot M (2010) *Fair Society, Healthy Lives.* (Accessed 10 June 2010) www.ucl.ac.uk/gheg/ marmotreview/FairSocietyHealthyLivesExecSummary.

Nursing and Midwifery Council (NMC) (2010) *Advice and Supporting Information for Implementing NMC Standards for Pre-registration Nursing Education.* London: NMC.

Pilgrim D, Tomasini F and Vassiley I (2011) *Examining Trust in Healthcare.* Basingstoke: Palgrave MacMillan.

Poulton BC (2008) Barriers and facilitators to the achievement of community-focused public health nursing practice: a UK perspective. *Journal of Nursing Management* 17:74–83.

Poulton BC, Mason C, McKenna H, Lynch C and Keeney S (2000) *The Contribution of Nurses, Midwives and Health Visitors to the Public Health Agenda.* Belfast: DHSSPS.

Prochaska JO and DiClemente CC (1983) Stages and processes of self change of smoking: toward an integrative model of change. *Journal of Consulting and Clinical Psychology* 51:390–5.

Raymond B (2005) Health needs assessment, risk assessment and public health. In Sines D, Appleby F and Frost M (eds) *Community Health Care Nursing*, 3rd edn. Oxford: Blackwell, pp. 70–88.

Reading S (2008) *Research and Development: Analysis and Interpretation of Evidence*. In Coles L and Porter E (eds) *Public Health Skills: A Practical Guide for Nurses and Public Health Practitioners*. Oxford: Blackwell, pp. 170–89.

Rollnick S, Mason P and Butler C (1999) *Health Behaviour Change: A Guide to Practitioners*. London: Churchill Livingstone.

Seedhouse D (2001) *Health: The Foundations for Achievement*, 2nd edn. Chichester: John Wiley & Sons.

Skills for Health (2008) *Skills and Career Framework*. (Accessed 5 November 2010) www.skillsforhealth.org.uk/workforce-design-development/workforce-design-and-planning/tools-and-methodologies/career-frameworks/~/media/Resource-Library/PDF/Public_Health_Report_Web-April_09.ashx.

Stevens A and Raftery J (1994) *Introduction to Health Care Needs Assessment*, vol. 1. Oxford: Radcliffe Medical Press, pp. 1–30.

Sustainable Development Research Network (2005) *Wellbeing Concepts and Challenges: Discussion Paper* by Fiona McAllister for SDRN. DEFRA.

Tannahill A (1985) *What is Health Promotion? Health Education Journal* 44:167–8.

Tonnes K and Tilford S (2001) *Health Promotion Effectiveness, Efficiency and Equity*, 3rd edn. Cheltenham: Nelson Thornes.

Tudor-Hart J (1971) The inverse care law. *Lancet* 1:405–12.

Wanless D, HM Treasury (2004) *Securing Good Health for the Whole Population: Final Report*. London: The Stationery Office.

Whitehead D and Irvine F (2010) *Health Promotion and Health Education in Nursing*. Basingstoke: Palgrave Macmillan.

Wilkinson R and Marmot M (2003) *Social Determinants of Health. The Solid Facts*, 2nd edn. Geneva: WHO Europe International Centre for Health and Society.

Wilkinson R and Pickett K (2009) *The Spirit Level. Why More Equal Societies Almost Always Do Better*. London: Allen Lane.

Williams R and Wright J (1998) Epidemiological issues in health needs assessment, *British Medical Journal* 316:1379–82.

Wills J and Earle S (2007) Theoretical perspectives on promoting public health. In Earle S, Lloyd C, Sidell M and Spurr S (eds) *Theory and Research in Promoting Public Health*. Milton Keynes: Open University Press, Chapter 5.

World Health Organization (WHO) (1946) *Constitution*. Geneva: WHO, p. 2.

WHO (1984) *Health Promotion: A Discussion Document on the Concepts and Principles*. Copenhagen: WHO.

WHO (1986) *Ottawa Charter for Health Promotion*. Canada: WHO.

WHO (2001) *Public Health Nursing: Past and Future. A Review of the Literature*. Copenhagen: WHO.

WHO (2006) *Engaging for Health: A Global Health Agenda 2006–2015*. WHO Library Cataloguing-in-Publication Data.

Wright J (2001) Assessing health needs. In Pencheon D, Guest C, Melzer D and Gray JAM (eds) *The Oxford Handbook of Public Health Practice*. Oxford: Oxford University Press.

CHAPTER 3

Professional approaches to care

Jo Skinner

> ## LEARNING OUTCOMES
>
> - Discuss the factors that influence being a professional in the context of current healthcare practice
> - Analyze and apply ethical principles drawing on codes of practice in relation to providing care in the community
> - Reflect critically on professionalism in relation to service user and carer involvement and partnership working

INTRODUCTION

The relationship between professionals and clients has been the central feature of professional practice throughout history. Professionalism has never been more important regarding public trust and care quality. The nature of professional practice in the community is particularly challenging given the complex care needs, diverse organizations and professions, as well as the need to demonstrate cost-effective health outcomes. The relationship between service users and professionals is changing radically.

This chapter explores the transition in professional practice from a traditional, hierarchical and individualistic model to a more inclusive partnership model. The partnership model includes extended service user and carer involvement, interprofessional working and a wider public health approach. Throughout the chapter, issues relating to both models and ethical principles underpinning practice are highlighted; and a case study and examples from different areas of community practice are used to illustrate principles. There are three sections: the first presents an overview of the traditional model of professional practice, followed by principles informing professional practice and finally factors influencing the development of a new extended partnership model of professional practice.

CASE STUDY

Marjory Davies is 85 years old and lives alone in a three-bedroom house with four flights of stairs. Miss Davies has had a series of falls; the most recent fall required several weeks in hospital. Ahmed, her neighbour, had noticed her curtains were not drawn and he alerted Miss Davies' GP. Miss Davies has returned home and the district nurse has assessed Miss Davies to plan her rehabilitation. Her social worker has advised Miss Davies about her options for residential care. Miss Davies has consistently refused any suggestions that she should move out of her home.

THE TRADITIONAL MODEL OF PROFESSIONAL PRACTICE

It is not easy to define precisely what a *professional* is or indeed what *professionalism* is–both concepts are fluid and contested areas (Evetts, 1999). Traditionally, a professional is someone who is associated with being part of an élite group of experts with claims to specialist knowledge and skills that license their practice. The nature of the work is vocational and like professional roles, such as law and medicine, is valued within society. Professionals exercise their duty in the best interests of their clients and thereby their approach is intentionally altruistic. In that sense professionals may see themselves as the ideal advocates for their clients, being able to define their clients' needs and determine any solutions based on their expertise. Such attributes result in a high degree of professional autonomy and particular trusting relationships with their clients. In healthcare, licensed practitioners are permitted access to the human body in order to undertake intimate or intrusive assessments, clinical examinations and treatments. Thus, higher moral standards are expected of professionals to do what is best for patients; this is enshrined in law as *a duty of care* owed to patients (Dimond, 1997). In the case of Miss Davies (case study), she is owed a duty of care by all three professionals: district nurse, social worker and GP. Therefore, all professionals, and those who are members of recognized professions, share certain characteristics (Box 3.1).

Box 3.1 Characteristics of professions
A distinct body of specialist knowledge and skills (often rooted in ancient practice or tradition)
A lengthy and exclusive training leading to registration
Altruism
Code of practice
Duty of care
Autonomy
Accountability
Privileged access to and trusting relationship with clients
Public trust and good standing
Higher social status, pay, reward and career structure

Control over who may enter these elite professions is strictly governed, usually through a rigorous selection process. This keeps up demand for such skills by reinforcing their status, value and power (Finlay, 2000). Professionals can make certain demands, including control over the way they practise, in recognition of their unique skills and status. The process of becoming a professional entails lengthy and rigorous training validated by peers. Historically, those élite professions were male dominated and *patriarchal* in nature. Specialist literature and technical language reinforce 'membership of the club', thus excluding others, particularly their clients. As Williams (2000: 99) noted, professional autonomy 'empowers the strongest at the expense of the weakest'. Professional networks and associations, like membership of Royal Colleges, reinforce entitlement. Regulatory bodies protect the public, policing entry onto and removal from professional registers, e.g. the Nursing and Midwifery Council (NMC), the General Medical Council (GMC) and the Health Professions Council (HPC).

ACTIVITY 3.1

Reflection point
Do you consider yourself a professional? What defines you as a professional? How is this different to acting in a professional way?

Many of these features reflect an 'old' model of professional practice associated with what is known as a *medical model of health* (Box 3.2). This model is particularly problematic from a community and public health viewpoint as the focus is on the body, acute illness and the disease process such that social or economic causes of illness are omitted. Concepts within the medical model are informed by and reinforce values, attitudes and practice.

Box 3.2 Features of the medical model of health

Focus on the disease process and cure
Scientific rational approach
Professional as expert
Task focused
Illness model of health: little emphasis on prevention or public health

Becoming 'a professional' is a process of acculturation and socialization where new recruits are exposed to the norms and values that pertain to a particular profession, including language and how to relate to clients. Professional education exposes students to role models or mentors with particular placement experiences that serve to define and reinforce attitudes, values and behaviours as much as the specialist knowledge. Training is separate from other professions, and patients do not play an active role in the curriculum, other than permitting students to practise their skills on them. At the end of this acculturation process, there has been a transformation from student to a fledgling practitioner. Benner (1984), cited by Gatley (1992), describes this process in nursing as a continuum 'from novice to expert' whereby experiential learning is central to developing intuitive knowledge and skills. So while professions share certain common characteristics (Box 3.1), not necessarily all, there remain differences in the way that professionals interact with clients, conceptualize their practice and relate to other professionals.

Training establishes professional identities and it is easiest to make distinctions between or within professions where practice is highly specialized, e.g. neurosurgery. Such distinctions may be codified by legislation and regulations–for example, except in an emergency, it is a criminal offence for anyone other than a UK registered midwife or doctor to attend a woman in childbirth (Dimond, 1990). Such codification has led to the creation of hierarchies even within professional groups and characterizing some groups as semi-professions, particularly along gender lines. Boundaries between professionals have emerged such that they jealously guard them in order to protect their roles. This can lead to resistance to change, defensive practice or tribalism (Dalley, 1989). This reflects the traditional view of professions in terms of historical claims to knowledge and expertise and is ultimately an issue of power.

ACTIVITY 3.2

Discussion point
Which professions are legally entitled to prescribe? What are the boundary issues?

You may find Radcliffe (2008) helpful to your discussion.

Differences between professions are frequently reinforced through traditions, training and to some extent stereotyping (Pietroni, 1991). Theoretical perspectives also underpin this, for example in social care the concept of anti-oppressive practice (Ward, 2009) is key to explaining social work practice as well as a driver to empower clients. This reflects the *social model of health* (Box 3.3). Doctors are associated with adopting a purely medical model of health while other professional groups across health and social care adopt the social model of health (Brechin *et al.*, 2000) (Box 3.3) that takes in the wider determinants of health and health inequalities (Wilkinson and Pickett, 2010; Marmot, 2010). This is particularly important when taking a public health approach that is population based (Dawson, 2006). These stereotypes or archetypes are too crude and do not take account of the huge variation across practice areas, different care settings and individual philosophies. In the community, it would be difficult, not to say unethical, for any health or social care practitioner working with service users to ignore wider psychosocial and environmental factors impacting on care. For example, in occupational health nursing the work environment is a critical aspect of any care (Black, 2008) and must be balanced with the scientific explanations of occupational exposures to noise, dust or other hazards to health (Harrington *et al.*, 1998). However, these concepts and models are useful starting points for challenging assumptions about professions and the extent to which practice is task oriented.

Box 3.3 Features of the social model of health

Health is holistic and not just the absence of disease
Wider determinants of health as causes of ill health and health inequalities
Holistic approach to assessment and sources of evidence
Service user as expert in own health
Emphasis on health and wellbeing
Service user participation in health/community as full citizen
Emphasis on prevention and public health

ACTIVITY 3.3

Discussion point
List the advantages and disadvantages of having different professionals involved in Miss Davies' care.

Would your list be different if the service user were a child or an employee?

For many years boundaries between professions were fairly rigid and the number of professional groups relatively stable. In primary care, the professional hierarchy was well established (Peckham and Exworthy, 2003), with GPs at the apex. Using prescribing as an example (Activity 3.2), traditionally doctors and dentists were legally empowered to prescribe; in 1992 the Medicines Act (1968) was amended so that all district nurses and health visitors were enabled to prescribe from a community prescribing formulary with training integrated into specialist programmes (Dimond, 1997; NMC, 2006). However, nurse prescribing was hard won; it followed extensive pilots to address the sceptics (Brew, 1997) and was not fully introduced until 1999. This has paved the way for prescribing rights to be extended across nursing and midwifery and to other professional groups such as pharmacists and physiotherapists (Radcliffe, 2008). Interestingly, not all prescribers were granted the same prescribing rights, so new boundaries emerge, and arguably maintain hierarchies (Williams, 2000). There is some contention about whether such developments are *extended roles* or whether this is really *skill substitution*. In the case of nurses they have taken on the work others, namely doctors, no longer wish to do (Williams, 2000); however, increasing the skill mix among the workforce has also been an important mechanism for health service managers to reduce costs. In reality, it is a fusion of all these aspects with some degree of compromise between the various vested interests. Boundaries for professional practice are shifting and encompass the legal and policy frameworks within which all practitioners operate (Dimond, 1997).

PRINCIPLES INFORMING PROFESSIONAL PRACTICE

Ethical principles and legal and policy frameworks direct the practice of all professionals. In the community, it is important to understand these principles and be able to apply them in different situations as part of professional decision-making. Values encompass personal, societal and professional domains and importantly influence practice. These values are socially constructed and thereby liable to change.

Professionals make decisions with or on behalf of others and need to have clear reasons to justify them. Being accountable is a key element of professional practice and clinical reasoning. Moral reasoning informs decisions, for example whether or not to treat. A recent feature of professional practice has been the development of *evidence-based practice*, whereby decisions about treatment and care are neither subjective nor capricious. Using research evidence to underpin professional practice has come to be viewed as best practice, being both rigorous and objective following the scientific tradition. The standard by which professionals are judged is in relation to their peers (Dimond, 1997; Greenhalgh, 2006). Steel (2006: 57) makes the point that, 'The development of a more open and evidence-based approach to decision making in healthcare has shown how much personal values influence professional behaviour'. Referring to public health, he warns that science is far from being value free but that it is important to make values clear and decisions explicit (Steel, 2006).

However, the plethora of research published means that professionals need to be able to access, appraise and use research findings to underpin their practice (Greenhalgh, 2006). Given the complexity of research findings, particularly weighted towards quantitative research, this needs to be translated into guidance for practice. Organizations such as the National Institute for Health and Clinical Excellence (NICE), NHS evidence, public health observatories, professional bodies and peer-reviewed journals often mediate and disseminate guidance. The wholesale adoption of the scientific rational model undermines the 'art' of professional practice, which encompasses tacit knowledge, narrative-based approaches, service user individuality and professional autonomy. Greenhalgh (2006) points out that professionals may be profoundly influenced by their own experiences but this may not always be a good basis for making decisions. It is clearly important to recognize the value of and difficulty in managing both evidence- and narrative-based approaches. For example, an experienced practice nurse may intuitively understand that a woman's reluctance to have cervical screening is due to past sexual violence. A solely evidence-based practice approach may lead to task-focused care to obtain consent for a cervical smear and omit the importance of human interaction and relationships as an integral part of therapeutic care and may transgress patients' values.

Decision-making is influenced by many factors (Box 3.4) including the context and clinical and ethical aspects (Grundstein-Amado, 1992). Access to high-quality information is required from multiple sources, with interplay between them to draw rational conclusions which can be justified.

Box 3.4 Decision-making factors

Comprehensive assessment includes different stakeholder perspectives
Wider determinants of health
Ethical and legal guidance
Evidence base
Clinical reasoning
Options and preferences
Evaluation
Accountability
Safety
Concordance
Cost and sustainability

Principles of ethical practice

There is a common set of principles that guides ethical practice in health and social care (Beauchamp and Childress, 2008; Adams *et al.*, 2009). Decisions are based not just on clinical evidence but on a set of moral principles. Health itself is enshrined within human rights values (Nygren-Krug, 2002). In order to do what is right in the particular circumstances, different stakeholders will have different views which need to be considered when making decisions. In the community, value-based decisions impact not only the service user but their families and social networks and also their property, for example the impact of converting a living room into a bedroom. Four ethical principles inform decision-making in healthcare practice (Beauchamp and Childress, 2008):

- respect for autonomy
- non-maleficence
- beneficence
- justice.

   Respect for autonomy: individuals have the right to make their own decisions. Professionals must respect the decisions that service users make and ensure their practice is consistent with this, e.g. informed consent. There are exceptional circumstances where individuals are unable to make decisions; professionals must understand the circumstances and legislation that override this self-rule principle.

   Non-maleficence: practitioners should cause no harm, whether intentional or unintentional. Any resulting harm due to a breach in the duty of care owed to that person may be considered negligence, leaving the practitioner open to a charge of professional misconduct and subject to action for compensation through the courts (Dimond, 1997).

   Beneficence: it may seem obvious that care offered should be beneficial to service users but this may not always be the case. There may a clash between the service or policy objectives and the individual, as we saw with the practice nurse. Professionals need to ensure that decisions about care and treatment offered are considered safe and effective (Box 3.4). In the community professionals need to consider the viewpoints, preferences and needs of patients and carers: it must not be assumed that patients' and carers' needs are the same.

   Justice: care must be equitable in terms of need and access to resources. In the community this may be a challenge as there will be unequal circumstances and resources affecting quality of care, for example housing, access to family support or respite. This does not mean that equal time or care has to be allocated among service users but that there should be equitable provision relative to the assessed needs (Thompson *et al.*, 1990). For example Gerrish's (1999) research showed that there was unequal access to district nursing services for ethnic minority patients because of the way district nursing services were aligned to different GP practices.

Professional practice requires decisions and choices to be made to achieve what is best *and* what is right – though sometimes such choices lead to a moral dilemma. This is where there is conflict between moral principles, in choosing one principle in preference to another (Thompson *et al.*, 1990). In the case of community mental health nursing, where a service user declines treatment but the nurse is aware of the potential harm if the patient does not take his medication, the principle of autonomy conflicts with beneficence, unless the patient is deemed incapable of making such a decision under the Mental Capacity Act (2005).

Having considered Miss Davies' case regarding her autonomy, she may withhold consent to alternative accommodation or rehabilitation, which she is perfectly entitled to do, providing she is deemed capable of making such decisions. This is at the heart of giving informed consent to treatment. There are four important conditions that need to be in place for informed consent.

ACTIVITY 3.4

Discussion point
Using the four principles of ethical practice above, discuss Miss Davies' case from each person's perspective. What do you think are the key ethical principles here and why? Do you think district nurse and social worker views will be different? What is guiding their practice?

INFORMED CONSENT

The following conditions need to be present in order for consent to be informed and thereby valid.

1　Sufficient information is made available in order to make a decision, including the potential risks and benefits.
2　Understands the information relevant to the decision.
3　Uses or weighs up that information as part of the decision-making process.
4　Consent must be voluntary and without any undue pressure.

In law anyone over 18 years is deemed to be capable of giving consent unless there is evidence to the contrary (Dimond, 1990). In the case of Miss Davies, staff may wish to ensure that she is not only capable of making the decision under the Mental Capacity Act (2005) but also that there is no undue pressure placed on her to comply with professional advice. Vulnerable people may be susceptible to others' suggestions, feeling they have to comply for fear of losing services or because they wish to be helpful. It may also be the case that older people are used to a paternalistic approach where professionals are seen as expert, not to be challenged, and it is assumed that they always act in the patient's best interest. In Miss Davies' case both the district nurse and social worker will need to work collaboratively to ensure that the service user feels supported in whatever decisions she makes and that there are no mixed messages coming from them.

Children are also vulnerable: those 16 years and over are deemed as having the capacity to give their consent. However, the legal position is different for those under 16 years and the Gillick competency must be applied (Dimond, 1997). This is where 'minors who are capable of understanding the significance of the proposed treatment can, in exceptional circumstances, be regarded as competent in law to give consent' (Dimond, 1997: 41). For example, where a school nurse is asked for contraceptive advice by a young person under the age of 16 years, in making her assessment the nurse would need to satisfy herself not only that the young person understood the significance but also that exceptional circumstances applied. Assumptions should not be made that informed consent cannot be given purely on the basis of age or condition such as learning disabilities or dementia.

PROFESSIONAL VALUES

Alongside these ethical principles, all professions have their own values and concepts that guide and shape practice, providing a means to explore with others the nature of practice and need to be shared (Dominelli, 2009) (Box 3.5). An important aspect of working in the community is the quality of the service user–practitioner relationship, which is key to providing care that is personalized and effective.

Community nurses get to know well service users, families and their circumstances over a period of months and years, providing care continuity. Luker (2002) study on community nurses' construction of quality demonstrates where the 'centrality of knowing the patient and his/her family was an essential antecedent to the provision of high quality palliative care' (Luker, 2002: 775). This value of *knowing the patient* is held in high regard in the community. For example, in Miss Davies' case, the district nurse should seek to establish a relationship stemming from the *first assessment* and subsequent planning care.

Box 3.5 Common professional values
Respect and dignity Caring Autonomy Holism Confidentiality Empowerment Partnership Equity Social justice Human rights Advocacy

Values need to be shared; at the abstract level they are less problematic but the context in which they apply is where conflict may arise (Dominelli, 2009). Williams'

(2000) research showed that despite shared values of caring, compassion and holism between GPs and community nurses, these values were perceived differently by both professional groups, which fuelled communication difficulties. Thompson *et al.* (1990) state that what appears to be a moral dilemma is more due to inadequate information or a breakdown in communication. Communication is central to all aspects of professional practice and is an area that has warranted numerous policy and practice initiatives to enhance it. For example, the *Single Assessment Process* (SAP) was designed to overcome difficulties in sharing information and duplication for service users (Miller and Cameron, 2011; Worth, 2001). In the case of Miss Davies' a joint assessment ought to result in a comprehensive plan addressing her preferences. There is variable support for SAP, which may indicate a failure to understand the values of those who need to use it. Conversely, the learning disabilities *hospital passport* identifies the individual's needs and preferences in advance and crucially is owned by them; it has proven to be an essential document that has saved lives (Skinner, 2011).

PROFESSIONAL CODES OF PRACTICE

These values are expressed in professional *codes of practice*, for example NMC (2008) and GSCC (2010), setting out the ethical standards to which practitioners are held to account, guiding day-to-day practice decisions. Having privileged access to service users, codes are an important way of assuring the public that professionals are regulated so that they can have confidence in them as part of the social contract.

ACTIVITY 3.5	**Discussion point**
	Analyze a professional code of practice from a professional group in relation to the four ethical principles above.

The traditional model pre-dates formal codes of practice; it reflects the utilitarian principle of best interest that bypasses the service user undermining the principle of autonomy. Autonomy is further codified in the Human Rights Act (1998). Conflict may arise between service users' rights and the professionals' duty of care, that is confidentiality, right to privacy or freedom from discrimination (Thompson *et al.*, 1990; O'Keefe *et al.*, 1992).

Box 3.6 Excerpts from GSCC, NMC and GMC codes

GSCC (DH, 2002)

1.3 Supporting service users' rights to control their lives and make informed choices about the services they receive;

3.1 Promoting the independence of service users and assisting them to understand and exercise their rights;

4.1 Recognising that service users have the right to take risks and helping them to identify and manage potential and actual risks to themselves and others;

NMC (2008)

You must make the care of people your first concern:

1 You must treat people as individuals and respect their dignity
2 You must not discriminate in any way against those in your care
3 You must treat people kindly and considerately
4 You must act as an advocate for those in your care, helping them to access relevant health and social care, information and support

GMC (2006)

Make the care of your patient your first concern

Treat patients as individuals and respect their dignity

• Treat patients politely and considerately

• Respect patients' right to confidentiality

Work in partnership with patients

• Listen to patients and respond to their concerns and preferences

• Give patients the information they want or need in a way they can understand

• Respect patients' right to reach decisions with you about their treatment and care

• Support patients in caring for themselves to improve and maintain their health

While there has been increasing convergence in these codes (Box 3.6), there is a need for a shared code of practice for health and social care professionals based on common ethical principles and values, reflecting a human rights approach. Health and social care professionals are required to keep confidential service users' information, which is reinforced in the respective professional codes of practice (NMC, 2008; GSCC, 2010; GMC, 2006) and legislation (Data Protection Act, 1998). However, failure to share vital information with other professions about service users may not only be inefficient but harmful and in some cases fatal, most notably in child protection (Laming, 2003) and mental health (Cold, 1994). Paradoxically, professionals may use their codes of practice or legislation inappropriately, practising defensively and inhibiting partnership working. Such codes may inadvertently reinforce boundaries and stereotypes between professional groups and represent a conflict of values. Although confidentiality is a common value it does not mean that service users' information can be shared automatically. The Data Protection Act (1998) governs the way in which information is collected, stored and shared (Box 3.7).

Box 3.7 Data protection

Under the Data Protection Act, you must:

• only collect information that you need for a specific purpose;

• keep it secure;

• ensure it is relevant and up to date;

• only hold as much as you need, and only for as long as you need it;

• allow the subject of the information to see it on request.

Source: ICO (nd)

Although professionals must understand the law to ensure it is correctly implemented, it is essential that health and social care professionals share information in the best interests of service users. The Caldicott Principles (Newham Council, 2009) have been introduced to help practitioners determine what information should be shared and under what circumstances (Box 3.8).

Box 3.8 Caldicott Principles

Confidentiality and security of service users' information held by professionals and organizations should follow six general principles of good practice:
- A formal justification of purpose is required prior to sharing information
- Identifiable information is to be transferred only when absolutely necessary
- Information should be limited to the minimum required only
- Access to information should be on a need-to-know basis only
- All staff to understand their responsibilities in sharing information
- All staff should comply with and understand the law

Source: Newham Council (2009)

In the case of Miss Davies the district nurse and social worker may share information through the SAP, and in practice formal agreements are made between organizations with shared service responsibilities.

In the community professionals hold a great deal of power over service users due to the invisible nature of the work, staff must be completely trustworthy and uphold codes of practice. Staff too may be vulnerable to accusations that may be hard to defend, such as elder abuse or stealing from patients (Box 3.9).

Box 3.9 Critique of professions

Self-interested
Maintain status quo
Incapable of self-regulation
Retain power
Block change including policy implementation
Defensive practice: hiding behind rules and regulations or may flout them

---

Can professionals be trusted?

Trust and professionalism are closely associated (Evetts, 2006a,b). Service users want safe and effective treatment delivered by trusted professionals but there has been a profound loss of trust in professionals (Evetts, 2006b). Confidence was undermined after a series of scandals where public servants, including health professionals, breached standards; this was brought to a head when in 2000, Harold Shipman, a GP in Greater Manchester, was found guilty of murdering 15 patients and forging a will – most of his victims were elderly women living alone, killed by a lethal injection. A subsequent investigation revealed that he had murdered between 215 and 260 patients over a period of 23 years, despite being highly respected by many patients. This rocked the nation's trust in doctors, leading to questioning of the extent of their professional power and that of others.

Professional regulatory bodies have legal powers to regulate their respective professions. They set the standards for education and practice, maintain a register of eligible practitioners, have powers to investigate breaches in professional conduct and revoke the practitioner's licence to practise. Post Shipman, professional self-regulation has come under scrutiny and exposed the lack of transparency, complacency and the reluctance of peers to remove unfit practitioners from the register. This has been addressed through reappraisal of codes, changes to professional education, strengthening the requirements for fitness to practise, including re-registration, and ensuring that more lay people sit on the professional regulatory boards (King's Fund, 2007).

There is now greater convergence in the use of professional codes of ethics and revalidation of practice (Thistlethwaite, 2007). The hallmarks of professional practice are summarized in Box 3.10.

Box 3.10 Hallmarks of professional practice

Critical reflective practice
Effective communication
High standards set for safety and effectiveness
Accountability
Service users' and carers' feedback and evaluation sought
Peer review and feedback sought
Develops others: service users; families; team and students
Keeps up to date and lifelong learning; can access and use information
Upholds the code and practises ethically
Knowledgeable about legal and policy frameworks
Leadership
Influences change; research minded
Develops and maintains networks and partnerships

Service users are generally less reliant on professionals as sole experts or keepers of professional knowledge. Access to the Internet, promotion of self-care and the need to involve service users more means that professionals are less able to hide behind jargon or use terminology that excludes service users. However, for more vulnerable service users this should not be assumed and all patients have a right to be consulted (DH, 2009).

TOWARDS A NEW PARTNERSHIP MODEL OF PROFESSIONAL PRACTICE

Drivers for a new model of professional practice have been gathering momentum and have largely come from outside the professions, reflecting wider societal changes, policy, costs and a recognition of the complexity of health and social care problems. This has also influenced fundamentally professional education with much stronger service user and carer involvement.

The challenge to the old model of professional practice has brought in some radical changes reflecting the shift in societal values that are rights based within a post-modern pluralistic society.

Although the idea of partnership working with service users has developed over the past 20 years what is new is their role in professional socialization. The new model of professional practice is one of partnership between service users and professionals and interprofessional working. This is contained within the Nursing and Midwifery Council Standards for pre-registration nurse education (NMC, 2010).

New professionalism?

Although a number of changes have taken place following the reappraisal of professions, professionalism remains a fluid concept and a contested area (Evetts, 2006a). There is no consensus among researchers about what professionalism is but the attributes of professional behaviour have been easier to identify (Parker *et al.*, 2006). Parker *et al.* state that 'the attributes identified as most indicative of professionalism seem to be the subjective, value-laden types such as integrity, regard for the patient and interaction with others' (Parker *et al.*, 2006: 96). The notion that 'good practitioners' know what is quality care is a dated view (Katz *et al.*, 2007). Coulter's (2005) work identifies that patients want professionals who are good communicators, up to date in clinical knowledge and skills, enable participation in decisions about care and provide emotional support, empathy and respect. Communication skills are inextricably bound up with the quality of the patient's experience (Leatherman and Sutherland, 2007; Coulter, 2005).

The balance of power towards service users is changing (De Voe and Short, 2003) through a process of deprofessionalization and patient empowerment (Finlay, 2000); however, many accept that the 'traditional' concept of professionalism is anachronistic and that there has been a paradigm shift to a new norm which is just as problematic to articulate (Davies, 2007; Evetts, 2006a).

Indeed it is recognized that no single profession is able to meet the health and/or social care needs on their own. In the last half century, myriad new specialties and professions have emerged as healthcare becomes more complex. This has led to greater crossover of traditional roles like prescribing or approved social workers. In many cases this facilitates better access to health and social care services but highlights an increased need for partnership working.

The nature of partnership working

Even if it is agreed that no single profession has all the required knowledge and skills let alone capacity to meet the needs of today's clients, it could be questioned whether these professional differences enhance or complement the assessment of need and planning of care or lead to role conflict and poor teamwork. If there are perceived or actual differences between professional groups, with some seen as more powerful than others, there may be an impact on practice, for example a GP and a practice nurse, where the GP is also the practice nurse's employer.

Box 3.11 Characteristics of effective partnership working

Sharing a common vision and goals
Planning for the medium term
Sharing information
Sharing resources
Common understanding of need
Joint meeting of needs
Users experience partnership as coherence in care delivery
Equality and trust between partners
Common values for social justice
Leadership
Voluntary

Partnership working requires trust and reciprocity (Glendinning *et al.*, 2002) to counter traditional barriers (Hardy *et al.*, cited by Hudson, 2000), avoid blame and have clarity about roles and accountability. Interprofessional working in the community (Box 3.11) is essential to avoid gaps and duplication and to focus on agreed outcomes as discussed in Chapter 10.

INFLUENCE OF SERVICE USER INVOLVEMENT ON PROFESSIONAL PRACTICE

Service user involvement is central to healthcare practice whether in direct care, research or education. This represents a considerable philosophical and practical shift away from seeing the service user as a passive passenger in their journey of care. In refuting the medical model whereby the professionals do not always know best, the emergence of the service user as the expert in their own condition is new (DH, 2006, 2008). Indeed, the notion of being a professional is shifting too as access to 'elite' information is more readily available and there is greater emphasis on interprofessional working to combat complex health problems. This new paradigm may challenge the traditional hegemony of the medical model of health (Brechin *et al.*, 2000). In addition, service users may now hold special knowledge and experience different from the professionals. Partnership working is a key aspect of this and features strongly in service user involvement.

As professionals have changed so have service users. The move towards health consumerism recasts service users as citizens who must be consulted, offered choice and have a greater say in decisions (Hogg, 1999). By 'reclassifying' health within a wider public health model, the old orthodoxy's power has been challenged, especially in terms of discrimination. This challenge arose from different quarters, reflecting hard-won rights from various groups including women, people with disabilities and carers. For service users 'having a voice' is not confined to individual care decisions but more fundamentally extends to strategic decisions about the nature and shape of health provision. This involvement extends from policy-making and service design to involvement in professional education. Having said this, the reach of professional power in the community for vulnerable and *invisible* people, including carers, has the potential for abuse or disempowerment. Some professionals retain power to control their work, for example GPs were able to negotiate with the government not to provide *out-of-hours* services (Peckham and Exworthy, 2003), even though improving access to primary care is fundamental.

ROLE OF SERVICE USERS IN PROFESSIONAL EDUCATION

The role of professional education in shaping future practitioners is essential. Changes emphasize the importance of communication and partnership working (GSCC, 2010), recognizing that competence alone is not enough to constitute professionalism (Parker *et al.*, 2006). Professionals must balance their technical abilities with those that people value (Leatherman and Sutherland, 2007). These have been codified in the professional standards for education. In this vein, pre-registration nursing has been widely criticized and now an all-graduate qualification has been introduced to redress this imbalance (NMC, 2010). It is an increasing expectation that service users play an active role in all areas of professional education programmes from curriculum design to recruitment of students, teaching and assessment (DH, 2002; NMC 2010).

An evaluation of service user involvement in health and social care education spanning nursing, social work and allied health professions showed that in contrast to the traditional model service users are now part of the specializing and acculturation process (Skinner, 2011). Service users and carers then hold a new sort of power, manifested in the power of teaching through stories (Fraser and Greenhalgh, 2001). This brings a direct challenge to professional power as well as a rich reality to education whereby

> knowledge that comes from lived experience be re-valued not necessarily in opposition but alongside more specific professional discourses and bodies of knowledge.
>
> *(Brown, in Brechin et al., 2000: 101)*

This contrasts with the apprenticeship learning in the traditional model. In the new model of education (and practice) service users participate as *experts by experience* (Skinner, 2011). Service users in effect now have a quasi-regulatory function locally, by sanctioning aspects of professional education. This could lead to a new form of professional accountability which is shared with or 'controlled' by service users, though professionals decide which service users are involved (Skinner, 2011).

ACTIVITY 3.6

Discussion point

Can you identify service user involvement in your course or practice area? If so what is its nature?

If you were designing a new service from scratch, how would you go about involving service users? How would you ensure this was 'genuine' and not tokenistic?

There is no *uniform or single set of standards* or benchmarks for service user involvement across the health sector. However, professional regulatory bodies, including the General Social Care Council and the Nursing and Midwifery Council, require assurances about it (DH, 2002; NMC, 2008). Universities determine their own service users' and carers' involvement (SUCI) policy and practice (Skinner, 2011).

Table 3.1 highlights the dichotomy between the old and new models of professional practice, though in reality elements of both models co-exist and different professional groups are at different stages of transition. It may be the case that professionals are regrouping and professional power is still firmly with the professionals, although service users have more rights, powers and resources at their disposal to challenge practice.

Table 3.1 Professional practice old and new models

Then – old	Now – new
Patients/individuals	Service users; clients; partners; people/groups/community/population
Tradition/knowledge handed down/scientific discovery/experimental treatment	Evidence-based practice; treatment decisions determined externally by peer-reviewed research or regulatory authorities
Apprenticeship model of learning	Service users involved in training and lifelong learning
Expertise rests with professionals	Access to specialist knowledge widely available, e.g. Internet Service user as expert
Job for life/way of life/once qualified always qualified	Revalidation – proof of ongoing fitness to practise/maintain competence/lifelong learning
Clinical autonomy	Patient autonomy – shared decision-making with patients and in multidisciplinary teams
Roles distinct and hierarchical boundaries	Role overlap; blurred boundaries; skill mix
Focus on cure	Focus on care and experience of care
Focus on skills	Focus on academe; all-graduate profession
Paternalism/professionals define patients' needs	Client-centred care/autonomy/human rights/Patient and public involvement
Medical or social models of health	Hybrid holism
Self-regulation; lifelong registration	Lay regulation/regulatory bodies; licence to practise; proof of fitness to practise
High levels of trust	Less trust and more accountability required
Vocation	Vocation
Best interest; needs determined by professionals	Personal autonomy; rights-based care
Control of resources, e.g. unlimited prescribing	Variable control over resources
Consent	Informed consent
Accountability to peers	Accountability to public and policy-makers; codes of practice

CONCLUSION

The chapter highlights a shift in the balance of power towards service users by challenging and redefining what it means to be a health professional in the twenty-first century. Two models of professional practice, old and new, shape relationships between service users and professionals. These models are in a state of flux regarding the conceptualization of professionalism, role boundaries, core values and power.

Partnership with service users and carers may now play a significant role in the professionalization of health and social care practitioners. This process not only meets the expected quality and policy agendas to improve fitness to practise but also empowers service users. This is based on mutual respect, trust and reciprocity, which are fundamental to partnership working (Glendinning *et al.*, 2002). Service users and carers are not just being informed about decisions but are key to decision-making (Ovretveit, in Brechin *et al.*, 2000).

The professionalization of health and social care students is being shaped by service user involvement and this may be considered best practice, increasingly reflected in the regulation of professional education (DH, 2002; NMC 2010), although it is too early to judge the extent and permanence of this influence.

Professionals traditionally have wielded considerable power in relation to 'non-professionals' and especially service users. This is viewed as outmoded and undesirable, resulting in a shift in the balance of power towards service users and carers and interprofessional working. This chapter has reviewed the nature of professional practice in relation to two models and the application of ethical principles and values for professional practice within the community. It argues that professional practice has moved from a traditional model of practice towards a more inclusive partnership model involving service users and interprofessional working. The emerging role of service users in the professionalization process because of their involvement in professional training is explored as part of this new extended partnership model of practice, resulting in a redefinition of what it means to be a health professional in the twenty-first century.

REFERENCES

Beauchamp TL and Childress JF (2008) *Principles of Biomedical Ethics*, 6th edn. New York: Oxford University Press.

Black C (2008) *Working for a Healthier Tomorrow*. London: The Stationery Office.

Boyd KM, Higgs R and Pinching A (eds) (1997) *The New Dictionary of Medical Ethics*. London: BMJ Publishing Group.

Brechin A, Brown H and Eby MA (2000) *Critical Practice in Health and Social Care*, 2nd edn. London: Sage OUP.

Brew M (1997) Nurse prescribing. In Burley S, Mitchell EE, Melling K, *et al.* (eds) *Contemporary Community Nursing*. London: Arnold, pp. 229–43.

British Psychological Society (2006) *Code of Ethics and Conduct*. (Accessed 1 October 2011) www.bps.org.uk/sites/default/files/documents/code_of_ethics_and_conduct.pdf.

Cold J (1994) The Christopher Clunis enquiry. *Psychiatric Bulletin* 18:449–52.

Coulter A (2005) What do patients and the public want from primary care? *British Medical Journal* 351:1199–200.

Dalley G (1989) Professional ideology or organisational tribalism? The health service–social work divide. In Taylor R and Ford J (eds) *Social Work and Health Care*. Research Highlights in Social Work 19. London: Jessica Kingsley.

Davies C (2007) The promise of 21st century professionalism: Regulatory reform and integrated care. *Journal of Interprofessional Care* 21:233–9.

Dawson A (2006) Understanding ethics in public health. In Pencheon D, Guest C, Melzer D and Muir Gray JA (eds) *Oxford Handbook of Public Health*, 2nd edn. Oxford: Oxford University Press.

De Voe J and Short SD (2003) A shift in the historical trajectory of medical dominance: the case of Medibank and the Australian doctors' lobby. *Social Science and Medicine* 57:343–53.

Department of Health (DH) (2002) *Requirements for Social Work Training*. (Accessed 16 January 2012) www.dh.gov.uk/prod_consum_dh/groups/dh_digitalassets/@dh/@en/documents/digitalasset/dh_4060262.pdf.

DH (2006) *A Stronger Local Voice: A Framework for Creating a Stronger Local Voice in the Development of Health and Social Care Services*. London: Department of Health.

DH (2008) *Real Involvement Working with People to Improve Health Services Guidance to NHS*. London: Department of Health.

DH (2009) *The Handbook to the NHS Constitution for England*. London: TSO.

Dimond B (1990) *Legal Aspects of Nursing*. Hemel Hempstead: Prentice Hall.

Dimond B (1997) *Legal Aspects of Care in the Community*. Basingstoke: Macmillan.

Dominelli L (2009) In Adams R, Dominelli L and Payne M (eds) *Critical Practice in Social Work*. Basingstoke: Palgrave Macmillan.

Evetts J (1999) Professionalisation and professionalism: issues for interprofessional care. *Journal of Interprofessional Care* 13:119–28.

Evetts J (2006a) The sociology of professional groups: new directions. *Current Sociology* 54:133–43.

Evetts J (2006b) Trust and professionalism: challenges and occupational changes. *Current Sociology* 54:515–31.

Finlay A (2000) The challenge of professionalism. In Brechin A, Brown H and Eby MA (eds) *Critical Practice in Health and Social Care*. London: Sage, pp. 74–95.

Finlay L (2000) Understanding professional development. In Brechin A, Brown H and Eby MA (eds) *Critical Practice in Health and Social Care* London: Sage, pp. 48–69.

Fraser SW and Greenhalgh T (2001) Coping with complexity: education for capability. *British Medical Journal* 323:799–803.

Gatley E (1992) From novice to expert: the use of intuitive knowledge as a basis for district nursing. *Nurse Education Today* 12:81–7.

General Social Care Council (GSCC) (2010) *Codes of Practice for Social Care Workers*. (Accessed 16 January 2012) www.gscc.org.uk/cmsFiles/CodesofPracticeforSocialCareWorkers.pdf.

Gerrish K (1999) Inequalities in service provision: an examination of institutional influences on the provision of district nursing care to minority ethnic communities. *Journal of Advanced Nursing* 30:6.

Glendinning C, Powell M and Rummery K (2002) *Partnerships, New Labour and the Governance of Welfare*. Bristol: Policy Press.

General Medical Council (GMC) (2006) *Good Medical Practice*. (Accessed 1 October 2011) www.gmc-uk.org/static/documents/content/GMP_0910.pdf.

GMC (2006) *Good medical practice; duties of doctors*. (Accessed 14 March 2011) www.gmcuk.org/guidance/good_medical_practice/duties_of_a_doctor.asp.

Greenhalgh T (2006) *How to Read a Paper: The Basis of Evidence Medicine,* 3rd edn. Oxford: Blackwell.

Grundstein-Amado R (1992) Differences in ethical decision-making processes among nurses and doctors. *Journal of Advanced Nursing* 17:129–39.

Harrington JM, Gill FS, Aw TC and Gardiner K (1998) *Occupational Health,* 4th edn. Oxford: Blackwell Science.

Health Professions Council (HPC) (2008) *Standards of Conduct Performance and Ethics.* (Accessed October 2011) www.hpc-uk.org/aboutregistration/standards/standardsofconductperformanceandethics.

Hogg C (1999) *Patients, Power and Politics: From Patients to Citizens.* London: Sage.

Hudson B (2000) Inter-agency collaboration – a sceptical view. In Brechin A, Brown H and Eby MA (eds) *Critical Practice in Health and Social Care.* London: Sage, pp. 253–74.

ICO (nd) *Health Data Protection – Looking after the Information You Hold about Patients.* (Accessed 1 October 2011) www.ico.gov.uk/for_organisations/sector_guides/health.aspx.

Katz JN, Kessler CL, O'Connell A and Levine SA (2007) Professionalism and evolving concepts of quality. *Society of General Internal Medicine.* USA.

King's Fund (2007) *Professional Regulation. King's Fund Briefing.* London: King's Fund.

Laming Lord (2003) *The Victoria Climbié Inquiry Report.* London: Department of Health.

Leatherman S and Sutherland K (2007) *Patient and Public Experience of the NHS.* London: The Health Foundation.

Luker KA (2002) Nurse prescribing from the community: nurse's perspective. *International Journal of Pharmacy Practice* 10:273–80.

Marmot M (2010) *Fair Society, Healthy Lives: A Strategic Review of Health Inequalities in England Post-2010.* (Accessed 14 December 2010) www.marmotreview.org/english-review-of-hi: www.marmotreview.org/AssetLibrary/pdfs/chapters%20of%20fshi/FairSocietyHealthyLivesContents.pdf.

Miller E and Cameron K (2011) Challenges and benefits in implementing shared interagency assessment across the UK: A literature review. *Journal of Interprofessional Care* 25:39–45.

National Archives (2010) *Policy and Guidance Confidentiality*. Department of Health Publications. (Accessed 8 March 2011) http://webarchive.nationalarchives.gov.uk/+/www.dh.gov.uk/en/Publicationsandstatistics/Publications/PublicationsPolicyAndGuidance/Browsable/DH_5133529.

Newham Council (2009) *Caldicott Principles.* (Accessed 8 March 2011) www.newham.gov.uk/yourcouncil/informationmanagement/.

Nursing and Midwifery Council (NMC) (2006) *Standards of Proficiency for Nurse and Midwife Prescribers.* London: NMC.

NMC (2008) *The Code: Standards of Conduct, Performance and Ethics for Nurses and Midwives.* (Accessed 1 October 2011) www.nmc-uk.org/Nurses-and-midwives/The-code/The-code-in-full.

NMC (2010) *Standards of Proficiency for Pre-registration Nursing Education.* (Accessed 1 October 2011) www.nmc-uk.org/Educators/Standards-for-education/Standards-of-proficiency-for-pre-registration-nursing-education.

Nygren-Krug H (2002) *25 Questions and Answers on Health and Human Rights*. Geneva: World Health Organization.

O'Keefe E, Ottewill R and Wall A (1992) *Community Health Issues in Management*. Sunderland: Business Education.

Parker K, Moyo E, Boyd L, Hewitt S, Weltz S and Reynolds S (2006) What is professionalism in the applied health sciences? *Journal of Allied Health* 35:2.

Peckham S and Exworthy M (2003) *Primary Care in the UK*. Basingstoke: Palgrave Macmillan.

Pietroni PC (1991) Stereotypes or archetypes? A study of perceptions amongst health care students. *Journal of Social Work Practice* 5:61–9.

Radcliffe V (2008) Non-medical prescribing. In Neno R and Price D (eds) *The Handbook for Advanced Primary Care Nurses*. Maidenhead: Open University Press, pp. 78–88.

Ross F (2006) *The Professional Experience of Governance and Incentives: Meeting the Needs of People with Complex Conditions in Primary Care*. NCCSDO. (Accessed 1 October 2011) www.sdo.nihr.ac.uk/files/project/128-final-report.pdf.

Skinner J (2011) *VALUE: Valuing Users in Education*. An evaluation report. Unpublished.

Steel N (2006) Being explicit about values in public health. In Pencheon D, Guest C, Melzer D and Muir Gray JA (eds) *Oxford Handbook of Public Health Practice*. Oxford: Oxford University Press, pp. 56–62.

Thistlethwaite J (2007) A commentary from the editorial team. *Journal of Interprofessional Care* 21:2336–9.

Thompson IE, Melia KM and Boyd KM (1990) *Nursing Ethics*. Edinburgh: Churchill Livingstone.

Ward D (2009) Groupwork. In Adams R, Dominelli L and Payne M (eds) *Critical Practice in Social Work*. Basingstoke: Palgrave Macmillan, pp. 115–24.

Wilkinson R and Pickett K (2010) *The Spirit Level: Why Equality is Better for Everyone*. London: Penguin.

Williams A (2000) *Nursing, Medicine and Primary Care*. Buckingham: Open University Press.

Worth A (2001) Assessment of the needs of older people by district nurses and social workers: a changing culture? *Journal of Interprofessional Care* 15:257–66.

FURTHER RESOURCES

www.cqc.org.uk – Care Quality Commission

www.wales.nhs.uk/sitesplus/829/opendoc/167542 – Health and Social Care Working Together (2010) examples of good practice in Wales

www.evidence.nhs.uk – NHS evidence

www.nice.org.uk – NICE (the National Institute for Health and Clinical Evidence)

Managing risk

Dee Drew and Debra Smith

LEARNING OUTCOMES

- Explain the importance of preparation needed prior to visiting patients and clients in their homes
- Explore issues relating to the health and safety of nurses working in community settings
- Discuss the use of risk assessment tools to predict patients at risk of readmission and admission
- Consider the care of vulnerable individuals in the community

INTRODUCTION

Working in the community provides many challenges and opportunities. When placed in non-hospital settings as a student nurse or embarking upon a career as a community staff nurse, it is timely to reflect upon personal safety. Staff who are new to the community setting should be carefully mentored, especially if exposed to working as part of a large team (Drew, 2011). Therefore, the first section of this chapter explores the safety of nurses working in community settings. This includes preparation for home visiting, car safety and the principles of risk management. Risk assessment is crucial to support the health and safety of both patients and nursing teams (Reynolds, 2009).

The second part of this chapter focuses upon predictive risk, the use of tools to assess readmission and admission of patients and explores the care of vulnerable groups, including those with mental health problems, older people and children.

PERSONAL SAFETY

This section includes the considerations for preparation for home visiting, car safety and organizational support. These issues will be followed by an exploration of the principles of risk management.

Preparation and being streetwise

This includes developing knowledge of the area in which the nurse is to work, developing self-awareness and understanding why and how aggression can escalate.

First, learn the geography of the area, whether that is a town, clinic or surgery. Become familiar with the layout of rooms and buildings and note the position of exits. Find out what is known about the community. Without falling into the trap of stereotyping people, investigate what reputation the area has; for example, find out about crime rates. Talk to your colleagues about safety. It is strongly recommended that visible security measures, involving personnel and technology, should be evident in health centres and clinics.

ACTIVITY 4.1

Reflection point

The Ladybridge Estate is known to be a very deprived area with a high crime rate. Car theft and muggings are increasing. List the precautions that could be taken by the community staff nurse prior to visiting a patient on the estate. Reflect upon your own experiences to date.

Review your local policy for lone working. Then discuss your findings with an experienced colleague/mentor.

There may be areas within the surrounding locality that are considered to be high risk. Sometimes community staff visit these in pairs. Find out if the remit of the post involves visiting after dark.

It is good practice to gather as much information as is possible before setting off to a patient or client's house. A survey by the Royal College of Nursing (2007) highlighted that risk assessments are not always considered before first visits and this could potentially put individuals at increased risk. It is important to locate and become familiar with your own organization's Lone Working Policy.

Preparation for home visiting

This section will focus on home visits as there are particular features that could, potentially, compromise personal safety.

Bearing the above in mind, first read carefully any records or notes pertaining to the visit. Talk to colleagues who may know the situation and who should make sure that concerns are shared. Look at the location of the visit – think about how you will get there.

Always remember that home visits, however welcome by the patient or client, are an invasion of that individual's space (Table 4.1).

The community nurse is a visitor in the patient's home and must wait to be invited in. It is good practice to discourage patients from leaving notes (for example 'please come round to the back – door open') and hanging keys on strings behind letter boxes. These strategies, obviously, put patients at risk from unscrupulous opportunists and should be discouraged. In addition to these measures, the community nurse should offer personal identification.

The majority of home visits are very welcome to the patient or client. Relationships between community staff and the people they care for can be very positive and a rewarding aspect of working in primary care. With thought, observation and self-awareness many potential problems may be avoided.

Table 4.1 Upon arrival at a patient or client's home

Considerations	Rationale
Remember that you are the visitor	It is the patient or client's space that you are invading – it is unknown what is or has recently been happening within that person's home
State clearly who you are and why you have come. Show your identity badge	Don't assume that the person will recognize a uniform (if one is worn) or will be expecting the visit. It is good practice to encourage patients and clients to ask to see identification. This protects them as well as the professional
Wait to be invited into the house and ask which room the patient or client would like you to use for your visit	Being pushy can make people irritated and angry. It may not be convenient for the patient or client to allow you into a particular room. This may be for good reason, e.g. if an unpredictable dog is shut in there!
Note the layout of the house – exits, telephones	In case a speedy exit is required
Be careful with people's property – protect their belongings	Spillages, breakages or rough treatment of belongings will irritate – remember the visitor status
Be alert – monitor moods and expressions during the visit	Changes in the demeanour of the patient or client could indicate potential conflict developing
Be self-aware – monitor the manner in which information is given and care carried out. Do not react to conditions which may seem unacceptable – dirty, smelly environments, for example	The nurse should not provoke feelings of anger. Remember that this is the patient or client's home
Trust instinctive feelings. If you feel that leaving quickly is the thing to do – go	Often assessment of situations takes place on many levels. If uncomfortable feelings are building up don't wait until there is an incident
If prevented from leaving' try not to panic – see the section relating to interpersonal relationships	It may be possible for you to de-escalate the situation

Car safety

Working in a community setting involves being mobile (Griffith and Tengnah, 2007b). In some localities bicycles may be an entirely appropriate way to get around; in busy cities public transport is often the best option. For most community staff, however, it would be impossible to function effectively without a car.

Some practical measures need to be undertaken relating to car safety (Table 4.2) and areas between car parks and clinic/surgery buildings should be well lit.

In addition, it is helpful to plan the route to the destination with care. As the geography of the area becomes more familiar, this will become easier. Try not to give the impression that you are unsure of the way. Some police experts are now recommending that car doors are kept locked while driving in more dangerous areas. Good preparation for the journey makes it more likely that the nurse will arrive at the patient's home feeling calm. It is better to avoid road rage – especially if it is your own. Community nurses should appear purposeful, confident and in control when walking between car and house. Walk towards the kerb side of the pavement and away from alleyways and hedges. Footwear should be comfortable and allow for

Table 4.2 Car safety

Consideration	Rationale
It makes sense to ensure the vehicle is well maintained	Not only is it inconvenient, it may be hazardous to break down in a remote place after dark. Well worth the expense of servicing and looking after the car
Try not to run out of petrol	The car will not be happy and again this could leave you stranded in remote or unsavoury places
Park with thought	Look for safe parking places. In the dark it is helpful to find a street light to park underneath. Try to park near to the destination
Take out breakdown cover	At least someone is coming to assist you. Always state that you are alone and make it clear if you are female
Keep any nursing bags out of view – in addition to any personal valuables	Some people may believe that nurses carry drugs in their bags – prevent temptation

speed, if necessary. It is not a good idea to wear jewellery at work for many reasons. Chains may catch or be pulled; rings and wristwatches are a hazard to patients and clients if physical care is needed. In addition to these (well-known) considerations, jewellery could catch the attention of muggers.

It is important to remember that insurance cover from employers relates to the duration of the shift.

ORGANIZATIONAL SUPPORT

Organizations that fail to make sure that their employees drive safely may face prosecution. Police may investigate whether basic checks have been made by management (such as whether vehicles have MoT certificates and insurance for business use). There may also be issues around excessive demands being made on staff (Griffith and Tengnah, 2007b), such as driving when tired.

Under the 1974 Health and Safety at Work Act, employers have a duty to provide a safe working environment. Along with the responsibilities for employers there are requirements that need to be carried out by employees. First, locate any policies and procedures that exist locally relating to health and safety. Study these carefully and note the reporting arrangements that are laid down for staff to follow.

Nurses must work within the parameters of their professional Code of Practice (NMC, 2008), and this should be enabled by employers.

It is good practice to contact the work base at the end of the day to let someone know that visits are complete. The team leader will delegate visits to each member of staff and will coordinate the team. The order in which visits are carried out may not be predictable, but someone will know where each nurse should be visiting on a daily basis.

Many community nurses have the use of a mobile telephone, which can be useful in difficult situations. It may not be possible, however, to access the phone at the very time that you may need it. Mobile phones do not ensure safety, but they help. The use of personal alarms may be useful, to frighten, disorientate and debilitate an attacker. The Suzy Lamplugh Trust (see Further resources) offers information about personal safety and car travel.

Assessment of risk is a requirement to minimize potential harm and community nurses need to consider safety issues from both practical and professional perspectives.

PRINCIPLES OF RISK MANAGEMENT

Risk management is an analysis of what could potentially harm people, the environment, the organization and the public, and subsequently assessing measures of prevention (DH, 2007).

These apply to all situations that have potential for risk. It is the case that many interventions carried out by nurses carry risks of harm to patients, the nurse and the general public.

Identify the hazards

This includes reports of threats and abuse, not only physical violence, by patients, carers or others. Remember that this could be when the nurse is on or off duty. Incidents include falls, needlestick injuries and stress (Griffith and Tengnah, 2010).

ACTIVITY 4.2

Discussion point
Select one of the identified hazards above. Locate local policies and procedures relating to that hazard and read them. Work through the stages of risk assessment with the chosen topic in mind. Discuss your thoughts with your team leader.

Your discussions may lead you to consider those who may potentially be vulnerable and by working through the following principles you can be better prepared for visits.

Identify who is at risk – who might be harmed and how

Specify who could be harmed by the risk. This could include other members of the nursing team, other professionals and lay people.

Remember that employers have their own duty of care for personal health and safety.

Evaluate the risk and decide on precautions

Assess the seriousness of the situation. Identify what can be done to minimize or eliminate the risk to protect those who could be harmed. Senior nurses will carry out the assessment of the risk with contributing evidence from the team. However, it is everyone's responsibility to identify and report potentially hazardous situations.

Record the findings and proposed actions

Decisions taken and workable measures to minimize the risk must be documented.

This provides a working plan for staff and managers outlining all of the above in addition to steps that may still need to be taken. Be sure to record events accurately (NMC, 2008). Documentation needs to be comprehensive and accurate, containing a full account of intervention and assessment of the situation (NMC, 2008). Avoid the use of jargon and abbreviations. Incident-reporting systems exist to protect the safety of patients and staff (Armitage, 2005; Evans *et al.*, 2007).

Poor communication of risks can result in misunderstanding and failure to pass on vital information to other colleagues.

Review and revise the assessment as necessary

Assessment is a dynamic process. It is important to revisit the document, particularly after incidents are reported. Staff training and communications should also be reviewed.

Policies and procedures need to be current, available to those who need them and comprehensive. In order not to compromise patient care, care plans need to be regularly reviewed and updated so that staff are clear what has been found on assessment and what interventions are required.

ACTIVITY 4.3

Identify whose responsibility it is to review the health and safety policies in your area. Find out where these are kept and how often they are updated. Reflect on your own responsibilities in relation to health and safety.

A very useful publication by the National Patient Safety Agency is *Seven Steps to Patient Safety for Primary Care* (2006), a guide to best practice describing key areas of activity that primary care organizations and teams can work through to safeguard their patients.

THE SEVEN STEPS TO PATIENT SAFETY

Step 1 Build a safety culture

Create a culture that is open and fair

Step 2 Lead and support your staff

Establish a clear and strong focus on patient safety throughout your organization

Step 3 Integrate your risk management activity

Develop systems and processes to manage your risks and identify and assess things that could go wrong

Step 4 Promote reporting

Ensure your staff can easily report incidents locally and nationally

Step 5 Involve and communicate with patients and the public

Develop ways to communicate openly with and listen to patients

Step 6 Learn and share safety lessons

Encourage staff to use root cause analysis to learn how and why incidents happen

Step 7 Implement solutions to prevent harm

Embed lessons through changes to practice, processes

Patient safety concerns everyone in the NHS, and it is crucial that every member of staff is aware of these issues. The current government has stated its objective to reduce mortality and morbidity, increase safety and improve patient experience and outcomes (DH, 2010). This can be achieved only if professionals and organizations work within a culture of open information and take responsibility for their contribution to the patients they care for.

RAISING CONCERNS

The Nursing and Midwifery Council has produced useful guidance for nurses who are concerned (NMC, 2010). The booklet offers a step-by-step guide to raising and escalating concerns. It begins at Stage 1 by advocating that concerns are first raised internally with the respective line manager. These issues may be about the safety and wellbeing of people in the nurse's care or the environment in which nurses work.

Organizations must clearly enable nurses to raise concerns (RCN, 2010).

IDENTIFYING PATIENTS AT RISK OF READMISSION AND ADMISSION

There are a number of ways of seeking to identify patients who may become high risk, particularly in terms of admission or readmission to hospital. Three main strategies have been explored (King Fund, 2006) to ascertain the most effective way to do this. Evidence demonstrates that the most reliable method is that of predictive modelling.

Following on from this work, a number of tools have been developed to identify patients at risk of rehospitalization (PARR1 and PARR2, Scottish Patients at Risk of Readmission and Admission, SPARRA). Based upon prior hospital discharge data a case-finding algorithm identifies patients at high risk of rehospitalization, providing a mechanism to 'flag' those with a high probability of subsequent emergency admission. These patients may have their risk reduced with improved health and social care.

A risk score is generated from a range of information about the patient, including the reason for current admission, previous admissions within the past 3 years, conditions and diagnoses and geographical data.

The use of predictive modelling aims to help identify those not yet considered to be 'high risk' to help prevent deterioration in their conditions and hospitalization. High rates of previous admission to hospital in isolation do not necessarily indicate a continued high risk and the need for interventions. Keeping patients at home is a key aim for community services and largely viewed as the better outcome for most patients. Implementation of the long-term conditions agenda (DH, 2005) focuses upon helping patients to receive care closer to home (DH, 2005) by prevention of admission or by accelerated discharge. These tools may also be helpful in service delivery and prove cost-effective (Billings *et al.*, 2006).

Vulnerable groups

Within the community setting, it is difficult to offer any one single definition of the term 'vulnerable' and often the concept of vulnerability is open to interpretation by health professionals. Individuals who may come under the umbrella term of vulnerable include the young, old, unemployed, individuals with mental health problems, those suffering with long-term conditions or disabilities, and those from ethnic minority groups. It is important to highlight that patient safety issues when working with vulnerable groups are paramount and community nurses must ensure that they are aware of both national and local policies for the protection of their patients (Brammer, 2009).

From the above explanation, it is clear that community nurses frequently come into contact with individuals from vulnerable groups. However, for the purpose of this chapter, the issues of mental health, falls and child protection will be considered in respect of community nurses and their involvement in the care of vulnerable groups.

PEOPLE WITH MENTAL HEALTH ISSUES

It is acknowledged that the rising incidence of mental health disorders is a cause for concern for health service providers within the UK. Currently, up to 40% of elderly people who visit their GP will have a mental health problem. The figure rises to 60% for residents in care homes suffering from mental health issues. In the current climate of an ageing population, it is projected that up to one million people will be suffering with dementia by 2025 (Commission for Healthcare Audit and Inspection, 2009).

It is recognized that community nurses have an increased role in the care of patients with an established mental health problem or those who may be at risk of isolation, stress and other chronic conditions that may contribute to the development of mental health issues (Haddad, 2010). Indeed, Lord Darzi's review, *High Quality Care for All* (DH, 2008), identified the key public health promotion role of nurses working within the community environment. Many people visited by community nurses are elderly people, who by the nature of the ageing process, and other diseases including diabetes, hypertension and cardiovascular disease, can be predisposed to mental health problems, and subsequent alterations in their cognitive function and abilities (Manthorpe and Iliffe, 2007). This can have a major impact upon the individual and their family and carers, and may result in the need for provision of both social and physical care. Furthermore, when cognitive function and the ability to participate in self-care are so affected, it may become too difficult to support the individual within their own home. This can have a profound effect upon the long-term care of the individual. Community nurses can implement strategies which may include screening, assistance with medication, referral to other specialized mental health services as well as monitoring individuals with established mental health problems (Thompson *et al.*, 2008).

Of all of the mental health disorders, caring for patients with dementia can be one of the most challenging for community nurses (Sherrod *et al.*, 2010). Dementia can be defined as 'a combination of impairment in two or more aspects of cognition, for example, memory loss, orientation, and problems with managing everyday tasks' (NICE, 2006). For patients who are visited on a regular basis by community nurses, it may be that such problems are identified at an early stage, and appropriate interventions and referral can be made. It is suggested that there is a need for reliable screening tools to be utilized in practice in order to appropriately assess individual needs (Haddad, 2010), for example, the Mini Mental State Examination (Shenkin *et al.*, 2008). In addition, it is essential that community nurses are appropriately educated to enhance their ability and confidence to recognize and manage mental health problems.

Another common mental health problem within the community is depression. For many individuals this can be a lifelong chronic condition which can have far-reaching effects on morbidity and mortality (Shia, 2009). It has an effect on individuals' self-esteem, wellbeing and relationships, and it can affect an individual's ability to work. As such it then has an overall effect upon the national economy. It has been estimated that at least one in four individuals will suffer from an episode of depression at some point during their lives (Shia, 2009). It can be triggered by a variety of factors including bereavement, relationship problems, unemployment, stress or physical health problems and many individuals will experience loss of interest, feeling sad and tearful, feeling tired, restlessness, sleeping problems, and eating problems. In addition, women can experience post-natal depression following the birth of a baby.

Depression can be classified as mild, moderate, severe and chronic. The severity of the condition is determined by the number and severity of symptoms as well as the resulting degree of functional impairment (NICE, 2004). Consequently, it places a high demand on primary care services, in particular GP appointments, with a high proportion of consultations relating to patients with a mental health issue.

It is extremely important that community nurses are able to realize the crucial role that they have in recognizing those individuals with signs and symptoms of depression and making the appropriate referral to other health professionals. There are a number of risk assessment tools available that can be used in the assessment of depression, including the Edinburgh Postnatal Depression Scale (Cox *et al.*, 1987). Collaborative and interprofessional working practices are paramount in order for individuals to receive the appropriate level of support and treatment.

Furthermore, it is essential that community nurses are aware of their role in improving patient safety in the area of mental health. The National Patient Safety Agency (2008) provides guidance on how everyone working in the NHS can work collectively to improve the quality and safety of care they provide to their patients.

CARING FOR OLDER PEOPLE

Community nursing encompasses caring for people of all ages. However, a large proportion of the community nurses' caseload will involve caring for older people.

This section will focus on living in isolation and will cover falls.

The number of older people is set to increase. The fastest rise has been in individuals over the age of 85. In 2008 there were 1.3 million individuals aged 85 and over in the UK. By 2018 this number is projected to increase to 1.8 million and by 2033 to 3.3 million (ONS, 2009). Many of these people will be living alone.

In 2008, Age Concern (now Age UK) described the term 'social exclusion' as 'feeling detached from society, trapped at home, cut off from services, lonely and isolated and struggling to cope' (Age Concern, 2008: 2). Furthermore, it identified four specific groups which may need support. These are individuals who have been recently bereaved, those who are living in unfit housing, individuals who struggle to make their own decisions (for example, those with dementia and learning disabilities) and those aged over 80 years and living alone. It is essential that community nurses also recognize that individuals who have a sensory deficit, for example poor eyesight or hearing, also may experience social isolation and exclusion, particularly as they may have difficulties in participating in conversations, meetings and community social events (Jones and Rowbottom, 2010). Social isolation can also result in changes in nutritional status. The highest risk groups include the elderly housebound, especially men who live alone, those with a reduced income and those with additional chronic illness (Krondl *et al.,* 2008). Nutritional screening and assessment with an appropriate tool are required in order to address the needs of these individuals.

Community nurses need to be particularly aware of the needs of older people within these groups. It is important to know what support there is (both locally and nationally) in terms of health and social care. The range of voluntary services may vary across the UK, but can still provide valuable advice and resources to individuals and health professionals. Although the provision of advice and information is paramount, it is important to recognize the potential barriers that can exist in the provision of information to these individuals. Some of these barriers include an increasing reliance on the use of the Internet for information and transactions, and the use of language and communication styles. Community nurses need to work closely with these elderly people to assist them in accessing and understanding information (Hislop, 2010).

Falls

It is recognized that living alone and social isolation can also be risk factors for falls among the elderly population (Roe *et al.*, 2009). Although individuals of any age can fall, it is known that adults over the age of 70 years, especially women, have a significantly higher mortality rate from falls than younger people. Additionally, 50% of individuals over the age of 80 years will fall at least once each year, with a significant number of them having another fall within the same year. For individuals who live in residential care the number is even higher, with as many as 40% of residents falling at least twice each year (Oliver, 2007).

A fall can be defined as 'an event which results in a person coming to rest inadvertently on the ground or other level' (WHO, 2010).

Community nurses may come into contact with individuals who have sustained injuries, or who have lost mobility or have suffered a loss of function and are therefore at high risk of falling. As community nurses are in regular contact with older people, they are in a prime position to make a difference in the prevention and subsequent management of those who are at risk of falling or have actually fallen.

Falls in elderly people are a major cause of injury and disability. Injuries include soft-tissue damage, fractures and head injuries; sometimes as a result of lying on the floor for a prolonged period of time unable to get up, pressure damage, dehydration and hypothermia can develop (Oliver, 2007). The individual may require admission to hospital or to long-term care, and those who remain at home may subsequently have a fear of falling, which can have a significant impact upon their ability to perform their activities of daily living. Anxiety and loss of confidence can result in increasing dependency both on community services and on their family and carers. It is essential to promote a safe environment in order to prevent harm and accidental injury within the community, and this is a crucial element of the community nurse's role (Muir and Bennett, 2010).

An integrated falls service can provide care and treatment for individuals following a fall and promote prevention strategies to identify those at most risk and to reduce the incidence of falls.

The aim is to provide rehabilitation and long-term support to prevent further incidents and to promote individual confidence and independence (DH, 2001).

Key risk factors include a previous fall, recurrent falls within the past 12 months, balance and gait problems, recent fracture, and osteoporosis and/or low bone density (Muir and Bennett, 2010).

NICE (2004) recommends that older people who have had recurrent falls or who are assessed as being at a high risk of falling should be offered an individualized, multifactorial risk assessment. Many organizations will have approved documentation for recording the assessment (Robertson *et al.*, 2010). It is acknowledged that this assessment needs to be conducted by an appropriately qualified health professional. Many organizations have introduced a Falls Service to address the needs of this group. Following assessment, if appropriate, the individual may be offered a multifactorial intervention. The aim of this is to identify and address future risk, as well as promoting the individual's independence and improving their overall physical and psychological function. The following components are common to this type of intervention: strength and balance training, home hazard assessment and intervention, vision assessment and medication review (NICE, 2004). If nurses have not received specialized training to undertake this depth of assessment they are still in a position to give basic home safety advice, for example ensuring that loose carpets and rugs are removed or secured and that footwear is appropriate and fits well (Swann, 2010).

Until recently, prevention of falls had been considered low priority in service delivery, training and research (Oliver, 2007).

Community nurses and other health professionals working in the community environment need to take the opportunity to routinely ask elderly patients who they come into contact with about any falls they have had in the past 12 months. This needs to be recorded on appropriate organizational documentation using a recognized assessment tool. The next activity will enable you to consider the issues in relation to a specific patient.

ACTIVITY 4.4

Reflection point

Reflect upon an older person you have visited recently. Consider their home environment and identify any hazards. Discuss with a colleague ways that you can advise this person to keep themselves safe.

With the elderly population increasing, it is recognized that the consequences of frail individuals falling will pose a greater challenge to both health and social care services.

Find out about the falls prevention service in your area. Identify the criteria for referring a client.

SAFEGUARDING CHILDREN AND YOUNG PEOPLE

Child protection can be defined as 'the process of protecting individual children identified as either suffering or likely to suffer significant harm as a result of abuse or neglect' (Department for Children Schools and Families, 2010).

Children and young people are another important group for community nurses to focus upon in relation to risk assessment and safety. Child protection cannot be provided by one single discipline, it requires a multi-agency, collaborative approach. Community nurses are in a unique position to safeguard children as their contact with children, young people and their families allows them to deliver both proactive and reactive child protection approaches (DH, 2004). It is essential therefore that nurses are aware of and can recognize the predisposing factors of child harm. Maltreatment of children can manifest in many different ways, including signs of physical, emotional and sexual abuse, neglect and fabricated or induced illness (NICE, 2009). A child protection issue may arise in a variety of nursing encounters, even when the initial encounter has a completely different focus. It is possible that nurses who are new to the community environment may have received little training and preparation for this element of their role. Additionally, it is essential that nurses have the knowledge and skills to work collaboratively with other disciplines and agencies in order to protect and safeguard the health and wellbeing of children (Sheffield, 2008).

Community nurses who are involved in the care of patients with mental health problems are ideally situated to offer support and to identify the issues which suggest that a child may be at risk of neglect or harm. Often, these patients may be parents or relatives living in households alongside children.

If nurses suspect that a child is subject to harm or neglect, then they have a responsibility to refer their concerns to appropriate personnel (DH, 2006). This can be a very difficult area of nursing practice and needs to be addressed in a sensitive manner.

The Laming Report (2009) suggests that child protection training should be a mandatory element of GP initial education and continuing professional development. Additionally, all other members of general practice staff should receive mandatory training, as their roles often bring them into direct contact with children and young people. It is acknowledged that community staff will need support to develop their skills and confidence to be able to work in this important area (Laming Report, 2009).

It is the duty of the employer to ensure that the workforce is competent in the area of child protection and safeguarding. All staff should know what to do if they suspect a child is being abused or neglected, and should be able to recognize key indicators that suggest that a child or young person's welfare or development may be impaired or that they may be at risk of actual harm (Griffith and Tengnah, 2007a). Often, interagency training is delivered, as it is thought to improve collaborative working processes between professionals involved in child protection issues (Charles and Horwath, 2009).

Every Child Matters is a government initiative that was launched in 2003 following the death of Victoria Climbié. The policy provides guidance for those who deliver children's services, and includes children and young people up to the age of 19 or 24 years (for those who have any form of disability).

Working Together to Safeguard Children (2010) follows on from the report by Lord Laming and suggests that all training in safeguarding and promoting the welfare of children and young people should be child centred, promote the participation of children and their families in the process, value collaborative working, respect diversity and promote equality (DH, 2010). Other countries in the UK have equivalent policies and guidelines that can be accessed in further reading.

To understand and identify significant harm, it is necessary for health professionals to consider

- the nature of harm, in terms of maltreatment or failure to provide adequate care;
- the impact on the child's health and development;
- the child's development within the context of their family and wider environment;
- any special needs, such as a medical condition, communication impairment or disability, that may affect the child's development and care within the family;

- the capacity of parents to meet adequately the child's needs;
- the wider and environmental family context (DH, 2003).

Please carry out the next activity to supplement your developing knowledge in this crucial area of practice.

ACTIVITY 4.5

Find out who is the lead person for child protection issues in your organization. Identify the local policy and guidelines, read them and discuss the referral process with a colleague.

The above text and activities are designed to assist you in developing your professional practice with vulnerable groups. You will need to ensure that this aspect of your work is regularly updated in line with organizational processes and policies.

CONCLUSION

After careful consideration of the issues addressed within this chapter, turn back to the learning outcomes at the beginning and think about each one in turn. Look back and reflect upon the notes made for the first activity at the beginning of this chapter.

If this chapter has raised any concerns for practice, it is important that they are discussed with an experienced community nurse, either informally or through clinical supervision channels. Some useful addresses can be found at the end of this section.

Remember that the majority of staff working in community settings enjoy a close partnership with their patients and clients. The health centre or surgery is at the heart of the local community and relationships may build over a number of years. Visiting patients and clients in their homes is a privilege that greatly enhances the experience of community nursing. Taking practical precautions and taking time to think about the assessment of risk and preparation are crucial elements of nursing in the community.

REFERENCES

Age Concern (2008) *Out of Sight, Out of Mind: Social Exclusion Behind Closed Doors.* London: Age Concern.

Armitage C (2005) TRAIL: a model to promote active learning from adverse events. *Quality in Primary Care* 13:159–62.

Billings J, Dixon J, Mijanovich T and Wennberg D (2006) Case finding for patients at risk of readmission to hospital: development of algorithm to identify high risk patients. *British Medical Journal* 333:327–30.

Brammer A (2009) Legal developments since No Secrets. *Journal of Adult Protection* 11:43–53.

Charles M and Horwath J (2009) Investing in interagency training to safeguard children: an act of faith or an act of reason? *Children and Society* 23:364–76.

Commission for Healthcare Audit and Inspection (2009) *Equality in Later Life. A National Study of Older People's Mental Health Services.* London: The Stationery Office.

Cox JL, Holden JM and Sagovsky R (1987) Detection of postnatal depression. Development of the 10 item Edinburgh Postnatal Depression Scale. *British Journal of Psychiatry* 150:782–6.

Department for Children Schools and Families (2010) *Working Together to Safeguard Children*. London: The Stationery Office.

Department of Health (DH) (2001) *National Service Framework for Older People*. London: The Stationery Office.

DH (2003) *Every Child Matters*. London: The Stationery Office.

DH (2004) *National Service Framework for Children, Young People and Maternity Services*. London: The Stationery Office.

DH (2005) *Supporting People with Long Term Conditions: An NHS and Social Care Model to Support Local Innovation and Integration*. London: The Stationery Office.

DH (2006) *What To Do if You're Worried a Child is Being Abused*. London: The Stationery Office.

DH (2007) *Independence, Choice and Risk: A Guide to Best Practice in Supporting Decision Making*. London: The Stationery Office.

DH (2008) *High Quality Care for All*. London: The Stationery Office.

DH (2010) *Equity and Excellence: Liberating the NHS*. London: The Stationery Office.

Drew D (2011) Professional identity and the culture of community nursing. *British Journal of Community Nursing* 16:126–31.

Evans A, Williams L, Wiltshire M, *et al.* (2007) Incident reporting improves safety: the use of the RAID process for improving incident reporting and learning within primary care. *Quality in Primary Care*1 5:107–12.

Griffith R and Tengnah C (2007a) Protecting children: the role of the law 2. Legal powers to safeguard children. *British Journal of Community Nursing* 12:175–80.

Griffith R and Tengnah C (2007b) Role of the law in ensuring work related road safety. *British Journal of Community Nursing* 12:574–8.

Griffith R and Tengnah C (2010) Health and safety at work: a guide for district nurses. *British Journal of Community Nursing* 15:77–80.

Haddad M (2010) Caring for patients with long-term conditions and depression. *Nursing Standard* 24:40–9.

Hislop C (2010) Improving access to information: a key requirement for reducing social exclusion. *Working With Older People* 14:38–43.

Jones M and Rowbottom C (2010) The role of telecare in overcoming social exclusion in older people. *Journal of Assistive Technologies* 4:54–9.

King's Fund (2006) *Case Finding Algorithms for Patients at Risk of Re-hospitalisation. PARR1 and PARR2*. London: King's Fund.

Krondl M, Coleman P and Lau D (2008) Helping older adults meet nutritional challenges. *Journal of Nutrition for the Elderly* 27:205–20.

Laming Report (2009) *The Protection of Children in England: A Progress Report*. London: The Stationery Office.

Manthorpe J and Iliffe S (2007) Timely recognition of dementia: community nurses' crucial roles. *British Journal of Community Nursing* 12:74–6.

Muir N and Bennett C (2010) Prevention of unintentional injury in the community setting. *Nursing Standard* 24:50–6.

National Institute for Health and Clinical Excellence NICE (2004) *Falls. The Assessment and Prevention of Falls in Older People*. Clinical Guideline 21. London: The Stationery Office.

NICE (2004) *Depression: Principles of Care*. Update of Clinical Guideline 23. London: The Stationery Office.

NICE (2006) *Dementia: Supporting People with Dementia and their Carers in Health and Social Care*. Clinical Guideline 42. London: The Stationery Office.

NICE (2009) *When to Suspect Child Maltreatment*. London: The Stationery Office.

National Patient Safety Agency (NPSA) (2006) *Seven Steps to Patient Safety for Primary Care*. London: NPSA.

NPSA (2008) *Seven Steps to Patient Safety in Mental Health*. London: NPSA.

Nursing and Midwifery Council (NMC) (2008) *The Code: Standards of Conduct, Performance and Ethics for Nurses and Midwives*. London: NMC.

NMC (2010) *Raising and Escalating Concerns: Guidance for Nurses and Midwives*. London: NMC.

Office for National Statistics (ONS) (2009) *National Population Projections. 2008-Based*. Newport: ONS.

Oliver D (2007) Older people who fall: why they matter and what you can do. *British Journal of Community Nursing* 12:500–7.

Reynolds J (2009) Undertaking risk management in community nursing practice. *Journal of Community Nursing* 23:24–8.

Robertson K, Logan PA, Conroy S, Dods V, *et al.* (2010) Thinking falls – taking action: a guide to action for falls prevention. *British Journal of Community Nursing* 15:406–10.

Roe B, Howell F, Konstantinos R, *et al.* (2009) Older people and falls: health status, quality of life, lifestyle, care networks, prevention and views on service use following a fall. *Journal of Clinical Nursing* 18:2261–72.

Royal College of Nursing (RCN) (2007) *Lone Working Survey*. London: RCN.

RCN (2010) *Pillars of the Community: The RCN's UK Position on the Development of the Registered Nursing Workforce in the Community*. London: RCN.

Sheffield M (2008) Safeguarding children: the case for mandatory training. *Community Practitioner* 81:27–30.

Shenkin SD, Starr JM, Dunn JM, *et al.* (2008) Is there information contained within the sentence-writing component of the Mini Mental State Examination? A retrospective study of community dwelling older people. *International Journal of Geriatric Psychiatry* 23:1283–9.

Sherrod RA, Collins A, Wynn S and Gragg M (2010) Dissecting dementia, depression and drug effects in older adults. *Journal of Psychosocial Nursing* 48:39–47.

Shia N (2009) The role of community nurses in the management of depression. *Nurse Prescribing* 7:548–54.

Swann J (2010) Simple ways to prevent falls. *British Journal of Healthcare Assistants* 4:166–9.

Thompson P, Lang L and Annells M (2008) A systematic review of the effectiveness of in-home community nurse led interventions for the mental health of older persons. *Journal of Clinical Nursing* 17:1419–27.

World Health Organization (2010) Fact Sheet 344. (Accessed 22 December 2010) www.who.int/mediacentre/factsheets/fs344/en/.

FURTHER READING

Beckett C (2007) *Child Protection: An Introduction*, 2nd edn. London: Sage.

Corby B (2006) *Child Abuse: Towards a Knowledge Base*, 3rd edn. Berkshire: Open University Press.

Powell C (2007) *Safeguarding Children and Young People. A Guide for Nurses and Midwives.* Berkshire: Open University Press.

Scottish Government (2008) *Getting it Right for Every Child.* Edinburgh: Scottish Government.

FURTHER RESOURCES

www.cqc.org.uk – Care Quality Commission

www.dh.gov.uk – Department of Health

www.suzylamplugh.org – The Suzy Lamplugh Trust

www.nmc-uk.org – Nursing and Midwifery Council

www.npsa.nhs.uk – National Patient Safety Agency

www/rcn.org.uk/raisingconcerns – The Royal College of Nursing

www.unison.prg.uk – Unison

www.unitetheunion.org-cphve – CPHVA/Unite

CHAPTER

5

Therapeutic relationship

Patricia Wilson and Sue Miller

LEARNING OUTCOMES

- Identify the features of a therapeutic relationship
- Discuss some of the challenges for community nurses in establishing a therapeutic relationship
- Recognize some of the issues that may arise when trying to establish a therapeutic relationship with specific patients
- Explore some of the possible consequences of failing to establish a therapeutic relationship
- Analyze the impact of changes in policy on the development of therapeutic relationships

INTRODUCTION

This chapter will focus upon the relationship that exists between the nurse and the patient and their family. It is recognized that such a relationship should be therapeutic, and indeed this seems essential to the delivery of effective nursing care. However, it is unwise to assume a therapeutic relationship will automatically occur, as there are many challenges in establishing and maintaining such a relationship in community settings. In this chapter the key features of a therapeutic relationship will be identified, and some of the challenges of maintaining that relationship in a community setting will be discussed. This will lead the reader to consider some of the issues of particular relevance to his/her patient group, and to explore some of the consequences of failing to establish and maintain relationships. In conclusion, the current and potential changes in healthcare delivery will be reviewed with particular reference to the way these changes might impact on the nurse/patient/family relationship.

THE FEATURES OF A THERAPEUTIC RELATIONSHIP

The recognition of the importance of the therapeutic relationship is not a new phenomenon. Peplau's (1952) theory of nursing is based upon the importance of the relationship between the nurse and the patient, and she asserts this is the way in which all nursing care is delivered. The importance of this relationship has continued to be widely acknowledged and indeed Foster and Hawkins (2005) assert that it is central to advancing the best interest and outcomes for the patient. Since a therapeutic relationship is so important, it is essential to consider what features characterize such a relationship. In reviewing various definitions it becomes apparent that the important factors are:

- maintaining appropriate boundaries
- meeting the needs of the patient
- promoting patient autonomy
- positive experience for the patient.

Appropriate boundaries are maintained

A boundary as defined in the dictionary is '*a real or imagined line that marks the edge or limit of something*' (*Cambridge Dictionary Online,* 2010). Within the therapeutic relationship boundaries define how far the nurse is willing to go to meet the needs of the patient and his/her family. Therefore, it is important that the nurse, patient and family are clear regarding their relationship and what is reasonably expected of each party. This will protect all those involved in the relationship. The NMC Code (2008) states that nurses and midwives should 'maintain clear professional boundaries'. Additional guidance states 'boundaries define the limits of behaviour which allow a nurse or midwife to have a professional relationship with a person in their care' (NMC, 2009).

However, the process of finding the boundaries of care is far from automatic (Stone, 2008), as will be discussed later in this chapter.

Meets the needs of the patient

The purpose of the relationship between the nurse and patient is to meet the nursing needs of that patient. It is therefore important that the nursing needs of the patient are discussed at the outset of the relationship in order that mutually identified goals can be set and each person within the relationship can be clear about their role in achieving these goals. This might include the nurse, patient, family members, other professionals and carers. This will require expert communication skills on the part of the nurse in order that a relationship of trust can develop. Although the relationship exists to meet the needs of the patient, it is likely that the nurse will experience satisfaction in helping the patient to meet those needs. This is entirely appropriate. However, it is important that nurses do not allow their personal needs for positive self-esteem, control and belonging to undermine the professional relationship (Milton, 2008). This requires the nurse to be self-aware and open to seeking support from others when the need arises (Foster and Hawkins, 2005).

Promotes patient autonomy

Autonomy is the right to self-determination. Self-determination can be defined as an ability to understand one's own situation, to make plans and choices and to pursue personal goals (McParland *et al.*, 2000). This further supports the need for excellent communication skills on the part of the nurse in order to assist the patient to understand their own situation (Collins, 2009). Within a relationship that promotes patient autonomy the patient will contribute to the achievement of personal goals and will move towards independence.

Positive experience for the patient

The experience of participating in a therapeutic relationship will be positive for the patient as nursing needs will be met in a way that is most appropriate to the patient and their family. Truly therapeutic relationships can empower the patient, the family and the nurse.

These features are evident in guidance provided by the NMC (2009) – which states

> The relationship between a nurse or midwife and the person in their care is a professional relationship based on trust, respect and appropriate use of power. The focus of the relationship is based on meeting the health needs of the person in their care.

ACTIVITY 5.1

Reflection point
Think about entering a patient's home and establishing a therapeutic relationship. What skills do you have that would enable you to achieve this? What skills need further development? How can you develop your skills further? Discuss your ideas with your mentor/preceptor.

CHALLENGES OF DEVELOPING THERAPEUTIC RELATIONSHIPS IN COMMUNITY SETTINGS

Having considered the features of a professional relationship, some of the challenges of achieving such a relationship in the community setting will be discussed. Professional relationships with the patient are influenced by a number of factors that are illustrated in Fig. 5.1.

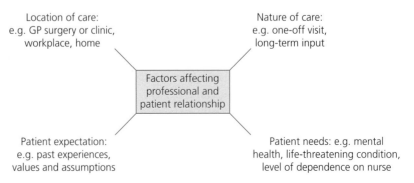

Location of care:
e.g. GP surgery or clinic, workplace, home

Nature of care:
e.g. one-off visit, long-term input

Factors affecting professional and patient relationship

Patient expectation:
e.g. past experiences, values and assumptions

Patient needs: e.g. mental health, life-threatening condition, level of dependence on nurse

Figure 5.1 Factors affecting the therapeutic relationship.

Location of care

The delivery of care within the home can provide a feeling of security for the patient and his/her carer/s as they are on familiar territory. This can make it easier to develop a good relationship, such that they are able to share their concerns and worries. It is also probable that patients and carers will be able to learn new skills more readily as they are likely to feel more relaxed within their 'normal' environment.

Example 5.1

Consider Mrs Patel whose 2-year-old son has recently been in hospital suffering from an asthmatic attack. Mrs Patel speaks some English but found the experience of her son being in hospital very stressful. When the health visitor made a visit to the home Mrs Patel was unsure how to use the prescribed medication, particularly the spacer device to administer the inhalers. Teaching within Mrs Patel's home is likely to be more successful as she will be more relaxed and it will be possible for the health visitor to reinforce any aspects of the care at a later date if this is necessary.

However, caring in the home environment can leave the nurse feeling vulnerable. A nurse who has recently left a hospital-based job to work in the community can feel very isolated (Drennan *et al.*, 2005). Despite the use of mobile phones and pagers it is more difficult to seek the advice of a colleague, and help may not be instantly at hand. A nurse who feels vulnerable and isolated will find it more difficult to inspire the confidence of patients.

Working in the relative isolation of the home can provide challenges to nurses in maintaining standards of care. If the relationship is not 'therapeutic' it can be difficult for the nurse to identify this his/herself, particularly if the situation has developed over time. The support and guidance of colleagues is essential, as is the willingness of the nurse to be open to that support. It is important that peers recognize unhealthy situations that colleagues are involved in (Halter *et al.*, 2007), but many find it difficult to discuss the situation with their colleagues (Totka, 1996).

Care given by the nurse within the patient's workplace will also be different from the more traditional hospital setting. The occupational health nurse has a pivotal role in keeping people healthy at work, or helping them to return to work as soon as possible (Oakley, 2008).

Example 5.2

Although work-related mental ill health is being increasingly recognized as a legitimate occupational health issue (Health and Safety Executive, 2007) many employees will still consider it detrimental for their career prospects to report mental health needs to their occupational health nurse. The challenge for the nurse within this context is to promote trust with the employees in order to facilitate a therapeutic relationship.

Developing therapeutic relationships may also be affected by a clinic or surgery setting, where the patient may gain the impression of busy workloads inhibiting the time they spend with the nurse. Paterson (2001) identified lack of time as a major inhibitor in developing a participatory relationship between professional and patient, and although the nurse is likely to be as busy, if not more so, when undertaking home visits, there may be fewer distractions than in a busy clinic.

Example 5.3

Consider the scenario of the new mother trying to explain her depression to the health visitor and how much harder this might be in a busy baby clinic rather than in the privacy of her own home.

In other cases the relative anonymity the surgery or clinic provides may be of benefit in facilitating the development of a therapeutic relationship. Initial assessments are often the first point of contact between community nurse and patient, and the nurse must develop skills to enable a conducive environment in order to establish the start of a therapeutic relationship (Hagerty and Patusky, 2003).

ACTIVITY 5.2

Reflection point

Do you wear a uniform when working in the community? What are the advantages and disadvantages of wearing a uniform? If you had a choice would you wear a uniform?

Working in the community many nurses find not wearing a uniform removes an unnecessary barrier and makes the development of a therapeutic relationship an easier task. It does however require skills on the part of the nurse to gain access to the patient's home, gain the patient's trust and explain her nursing role since a symbol, which for many carries some degree of status, has been lost (Shaw and Timmons, 2010).

For those community nurses who do wear a uniform other challenges arise. Wearing of a uniform can enable almost instant entry to some homes, but may present a barrier to acceptance by some people. This may be especially apparent with children who have perhaps learnt to associate uniforms with pain and discomfort. In these situations it will take time to address prior conceptions before a therapeutic relationship can be established.

If nurses do not wear a recognized uniform it is particularly important to consider the appropriateness of the clothing that is worn. Entering a home inappropriately dressed may cause offence and prevent establishment of a relationship. Perhaps this might require the nurse to cover her arms and legs if visiting Asian families, or maybe to remove shoes prior to entry into some homes. In order to meet the needs of individual families the nurse must enquire about family preferences and be willing to adapt behaviours to respect values different from her own in order to facilitate good relationships.

A final point about dress code: whether wearing uniform or not it is essential to carry identification at all times in order to protect the wellbeing of patients.

Nature of care

ACTIVITY 5.3

Discussion Point
Have you cared for a patient over a long period of time? How did your relationship with the patient develop? Did you find yourself becoming 'closer' to the patient? How did this make you feel? Discuss this with your mentor/preceptor.

A key element in the nature of the therapeutic relationship with all patient groups is the duration of the relationship. Morse (1991) describes three appropriate relationships. First, she describes the one-off clinical encounter that, for example, a practice nurse may have with a patient in a travel clinic. There are also encounters that last longer but focus on a specific need, such as maintenance of hormone replacement therapy. Both of these relationships are mutual and appropriate to certain situations, but Morse argues that within a much longer term nurse–patient relationship there should be a different focus, with the development of what Morse terms a connected relationship. Morse suggests that the key characteristic of a connected relationship is that the nurse views the patient as a person first rather than a patient.

Example 5.4

A district nurse has been visiting an elderly lady for several years. The visits now may often include a chat over a cup of tea about how the grandchildren are progressing or other issues in the patient's life that the nurse has developed a wealth of knowledge on over the years. Although it may be a venous ulcer that initiated the referral to the district nurse, the connected relationship that has developed with time allows the nurse to deal with other issues that may be far more important to the patient, such as feelings of loneliness. During the chat a skilled nurse will be able to assess for signs of depression or other psychosocial needs that are common in chronic illness.

Although for many families and professionals this can only be positive, there is a potential to step over the professional boundary and it is essential to maintain the appropriate balance within the therapeutic relationship. The consequences of not maintaining the balance will be explored later in the chapter.

ACTIVITY 5.4

Reflection point
Have you ever cared for a patient who did not follow the recommended treatment programme? Why did the patient not adhere to the treatment regimen? How did it make you feel?

In the home environment the patient and his/her carer could be perceived to have greater control within the relationship. Should the patient decide not to concur with recommended treatment, this may not be immediately evident as the nurse is spending only a short period of time within the home environment. Parkin (2001) notes that professionals are unable to control the home environment. If unbeknown to the nurse the patient has not adhered to the recommended treatment, the therapeutic relationship is threatened, since a relationship based on trust no longer exists. Within a therapeutic relationship the patient should be able to tell the nurse of his/her intentions. This might allow treatment to be modified such that the patient feels able to follow the regimen, but even if this is not the case at least the nurse is aware of the true situation and can modify the nursing care accordingly.

Example 5.5

Susie is 14 years old and has been diabetic for 3 years. She is supposed to record her blood glucose levels once daily, varying the time of day she takes the readings, but she finds this requirement tiresome and does not do it. Prior to the community children's nurse's visit she wonders what to do – should she make up some values to keep the nurse happy or should she tell the truth? Hopefully if Susie and the nurse have a good relationship she can be truthful and they can work together on what care Susie can reasonably be expected to give herself.

A study by Schaeuble *et al.* (2010) found teenagers felt it took time to develop trust in healthcare providers, with respect from the provider being a paramount issue. Some of the adolescents in the study stated that they withheld information out of fear of a provider's reactions; however, they still wanted to know the consequences of refusing or delaying treatment. Further exploration of the current and future context of concordance can be found in the last section of this chapter.

Patient expectations

Expectations of the nurse and community nursing service may also impact on the relationship between the nurse and adult patient. Over the past 25 years there has been a rapid rise in consumerism (Mills, 2005) with a corresponding rise in expectations of the Health Service. Recent health policy emphasizes patient choice and involvement (Wilson *et al.*, 2009). Many patients have clear ideas on the service they expect from community nurses, with a consequential detrimental effect on the therapeutic relationship when these expectations either are not met or are unrealistic. However, despite trends in healthy ageing and participation in healthcare (Healthcare Commission, 2006), many older adults were brought up in a society where medicine was seen to have all the answers and the public was expected to be the passive recipient of care (Coulter, 1999). There is some evidence that not all adult patients wish to be an active partner in the therapeutic relationship (Davis *et al.*, 2007), and there may be a significant number of patients who feel more comfortable with the paternalistic model of care (Roberts, 2001). The nurse 'doing for' the patient rather than enabling them to self-care contradicts current trends such as empowerment (Wilson *et al.*, 2007), which is a central theme in the *National Service Framework for Older People* (Healthcare Commission, 2006). The community nurse may find a challenge in helping some patients in developing the confidence and ability to self-care, and again the therapeutic relationship will be focused on trust and the facilitation of realistic independence.

Patient needs

The main purpose of the nursing or health-visiting intervention may also have a significant impact on the therapeutic relationship. The patient within the relationship may have significant physical and emotional needs such as in palliative care. The relationship developed within these cases may be based on intensive input by the nurse (Dunne *et al.*, 2005). In contrast, the practice nurse or occupational health nurse may see a patient for health screening with less obvious health needs as the focus of the intervention.

The substantial shift of care from hospitals to the community for those with mental health needs (Malone *et al.*, 2007) has resulted in a rapidly developing role for community nurses in supporting this patient group. With approximately one in six people at any one time suffering from mental illness in the UK (DH, 2009) the role is constantly evolving. Over the last decade, the mental health reforms outlined in the *National Service Framework for Mental Health* (DH, 1999a) have been firmly underpinned by focusing on the patient. However, empowering patients with mental health needs is often challenging, not least because of concerns from society and professionals as to whether some patients have the capability of making decisions over their care and treatment (Feenan, 1997). The therapeutic relationship with this group is essential in empowering patients to actively participate in decisions about their care. Peplau's (1952) developmental model is often used as the framework for developing a therapeutic relationship (Merritt and Procter, 2010), with the assessment (or orientation) phase focusing on the development of mutual trust and regard between nurse and patient, as well as data gathering. Developing a therapeutic interpersonal relationship is the foundation stone of quality nursing care (McKenna and Cutcliffe, 2008), and the community nurse may take on a number of roles to facilitate this, including that of counsellor, resource, teacher, leader or surrogate. All nurses working in the community develop knowledge of local resources and other agencies and facilitating the patient to access these may be the key component within this relationship.

It should also be acknowledged that the therapeutic relationship in the community setting is not only formed between nurse and patient, but will often encompass a family carer. In the UK there are approximately six million family carers who are the primary carers for a range of patients, ranging from young people with learning disabilities to frail elderly people (Carers UK, 2009). The *Carers Recognition and Services Act* (DH, 1995), the *Carers and Disabled Children's Act* (DH, 2000), and the *Carers (Equal Opportunities) Act* (England and Wales) (DH, 2004) enshrined the principle that a carer should be assessed and acknowledged as an individual rather than simply an adjunct to the patient, and be informed of their right to an assessment. For the community nurse this reinforces that an individual therapeutic relationship must also be developed with the family carer, but this poses a number of challenges.

First, a significant number of family carers are unknown to the community nurse (Simon and Kendrick, 2001), with Henwood (1998) estimating that only half of carers receive any support from community nurses. Second, the more a family carer does for the patient, the less intervention there will be from the community nurse

(Gerrish, 2008). Consequently, the family carers most likely to benefit from a therapeutic relationship are less likely to be visited by the community nurse. There is also evidence that despite legislation focused on carers' rights, community nurses are unlikely to proactively identify family carers and assess their needs as individuals (Simon and Kendrick, 2001; Gerrish, 2008). Third, there are often misguided assumptions by many professionals that family carers should undertake the caring role and that the role is taken on very willingly (Proctor *et al.*, 2001). Lastly, studies have shown that many family carers have significant health needs of their own, which often are unrecognized (Henwood, 1998), and undertake very complex and technical tasks (Pickard *et al.*, 2000). All too frequently, community nurses first meet a family carer when there is a crisis and the physical input and support is limited to when the crisis is over or the patient has been admitted to hospital. The therapeutic relationship with family carers should ideally be long term, with the nurse aiming to provide information and acting as a resource (Seddon and Robinson, 2001) and responding to the role the carer is happy to undertake. Twigg and Atkin (1994) describe three different responses by individuals to the informal caring role (Table. 5.1).

Table 5.1 Responses to caring role (adapted from Twigg and Atkin, 1994)

Response to Caring Role	Features of Response
Engulfment mode	Cannot articulate needs as a carer No other occupation Generally female spouse Total sense of responsibility and duty
The balancing/boundary setting mode	Have a clear picture of themselves as carers (e.g. how they save nation money) Generally male Often adopt language of an occupation – treat role as a job May emotionally detach themselves from recipient
Symbiotic mode	Positive gain by caring Does not want role taken away

It is important for the community nurse to recognize the carer's response to their situation and not take the carer for granted as a readily available resource (Manthorpe *et al.*, 2003).

Example 5.6

Imagine the case of Lily, a 75-year-old mother caring for her son Ted, who has Down's Syndrome. She is devoted to her son and has no other life than caring for him. The GP has referred Ted for a wound assessment, but when the nurse arrives it is apparent that Lily is exhausted by her role. The challenge for the nurse is to establish a relationship which enables Lily to acknowledge her individual needs and helps her to accept help without feelings of guilt. This may involve developing a long-term relationship and not simply the organizing of respite, which many informal carers do not want (Pickard *et al.*, 2000).

Another frequently met scenario is that of the husband caring for his wife. He has every detail organized and is business-like in his approach to the community nurse. Again, this may hide a number of physical and emotional needs for which the community nurse must develop a therapeutic relationship in order to enable him to express these. The needs of family carers should be recognized, and the community nurse must develop a relationship and provide interventions appropriate to both the patient and the carer as individuals.

WHEN THE BALANCE IS NOT MAINTAINED: FAILURES IN THERAPEUTIC RELATIONSHIPS

ACTIVITY 5.5

Discussion point
How do you define friendships? Have you ever been in a situation when a patient wanted to be your friend? What would you do if a patient wanted to develop a friendship with you? Discuss your ideas with a professional colleague.

In reality it is hard to learn about boundaries unless one is involved in setting them, and extending beyond the therapeutic boundary may only be apparent once it has been breached.

Example 5.7

Consider the case of Ann, who is John's community children's nurse. Ann has cared for John, aged 5, for the last 2 years and supported Gill, his single mother, through some difficult times while John has received treatment for acute lymphoblastic leukaemia. During Ann's recent visit to the home Gill and John invite her to John's sixth birthday party the following weekend. Ann considers this briefly and agrees to come. At the end of the party Gill asks Ann if she would be willing to babysit for John, as 'she's the only person she feels she can trust to care for John'. What should Ann do now? It would appear the edges of the professional boundary have become significantly blurred such that Gill feels it is appropriate to ask Ann to babysit.

It may be that it is in the interests of the patient and his/her carer to encourage the professional to develop a relationship of friendship since this has the potential to 'normalize' the patient, as it is 'normal' to have friends who visit. This is perhaps more likely to occur if nurses do not wear uniforms. Families may be keen that friendships do develop since a friend is likely to respond to requests for help, perhaps more swiftly than a detached professional. Therefore, nurses must consider their actions carefully in case actions are misinterpreted, as perhaps was the case when Ann attended John's party.

Hylton Rushton *et al.* (1996) describe over-involvement as a lack of separation between the nurse's own feelings and those of the patient. Typically the nurse may spend off-duty time with this patient, appear territorial over the care or treat certain patients with favouritism (Parkes and Jukes, 2008). Consequences for the patient are an overdependence on that particular nurse and a lack of support in reaching therapeutic goals (Moyle, 2003). For the community nurse the implications are often significant stress and deterioration in job satisfaction (Hylton Rushton *et al.*, 1996) and an inevitable detrimental effect on team working.

Of course, the balance in the therapeutic relationship may be tipped the other way. The detached, cold nurse who seems indifferent to his/her patient's emotional needs may be familiar to the reader. The results of under-involvement are a lack of understanding by the nurse of the patient's perspective, conflict and standardized rather than contextually dependent care (Milton, 2008). It has been suggested that the overwhelming feelings that a nurse may have for a patient's situation can lead to dissociation by the nurse within the therapeutic relationship (Crowe, 2000). Within the community setting the feeling of being the last resort in care has also been linked to under-involvement within the therapeutic relationship (Wilson, 2001a). The consequence of under-involvement for the patient is that the nurse has a lack of insight into the patient's perspective and is unable to facilitate the patient in meeting therapeutic goals.

ACTIVITY 5.6

Reflection point
Think of a likeable patient with whose care you have recently been involved. Reflect on the following: What were the characteristics of this patient and their care that made it a positive experience for you? If other colleagues were involved, do you think they felt the same way? Was the care you gave this patient affected by these feelings? Are there any consequences for yourself, the patient, and your other patients?

Maintaining a therapeutic relationship is particularly challenging within the community because of the commonly intense nature of care, duration of contact and the non-clinical environment. Reflection with colleagues and clinical supervision become invaluable tools to facilitate the nurse in developing the appropriate relationship with patients.

THE INFLUENCE OF THE CURRENT AND FUTURE CONTEXT ON THERAPEUTIC RELATIONSHIPS

Long-term interventions within the community setting will continue to increase with an ageing population (WHO, 2002) and rise in chronic illness (DH, 2010a), and this chapter has already explored the impact of duration of care on the therapeutic relationship. One response by policy-makers to the rise in long-term conditions is the facilitation of individuals to self-manage their own conditions. The Expert Patient Programme (DH, 2001) recognizes that individuals often have significant expertise about their chronic illness which has developed over years through experience, and the aim of the programme is to further develop this expertise in order to promote symptom control, quality of life and effective use of health resources (Wilson, 2001b, 2008; Wilson *et al.*, 2007). Within all spheres of community nursing, nurses are now dealing with far more knowledgeable patients, not least because of the readily available access to information via the Internet (Timmons, 2001). Therapeutic relationships in the current climate must be based on an acknowledgement that the patient may have considerable expertise in their own condition, exceeding the nurse's. There has been some debate as to how comfortable community nurses are with this (Wilson, 2002; Wilson *et al.*, 2006), but there can be little doubt that a therapeutic relationship that fails to take into account the knowledge that both nurse and patient bring will fail.

The Expert Patient Programme is one example of a policy that is based on partnership and responsibility (Wilson, 2001b). There has been an acknowledgement that healthcare professionals need appropriate training and support in order to develop partnership approaches (Health Foundation, 2008). The partnership approach is based on the principle of concordance (RPSGB, 1997) where the patient's views are considered of equal importance in treatment plans.

ACTIVITY 5.7

Discussion point
A child has severe eczema that has not responded well to normal treatments. The parents insist on trying a homeopathic remedy recommended to them by a self-help group. How would you feel about this? What issues would you need to take account of? What are the implications for the therapeutic relationship?

Community nurses are required to demonstrate evidence-based practice (Woodward, 2001) and the challenge of today's therapeutic relationship is to balance this with informed choice by the patient (Wilson, 2002). There is a balance to be maintained between the rights of the child (dependent on their age and understanding) and the rights of the parents in decision-making, against the risks of significant harm that might result from the treatment. The parents in the above scenario should be advised to ensure the advice regarding the complementary treatment comes from a registered practitioner. Community nurses need to assess their own knowledge base regarding complementary therapy and seek specialist advice if necessary. Within a therapeutic relationship the nurse will be aiming to facilitate an atmosphere where the parents feel able to be honest about the treatments the child is currently receiving, and should be able to direct patients and their families to sources of appropriate information.

A final feature of the current context of care that may have an effect on the therapeutic relationship is the fragmentation of care. Despite the move towards integrated care (DH, 2010b), the division of health and social care (Wilson *et al.*, 2009) means that patients within the community often have to deal with a vast array of professionals, which can be an inhibitor in the development of a therapeutic relationship (Hyde and Cotter, 2001).

CONCLUSION

In this chapter features of a therapeutic relationship have been identified, leading to an exploration of some of the challenges community nurses face in establishing therapeutic relationships. In future community healthcare provision, challenges will be shaped by an increasingly multicultural, ageing and informed population. The growing provision of healthcare in the community only serves to reinforce the need to establish appropriate relationships with patients, their families and other carers. Current government policy emphasizes partnership in care at all levels; the challenge for the community nurse is to develop this opportunity in everyday working practice.

REFERENCES

Cambridge Dictionary Online (2010) (Accessed 3 December 2010) http://dictionary. cambridge.org/dictionary/british/boundary.

Carers UK (2009) *Facts about Carers.* London: Carers UK.

Collins S (2009) Good communication helps to build a therapeutic relationship. *Nursing Times* 105:11.

Coulter A (1999) Paternalism or partnership? *British Medical Journal* 319:719–20.

Crowe M (2000) The nurse–patient relationship: a consideration of its discursive context. *Journal of Advanced Nursing* 31:962–7.

Davis RE, Jacklin R, Sevdalis N and Vincent C (2007) Patient involvement in patient safety: what factors influence patient participation and engagement? *Health Expectations* 10:259–67.

Department of Health (DH) (1990) *The NHS and Community Care Act.* London: HMSO.

DH (1995) *Carers Recognition and Services Act.* London: Stationery Office.

DH (1999a) *National Service Framework for Mental Health.* London: Stationery Office.

DH (1999b) *Our Healthier Nation – Saving Lives.* London: Stationery Office.

DH (2000) *Carers and Disabled Children's Act.* London: Department of Health.

DH (2001) *The Expert Patient – A New Approach to Chronic Disease Management for the 21st Century.* London: Stationery Office.

DH (2004) *Carers (Equal Opportunities) Act.* London: Department of Health.

DH (2009) *New Horizons. A Shared Vision for Mental Health.* London: Department of Health.

DH (2010a) *Long Term Conditions.* www.dh.gov.uk/en/Healthcare/Longtermconditions/ index.htm.

DH (2010b) *Improving Care for People with Long Term Conditions: 'At a Glance' Information Sheets for Healthcare Professionals. Care Co-ordination.* www.dh.gov.uk/en/ Publicationsandstatistics/Publications/PublicationsPolicyAndGuidance/DH_121603.

Drennan V, Goodman C and Leyshon S (2005) *Supporting Experienced Hospital Nurses to Move into Community Matron Roles.* London: Primary Care Nursing Research Unit, UCL.

Dunne K, Sullivan K and Kernohan G (2005) Palliative care for patients with cancer: district nurses' experiences. *Journal of Advanced Nursing* 50:372–80.

Feenan D (1997) Capable people: empowering the patient in the assessment of capacity. *Health Care Analysis* 5:227–36.

Foster T and Hawkins J (2005) Nurse–patient relationship. The therapeutic relationship: dead or merely impeded by technology? *British Journal of Nursing* 14:698–702.

Gerrish K (2008) Caring for the carers: the characteristics of district nursing support for family carers. *Primary Health Care Research and Development* 9:14–21.

Hagerty BM and Patusky KL (2003) Reconceptualizing the nurse–patient relationship. *Journal of Nursing Scholarship* 35:145–50.

Halter M, Brown H and Stone J (2007) *Sexual Boundary Violations by Health Professionals – an overview of the published empirical literature.* London: The Council for Healthcare Regulatory Excellence.

Health and Safety Executive (2007) *Managing the Causes of Work-related Stress.* London: HSE.

Health Foundation (2008) *Co-creating Health.* London: The Health Foundation.

Healthcare Commission (2006) *Living Well in Later Life: A Review of Progress against the National Service Framework for Older People.* London: Healthcare Commission.

Henwood M (1998) *Ignored and Invisible? Carers' Experience of the NHS.* London: Carers' National Association.

Hyde V and Cotter C (2001) The development of community nursing in the light of the NHS plan. In Hyde V (ed.) *Community Nursing and Health Care. Insights and Innovations.* London: Arnold, pp. 230–44.

Hylton Rushton C, Armstrong L and McEnhill M (1996) Establishing therapeutic boundaries as patient advocates. *Pediatric Nursing* 22:185–9.

Malone D, Marriott S, Newton-Howes G, Simmonds S and Tyrer P (2007) Community mental health teams (CMHTs) for people with severe mental illnesses and disordered personality. *Cochrane Database of Systematic Reviews* 3, CD000270.

Manthorpe J, Iliffe S and Eden A (2003): Testing Twigg and Aitkin's typology of caring: a study of primary care professionals' perceptions of dementia care using a modified focus group method. *Health & Social Care in the Community* 11:477–85.

McKenna H andCutcliffe J (2008) *Nursing Models, Theories and Practice.* Chichester: Blackwell Publishing.

McParland J, Scott P, Arndt M, *et al.* (2000) Autonomy and clinical practice 1: identifying areas of concern. *British Journal of Nursing* 9:507–13.

Merritt MK and Procter NG (2010) Conceptualising the functional role of mental health consultation-liaison nurse in multi-morbidity, using Peplau's nursing theory. *Contemporary Nurse* 34:140–8.

Mills C (2005) *NHS Reform: Consumerism or Citizenship.* Manchester: Cobbetts.

Milton CL (2008) Boundaries: ethical implications for what it means to be therapeutic in the nurse–person relationship. *Nursing Science Quarterly* 21:18–21.

Morse JM (1991) Negotiating commitment and involvement in the nurse–patient relationship. *Journal of Advanced Nursing* 16:455–68.

Moyle W (2003) Nurse–patient relationship: A dichotomy of expectations. *Journal of Mental Health Nursing* 12:103–9.

Nursing and Midwifery Council (NMC) (2008) *The Code: Standards of Conduct, Performance and Ethics for Nurses and Midwives.* London: NMC.

NMC (2009) *Clear Sexual Boundaries.* www.nmc-uk.org/Nurses-and-midwives/Advice-by-topic/A/Advice/Clear-sexual-boundaries.

Oakley K (ed.) (2008) *Occupational Health Nursing*, 3rd edn. Chichester: Wiley.

Parkes N and Jukes M (2008) Professional boundaries in a person-centred paradigm. *British Journal of Nursing* 17:1358–64.

Parkin P (2001) Covert community nursing: reciprocity in formal and informal relations. In Hyde V (ed.) *Community Nursing and Health Care: Insights and Innovations.* London: Arnold.

Paterson B (2001) Myth of empowerment in chronic illness. *Journal of Advanced Nursing* 34:574–81.

Peplau HE (1952) *Interpersonal Relations in Nursing.* New York: Putnam's Sons.

Pickard S, Shaw S and Glendinning C (2000) Health care professionals' support for older carers. *Ageing and Society* 20:725–44.

Procter S, Wilcockson J, Pearson P and Allgar V (2001) Going home from hospital: the carer/patient dyad. *Journal of Advanced Nursing* 35:206–17.

Roberts K (2001) Across the health–social care divide: elderly people as active users of health care and social care. *Health and Social Care in the Community* 9:100–7.

Royal Pharmaceutical Society of Great Britain (RPSGB) (1997) *Compliance to Concordance: Achieving Shared Goals in Medicine Taking.* London: RPSGB.

Schaeuble K, Haglund K and Vukovich M (2010) Adolescents' preferences for primary provider interactions. *Pediatric Nursing* 15:202–10.

Seddon D and Robinson CA (2001) Carers of older people with dementia: assessment and the Carers Act. *Health and Social Care in the Community* 9:151–8.

Shaw K and Timmons S (2010) Exploring how nursing uniforms influence self image and professional identity. *Nursing Times* 106, www.nursingtimes.net/nursing-practice-clinical-research/acute-care/exploring-how-nursing-uniforms-influence-self-image-and-professional-identity/5012623.article.

Simon C and Kendrick T (2001) Informal carers – the role of general practitioners and district nurses. *British Journal of General Practice* 51:655–7.

Stone J (2008) Respecting professional boundaries: What CAM practitioners need to know. *Complementary Therapies in Clinical Practice* 14:2–7.

Timmons S (2001) Use of the Internet by patients: not a threat to nursing, but an opportunity? *Nurse Education Today* 21:104–9.

Totka J (1996) Exploring the boundaries of paediatric practice: nurse stories related to relationships. *Pediatric Nursing* 22:191–6.

Twigg J and Atkin K (1994) *Carers Perceived.* Buckingham: Open University Press.

Wellard S (1998) Constructions of chronic illness. *International Journal of Nursing Studies* 35:49–55.

Wilson PM (2001a) *Being the Last Resort: A Critical Ethnography of District Nurses and their Patients with Long-term Needs.* University of Manchester, RCN Institute: unpublished MSc thesis.

Wilson PM (2001b) A policy analysis of the expert patient in the United Kingdom: self-care as an expression of pastoral power? *Health and Social Care in the Community* 9:134–42.

Wilson PM (2002) The expert patient: issues and implications for community nurses. *British Journal of Community Nursing* 7:514–19.

Wilson PM (2008) The UK expert patients program: lessons learned and implications for cancer survivors' self-care support programs. *Journal of Cancer Survivorship* 2:45–52.

Wilson PM, Bunn F and Morgan J (2009) A mapping of the evidence on integrated long term condition services. *British Journal of Community Nursing* 14:202–6.

Wilson PM, Kendall S and Brooks F (2006) Nurses' responses to expert patients: The rhetoric and reality of self-management in long-term conditions: A grounded theory study. *International Journal of Nursing Studies* 43:803–18.

Wilson PM, Kendall S and Brooks F (2007) The expert patients programme: a paradox of patient empowerment and medical dominance. *Health and Social Care in the Community* 15:426–38.

Woodward V (2001) Evidence-based practice, clinical governance and community nurses. In Hyde V (ed.) *Community Nursing and Health Care. Insights and Innovations.* London: Arnold, pp. 206–29.

World Health Organization (2002) *Innovative Care for Chronic Conditions.* Geneva: WHO.

FURTHER READING

Smith P (1992) *The Emotional Labour of Nursing.* Basingstoke: Macmillan.

Theodosius C (2008) *Emotional Labour in Health Care: The Unmanaged Heart of Nursing.* Abingdon: Routledge.

CHAPTER 6

Care across the lifespan

Helen McVeigh

LEARNING OUTCOMES

• Compare and contrast the different theories of growth and development
• Evaluate the issues that influence caring for clients across the lifespan
• Critically analyze how an understanding of a lifespan approach can enhance the quality of care provision

INTRODUCTION

This chapter explores the concept of a lifespan approach to healthcare. It is an approach that is able to reflect on and adapt to changes in demographics, society and the expectations of individuals within the community. The health of an individual is influenced by a complex interaction of a range of factors including physiological, psychological, social, cultural and environmental issues. A sound understanding of the factors that influence growth and development across the lifespan can enable the community nurse to adopt a truly holistic approach in the assessment, planning, implementation and analysis of healthcare interventions; however, it is recognized that health professionals may have distinct roles in the community, often focused on specific stages of the lifespan (e.g. Health Visitor – child health 0–5 years). The importance of developing a broad viewpoint and an awareness of all aspects of the lifespan continuum should underpin effective care provision.

THEORIES OF GROWTH AND DEVELOPMENT

There are many theories which explore the concept of human growth and development; however, it is beyond the scope of this chapter to consider them all. A basic understanding of these theories will enable the health professional to understand the individual, their illness and their reaction to illness.

Growth can be defined as an increase in physical size and maturity, whereas development describes an increase in functional ability (Cameron, 2006). Aspects of growth and development can be related to all stages of the lifespan, although it is suggested that growth and development applies to the period from conception to young adulthood whereas the notion of ageing is more readily applicable from middle age onwards (Taylor *et al.,* 2003).

It is useful to consider some of the theories which underpin growth and development and a lifespan approach. These theories can be grouped into several different categories and classified according to the following broad headings: biomedical, psychodynamic, cognitive, behavioural, humanist and sociocultural (see Box 6.1).

Box 6.1 Theories of growth and development

Biomedical – focus is on the change in body mechanics
Psychodynamic – focus is on development of personality traits and psychological challenges at different ages
Cognitive – focus is on the advancement and development of thinking
Behavioural – describes the development of human behaviour and behavioural learning changes
Humanist – describes the influence of human experiences such as love and attachment on personality development
Sociocultural – describes how culture and society influence behaviour.

Although exploration of the various theories can provide key information on the different life stages, it is important to recognize that a lifespan approach successfully combines aspects of all of these elements (Leifer and Hartshorn, 2004).

Utilizing a lifespan approach

The changes in physiology, psychology and behaviour that occur normally at different stages of the lifespan and how these are influenced by their interaction with other factors including life experience, social norms, culture, health status and the environment are explored in this chapter through the use of a multigenerational case history (Fig. 6.1). Aspects of need and healthcare at various life stages are considered and related to the different theoretical approaches. A wide range of healthcare professionals will input into this family's life history along their life span. Whichever professional you are, an understanding of the roles of others and how they may meet the needs of the clients is important, along with a holistic approach to healthcare reflecting not only knowledge of the individual but some understanding of how this is influenced by their environment, society and the relationships they are in. Most health outcomes are related to the choices made by the individual at each stage of the lifespan (Leifer and Hartshorn, 2004). For example, the elderly patient with chronic obstructive pulmonary disease (COPD) may well regret choices made as a teenager to adopt an unhealthy lifestyle and to smoke. Some understanding of why we behave in specific ways at certain life stages may help us in effectively targeting lifestyle choice and in providing health promotion and healthcare effectively tailored to meet the needs of our client group. We also need to remember that most individuals do not exist in isolation and healthcare needs will frequently impact on families and carers. The challenge for the community nurse is to recognize these influences and offer sensitive healthcare that reaches the client and their family/carers.

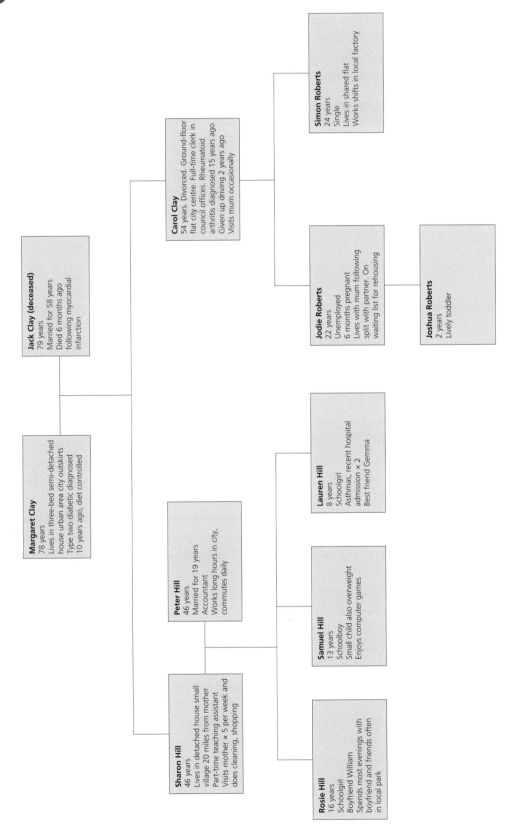

Figure 6.1 Case history genealogy.

BIOMEDICAL INFLUENCES

Historically the biomedical approach has dominated the organization and provision of healthcare (Taylor and Field, 2007). The biomedical approach ignores social and environmental factors and taken in isolation is essentially a reductionist method focusing on body mechanics, which assumes that the mind and body can be treated separately and that they can be repaired (Nettleton, 2006; Taylor and Field, 2007). Nurse education is underpinned by a sound understanding of human anatomy and physiology, and it is essential that nurses are able to recognize normal physiology. This knowledge should include knowing not only how the different organs and systems of the body work, but also how they grow and develop. An understanding of growth norms is useful when monitoring child health and in health surveillance. If we consider Samuel, who is rather small for his age, knowing there is an adolescent growth spurt which differs between the sexes, and that the male spurt although greater in intensity is usually on average 2 years behind that of females (Cameron, 2006) can enable us to determine whether this is normal variance or not. Tools such as human growth curve charts, which record the growth of an individual from 0–18 years, allow us to monitor and interpret recorded results.

A sound understanding of physiological changes and the normal patterns of ageing may aid us in the diagnosis and treatment of disease. An awareness of biomedical aspects such as genetic programming, wear and tear theory (cells having a specified life cycle), cell programming (cells divide until they are no longer able to), immune theory (immune response diminishing with age) (Taylor *et al.*, 2003; Grossmann and Lange, 2006) and how the body handles significant changes, e.g. drug administration, bacterial or viral invasion, is fundamental to effective healthcare.

Recognition that homeostasis (the ability of body systems to maintain equilibrium) may be impaired in the very young or elderly patient is essential knowledge for effective care provision. For example, individuals with the influenza virus are more likely to be seriously ill and at increased risk of mortality if they are at each end of the lifespan. Biologically this correlates with human development and physiology, lung function continues to increase and develop from birth until adulthood (around age 20 years) staying stable on average for around 15 years and then it begins to decline (Alder *et al.*, 2004).

ACTIVITY 6.1

Reflection point

Recently Margaret has had a fall resulting in a pre-tibial laceration to her lower leg which required the community nurse to visit and assess. Margaret has been self-treating for several weeks but the wound is not healing and the community nurse notes it appears to be infected. Her blood glucose levels are also elevated.

Using a biomedical approach, what is influencing wound healing for Margaret?

Samuel has also lacerated his leg playing football and Sharon has taken him to the surgery for advice.

What advice would you give to Samuel and his mother and how might that differ from the advice given to Margaret?

Knowledge of the stages of wound healing and the normal progression of wound healing should underpin nursing care for Margaret and Samuel. Samuel as a young healthy child will probably require little more than one or two simple dressing changes as we would expect his wound to heal within 4–7 days. Advice to Samuel and Sharon would focus on recognition of possible infection and risk management (playing football) while the wound heals. However, for Margaret decreased cell turnover, thinning of the epithelium, loss of collagen within the dermis and a diminished immune response, factors consistent with ageing, will result in prolonged healing and this may be further compromised by other physiological factors such as her diabetes. Advice and management will be more complex; establishing her understanding of why the wound is not healing and how this is influenced by her diabetes will be essential. Using a biomedical focus to guide practice can give the community nurse an indication of what to expect as the body ages, although patterns of decline will not necessarily follow a predictable sequence and may vary from individual to individual (Cameron, 2006). Although crucial to care provision it is important to recognize that biomedical factors will be overlaid by psychosocial influences.

PSYCHOSOCIAL INFLUENCES

Sociology can be defined as the study of social relationships; holistic healthcare recognizes that people's lives and behaviour cannot be divorced from the social contexts in which they participate (Taylor and Field, 2007). Psychosocial theory attempts to explain human development in terms of individual changes in cognitive function, behaviour, roles, relationships, coping abilities and social change, and as such it provides insight into individual personalities and attitudes across the lifespan. Life expectations and our understanding of health are not static but develop and evolve over time and are frequently linked to our socioeconomic circumstances.

The concept of health

The concept of health is important and it is essential to consider the individual's subjective interpretation of the meaning of health and illness. Health may be viewed negatively

- the absence of disease or illness

  Or positively

- a state of complete physical, mental and social well being, not merely the absence of disease or infirmity (WHO, 1946).

ACTIVITY 6.2

Reflection point
What is your interpretation of health?
Consider how Carol would define health.
How would this differ from Simon's definition?

The way in which we define health will impact on our life choices and subsequent behaviour. Simon's definition may reflect strength and fitness whereas Carol may focus on the ability to cope with life and the demands of work. Health perception will vary across the lifespan and genders. Nettleton (2006) suggests that for young men it may equal strength and physical condition whereas for young women it may equal vitality, energy and an ability to cope. As we age, the emphasis shifts from notions of mental and physical wellbeing and the ability to do things well in middle age, to wisdom, contentment and happiness in old age (Alder *et al.,* 2004). Perceptions will be influenced by physiological, social and environmental factors. For example, a working individual or young mother may consider that she has no time to be ill and Carol's perception will be influenced by her rheumatoid arthritis. It is important to recognize that views on 'what is health' are varied and those of our patients may well be different from our personal perspectives.

Health promotion

The promotion of health is an essential role for every community nurse, and strategies to support healthy behaviour and lifestyle are at the heart of improving the quality of life for individuals (Leifer and Hartshorn, 2004; Cox and Hill, 2010). The process of promoting health involves enabling individuals to take control of their own health and is focused on a proactive preventative approach. Individuals are encouraged to take responsibility and to be more knowledgeable about the behavioural and social factors that influence health (Nettleton, 2006). Current health policy supports patient empowerment and personal responsibility (DH 2010a,b). The community nurse needs to develop a reflective approach that combines knowledge of health promotion strategies with an understanding of lifespan influences. For example, the teaching style and strategy we might adopt for an adolescent may well be very different to that which would be effective for an older person, where a paternalistic approach of 'doctor knows best' may be expected. Objective analysis also suggests that there may be a tendency for health promotion to be targeted at those in younger age groups (Taylor *et al.,* 2003). However, it is important to remember that opportunities exist across the whole lifespan and that the effectiveness of any health message is reliant on how well it reaches the target audience. The Family Planning Association campaign 'Middle-age Spread' to encourage increased responsibility in the over 50s in relation to risky sexual behaviour in response to increasing incidence of sexually transmitted infection (STI) in older adults demonstrates the importance of differing approaches (FPA, 2010).

Children and families

Aspects of growth and development in childhood are rooted in the context of family life. The fundamental structure of the family in the UK has evolved from origins of the extended family group all living under one roof to more nuclear families living separately, divided by greater geographical mobility, and increasingly diverse family groupings, which include more single parents, remarriages and working families, which may well impact on child development. The family construct can be considered to have a growth and development lifespan originating in marriage/living together through having children, child rearing, separation and ageing family responsibilities (Leifer and Hartshorn, 2004). A sound understanding of the concept of family and its construct enables planning of individualized care for family members.

The basis of effectively meeting the needs of children is underpinned by an understanding of child development milestones (Smith and McSherry, 2004; Antai-Otong, 2007). Insight into emotional and behavioural development can enable us to respond effectively to children and family groups. At 2 years old, Joshua is developing social interaction and language skills (he has a vocabulary of around 100 words) and is mastering an element of self-control (he is toilet trained and dry through the day). However, the arrival of a new sibling may provoke regression as he struggles to adjust to the change in relationship with his mother. A sensitive approach and allowing him to participate in caring for the new baby may help with the process of adjustment.

It is important to recognize that children cannot be cared for in isolation from their families who will have an established health belief system (Smith and McSherry, 2004). Attitudes underpinning health belief are very hard to change, so the community nurse needs to understand what contributes to family decision-making about health. The Health Belief Model (Becker, 1974) highlights the purpose of beliefs in decision-making. The model suggests that behaviour change is underpinned by a cost–benefit analysis and evaluation of its feasibility (Naidoo and Wills, 2009).

ACTIVITY 6.3

Reflection point

Lauren has asthma; recently her symptoms have been much worse and she has had two severe attacks requiring overnight hospitalization.

Since the death of her father Sharon has visited her mother most days after work and Lauren has spent time with her best friend Gemma after school. Gemma has a pet cat; previous allergy testing revealed that Lauren is allergic to cat fur.

Using the Health Belief Model and a lifespan approach, consider how Sharon and Gemma will respond.

Sharon's concern about the increased risk to Lauren of further asthma attacks through spending time at her friend's house may be tempered by the needs of her elderly mother, work commitments and the tearful remonstrations of her daughter. Lauren's response is less rational and she is less likely to comprehend the consequences of continuing with the current arrangement. Understanding of chronic illness is dependent in some degree on the age of the child. Lauren is likely to have an understanding of the cause of her asthma but may not be able to relate this to cause and effect principles and coping mechanisms (Leifer and Hartshorn, 2004). As a community nurse supporting Sharon and Lauren, a holistic approach to care encompasses not only the needs of the individual but the family as well. Care delivery should recognize that the family has complex needs while encouraging both Lauren and her family to take an active role in healthcare decisions.

Adolescents

Adolescence is a time of significant changes marking the transition between childhood and adulthood. The characteristic physical changes of puberty are heightened by corresponding psychosocial development. There is increased emphasis on social conflicts and personal dilemmas during this time as the individual endeavours to identify their role within society (Erikson, 1980). This challenges and changes relationships between parents and peers, and there is often increased conflict in families as the individual experiments with a variety of roles and styles. Disputes are frequently related to difference of opinion around rights and responsibilities (Alder *et al.,* 2004). In our case history Rosie is frustrated by the attitude of her parents who consider her old enough to babysit for her younger siblings but not old enough for a sexual relationship, whereas from Peter and Sharon's perspective, Rosie wants sexual freedom without the responsibility of the potential consequences. The challenge of achieving a sense of self and independence may impact on healthcare, which may be particularly relevant for adolescents with a long-term condition. Peer pressure and the need for self-identity may mean that social logic replaces that of medical logic (Nettleton, 2006).

ACTIVITY 6.4

Reflection point

Rosie is not getting on very well with her parents and is frequently argumentative and confrontational. She has started going out in the evenings, often coming home late. Rosie has a boyfriend and a large circle of friends. There is very little to do in the village and they spend most of their evenings at the local park. She is very close to her cousin Jodie and confides in her that she is worried that she might be pregnant as she has been sleeping with her boyfriend.

Jodie has gone with Rosie to see the practice nurse. The pregnancy test is negative.

Consider the type of approach you might adopt in giving advice and support to Rosie.

It is important to take an approach which establishes a level of trust with Rosie. Rosie may be worried about the community nurse sharing information with her parents; therefore, an honest approach is important. It is important to take adolescents' psychosocial and cultural experiences and expectations into account (Briggs, 2010). Although Rosie's pregnancy test was negative, she needs advice on sexual health in the future as adolescents are likely to have a greater sense of invulnerability in relation to risk taking (Alder *et al.,* 2004). The emphasis should be on helping her to enjoy her teenage years while minimizing the risk of unwanted/unplanned pregnancy, STIs, HIV, cancer of the cervix and female infertility (Briggs, 2010). Providing health advice for adolescents can be challenging and requires an approach in which establishing trust and offering sound advice and respecting them as individuals is central.

Middle age and the world of work

Middle age is considered to be the period between 40 and 60 years of age. Physical growth and development has been replaced by aspects of ageing. The challenges of this period are often associated with work and maintaining roots within the community. Erikson (1980) noted that middle age is defined as a time of conflict between contribution to the family or community (generativity) and concern for self (stagnation). The consequences of ageing may be an emerging worry. Alder *et al.* (2004) highlight the concept of 'the mid life crisis' as a period of uncertainty and change that may be perceived as a last opportunity to achieve some of life's goals. Middle age may also be a time of re-evaluation and self-reflection, a time to focus on health behaviour and lifestyle choices. Opportunities exist for the community nurse to effectively manage risky behaviours.

ACTIVITY 6.5

Reflection point

Sharon and Peter are rather overweight. They both enjoy a glass of wine in the evenings, often eating late when Peter returns from work.

They feel that their busy lives do not allow them time to take regular exercise.

Consider how psychosocial factors will influence effective health promotion for Sharon and Peter.

It may be appropriate to identify how Sharon and Peter view their health and their ability to control it. Health promotion and changing behaviour may be easier if the individual has an internal locus of control where they feel they have some say in their future health rather than an external locus of control where individuals feel that their health is governed from the outside and would therefore not take responsibility for making changes to improve wellbeing (Niven, 2006). Decisions to change lifestyle may be based on weighing up any benefit against disadvantage highlighted in the Health Belief model (Becker, 1974). Concern for family (generativity) can be a positive influence; Samuel is an overweight teenager and an increased knowledge that childhood obesity will tend to carry over into adulthood (Larkin, 2009) may support behaviour changes. For the community nurse an understanding of social, cultural and environmental factors at this point in the family's lifespan is essential, and the emphasis should be on shared decision-making.

An individual may be challenged by chronic illness at any age, although the likelihood will increase with age. Chronic illness can confront our sense of self and reminds us that normal functioning is often central to social relationships and activities (Nettleton, 2006). The impact of chronic illness on life is twofold: its consequence, i.e. its effects, on the practical aspects of life (work and play) and its meaning as significant to our sense of self (Bury, 1991).

ACTIVITY 6.6

Reflection point

Carol has rheumatoid arthritis. Recently her symptoms have become much worse and she finds sitting for long periods very difficult. Although her employers have been very supportive Carol is finding it increasingly difficult to manage at work. She is frequently tired in the evenings and is finding it quite stressful living with her daughter and a lively 2 year old.

Consider the consequence and meaning of chronic illness for Carol.

It is important to recognize that expected norms across the lifespan may be challenged and changed by chronic illness. Carol's disability has resulted in her developing a set of coping mechanisms; however, recent exacerbation of symptoms has created new problems for her. The biomedical approach would emphasize the importance of maintaining mobility and minimizing resultant disability. However, her ability to cope is influenced by several psychosocial factors:

- social imagery associated with rheumatoid arthritis; limited mobility, severe disability and wheelchair use
- the individual sense of self
- the reaction of others.

The social model argues that attitudes and physical restrictions are often imposed by society and as a consequence opportunities and functional capability are decreased (Larkin, 2009). For Carol, increasing difficulties at work have resulted in the realization that she is less able to function in what might be termed socially accepted normality and that her increasing disability generates barriers in employment. Her capacity to cope may also be influenced by her mental health (many patients who suffer from a long-term condition may also suffer from depression (Alder *et al.*, 2004)), her health beliefs, and her perceived ability to overcome her disability, which may have been exacerbated by the demands of having her daughter and grandson living with her.

Ageing

Knowledge and understanding of the ageing process and the meaning of being old are essential for effective individualized care of clients in the community. Old age is often considered to begin at 65, but increasing life expectancy means we now have subgroups of young old, old and the very old (over 85 years) (Nilsson *et al.*, 2000). Our understanding of ageing is influenced by the concept of ageism, stereotypical ideas, social norms and expectations. We live in an ageist society, where physical change such as greying hair and loss of skin elasticity is viewed negatively, particularly in relation to women (Alder *et al.*, 2004). Many elderly individuals may hold stereotypical ideas of themselves; therefore, respect for individuality is vital (Taylor *et al.*, 2003). Some individuals may retain a view of the inner self which is younger than their body as a means of negating ageist expectations and preserving a sense of dignity (Nilsson *et al.*, 2000; Alder *et al.*, 2004).

As we age we carry an increasing wealth of health experiences with us, shaped by the cultural and social norms of the world we live in. Successful ageing may be marked by an ability to look back on life with a sense of fulfilment and wholeness, or the extent to which an individual is able to remain socially engaged (Wadensten, 2006; Antai-Otong, 2007). Erikson (1980) noted that individuals who could reflect on life with a sense of satisfaction achieved a sense of integrity rather than despair. Meaning in life is closely related to health and declining health often equates to a sense of loss (Grossman and Lange, 2006). Feeling old may relate to feelings of fear, helplessness, feeling different from peers and losing a sense of control over one's life (Nilsson *et al.*, 2000). Physical changes may restrict the capability for social involvement while factors such as changing role and status in the community or decline in mental ability will impact on the individual's experience of ageing.

ACTIVITY 6.7

Reflection point

On her visits to Margaret, the community nurse has noted that the house is rather untidy and that Margaret often looks unkempt and appears very uninterested. Carol is also concerned about her mother; she tells the nurse that prior to Jack's death her mother had enjoyed an active social life, as both her parents had been keen members of the local bowls club.

Critically consider how an understanding of ageing can influence the quality of care for Margaret.

Social aspects of ageing may be characterized by patterns of adjustment that result in a process of disengagement in which the older person gradually withdraws from society. Old age is also a time of increased losses and a period when the individual is less able to cope with crises and loss (Nilsson, 2000). Margaret is clearly struggling to maintain her emotions in the face of bereavement, which has also affected her role and social status within the community. She appears to have lost the social contact and network of support she had with Jack, and without an active social network she may be at increased risk of developing mental health problems (Taylor *et al.*, 2003). Strategies to enable Margaret to move through this period of loss and bereavement may include replacing the losses in some way with different roles or people (Wadensten, 2006).

Communication skills

How well we communicate with patients can influence the quality of the relationship we develop with them. Taking a lifespan approach to communication will enable us to utilize the most effective methods of communication with each client group. Communication with children requires concurrent dialogue with the family (Antai-Otong, 2007). How we explain illness to a young child needs to be thought through in light of their cognitive abilities; for example, Piaget noted that before the age of 7 years the child has an inability to distinguish between cause and effect (Leifer and Hartshorn, 2004). Communication with adolescents needs an engaging non-judgemental approach initiated through open dialogue. Good communication strategies will be based on a sound understanding of their needs and some insight into adolescent culture (Briggs, 2010). The types of resources used will be an important consideration in reaching certain groups; examples such as the successful YouTube video highlighting teenage pregnancy demonstrate effective communication with their target group (NHS Leicester City, 2009).

Older people may be hampered by age-related changes, such as hearing loss and decreased vision, that influence how they perceive and control external cues (Antai-Otong, 2007). Barriers to communication with older adults include ageism, hurried approaches, lack of respect and a lack of appreciation for the individual's life experience (Anatai-Otong, 2007). Intergenerational communication may be influenced by nurse assumptions and maintaining a professional, respectful approach which avoids overly familiar terms such as 'sweetie' and 'love' is of paramount importance (Knifton, 2009). Older people may need longer to retrieve learned material from their memory store and story-telling may be a valuable means of effective communication (Alder *et al.*, 2004); therefore, strategies that allow greater time for assessment may be useful.

Gender issues

Gender issues influence health across the lifespan. Life expectancy is greater for women than men in the UK by an average of 4.1 years (ONS, 2010). Biomedical factors indicate that males may be inherently more vulnerable and are less likely to survive the first year of life (Taylor and Field, 2007). However, it is the interaction between biological and social factors that is significant in relation to health. Boys are more likely to die from accidents or have an accidental injury; gender roles increase the health risk for males as boys are encouraged to be more active (Alder *et al.*, 2004). Female longevity may be linked to more positive health behaviours; for example, women are more likely to consume a healthy diet, although conversely more likely to develop an eating disorder (Taylor and Field, 2007). Into adulthood, male probability of early death is increased by risk-taking behaviour such as dangerous sports, fast driving, hazardous consumption of alcohol and illicit drug use (Taylor and Field, 2007). However, we should remember that this is not necessarily a static picture. Recent evidence shows there is a narrowing of the gap in life expectancy, which may in part be explained by increasing risk-taking behaviours in females (e.g. smoking and alcohol consumption) (ONS, 2009, 2010).

The Equality Act (DH, 2010c) supports gender-sensitive healthcare. The community nurse needs to recognize that men and women may access services and present symptoms differently, and this may impact on the accessibility of services. The likelihood of seeing a GP varies with age and gender; females and older individuals are more likely to access these services. Women are more likely to recognize symptoms of illness and seek help earlier (Taylor and Field, 2007). Women are also more likely to ask questions, be given information and be involved in shared decision-making than men (Antai-Otong, 2007). Although we could argue that female participation and uptake of services may be related in some part to need, i.e. reproductive years and increased morbidity in later life, this cannot be entirely explained by these factors, and issues such as masculinity and gender roles may be relevant (Banks, 2001). Access to services may also be linked to social factors such as employment. Peter's busy schedule means he is less likely to seek advice if he cannot attend in the evening, whereas Simon's choice may be guided by the impact on his salary. Understanding how age and gender may influence uptake and accessibility is important in the planning and delivery of services to effectively meet the needs of the local community.

CONCLUSION

This chapter has explored a lifespan approach to healthcare. Multidimensional views that take account of not only the biological and psychological but increasingly the social, cultural and environmental aspects of health and illness are essential. Age, gender and individual perceptions of health will all influence patient needs, assessment and care provision. It is important to recognize that each individual is part of a family system, and that the healthcare needs of the individual may well impact on the family. Proactive patient-centred approaches and developing positive health should underpin holistic healthcare provision. Understanding how aspects of the lifespan relate to the physical, psychological, social, environmental and spiritual elements of an individual's life can positively influence care provision and the quality of life for clients, their families and carers.

REFERENCES

Alder B, Porter M, Abraham C and van Teijlingen E (2004) *Psychology and Sociology Applied to Medicine*, 2nd edn. Edinburgh: Churchill Livingstone, pp. 8–45, 112–13.

Antai-Otong D (2007) *Nurse–Client Communication: A Life Span Approach.* Massachusetts: Jones & Bartlett, pp. 20–97.

Banks I (2001) No man's land: men, illness and help seeking. *British Medical Journal* 323:1058–60.

Becker M (1974) *The Health Belief Model and Personal Health Behaviour.* New Jersey: Slack Thorofare.

Briggs P (2010) Strategies for discussing sex with teenagers. *Practice Nursing* 21:71–4.

Bury M (1991) The sociology of chronic illness: a review of research and prospects. *Sociology of Health and Illness* 13:451–68.

Cameron N (2006) *Human Growth and Development.* California: Elsevier, pp. 1–20.

Cox CL and Hill MC (2010) *Professional Issues in Primary Care Nursing.* Chichester: Wiley Blackwell, 78–94.

Department of Health (DH) (2010a) *Equity and Excellence Liberating the NHS.* London: DH.

DH (2010b) *Healthy Lives, Healthy People: Our Strategy for Public Health in England.* London: DH.

DH (2010c) *Equality Act.* London: DH.

Erikson EH (1980) *Identity and the Life Cycle.* New York: Norton and Company, pp. 94–107.

Family Planning Association (FPA) *Sexual Health Week 2010: The Middle-age Spread.* www.fpa.org.uk/home.

Grossman S and Lange J (2006) Theories of aging as basis for assessment. *MEDSURG Nursing* 15:77–83.

Knifton C (2009) Dementia. In McVeigh H *Fundamental Aspects of Long Term Conditions.* London: Quay Books, pp. 153–76.

Larkin M (2009) *Vulnerable Groups in Health and Social Care.* London: Sage, pp. 29–46, 71–86.

Leifer G and Hartshorn H (2004) *Growth and Development across the Lifespan.* St Louis, MO: Saunders, pp. 50–65.

Naidoo J and Wills J (2009) *Health Promotion*, 3rd edn. Edinburgh: Elsevier.

Nettleton S (2006) *The Sociology of Health and Illness*, 2nd edn. Cambridge: Polity Press, pp. 3–75.

NHS Leicester City (18/05/2009) Leicester Teenage Pregnancy and Partnership. Available from: www.youtube.com.

Nilsson M, Sarvimaki A and Ekman SL (2000) Feeling old: being in a phase of transition in later life. *Nursing Inquiry* 7:41–9.

Niven N (2006) *The Psychology of Nursing Care*, 2nd ed. Basingstoke: Palgrave Macmillan, pp. 364–5.

Office for National Statistics (ONS) (2009) Alcohol-related deaths 2007. *Health Statistics Quarterly* 41:4.

ONS (2010) *Statistical Bulletin: Life Expectancy at Birth and at Age 65 by Local Areas in the UK 2007–09.* Newport: ONS, pp. 1–6.

Smith J and McSherry W (2004) Spirituality and child development: a concept analysis. *Journal of Advanced Nursing* 45:307–15.

Taylor R, Smith B and van Teijlingen E (ed) (2003) *Health and Illness in the Community.* Oxford: OUP, pp. 105–85.

Taylor S and Field D (2007) *Sociology of Health and Illness*, 4th edn. Oxford: Blackwell, pp. 3–44, 93–112.

Wadensten B (2006) An analysis of psychosocial theories of ageing and their relevance to practical gerontological nursing in Sweden. *Scandinavian Journal Caring* 20:347–54.

World Health Organization (WHO) (1946) *Constitution.* Geneva: WHO.

FURTHER READING

There is a vast amount of literature relating to the theories of growth and development and the application of these concepts to healthcare and your interest may well be guided by your professional role and client group focus. The following texts take a broad view.

Alder B, Porter M, Abraham C and van Teijlingen E (2004) *Psychology and Sociology Applied to Medicine*, 2nd edn. Edinburgh: Churchill Livingstone.

Crain W (2005) *Theories of Development: Concepts and Applications*, 5th edn. New Jersey: Pearson Education Ltd.

Leifer G and Hartshorn H (2004) *Growth and Development across the Lifespan.* St Louis, MO: Saunders.

Community nursing assessment

Helen Gough

LEARNING OUTCOMES

- Explore the meaning of assessment
- Analyze conceptual aspects of assessments
- Explore the concept of need
- Discuss assessment frameworks
- Critically reflect on decision-making

INTRODUCTION

The aim of this chapter is to examine community nursing assessment by defining terminology and identifying what constitutes a holistic assessment. The concept of need and its relationship to assessment will be explored along with existing assessment frameworks and models that have been developed to meet the wide range of assessment perspectives that exists within a community setting. Decision-making and its essential alignment with community nursing assessment will then be discussed, with opportunities to guide reflection on current practice.

EXPLORING THE MEANING OF ASSESSMENT

Assessment is a core skill for nurses, as any subsequent care depends on the accuracy of the assessment. This means that any mistakes in this process will inevitably lead to flawed care. Changes to UK health policy, which include improving the health of the population and providing healthcare locally, place the community nursing workforce at the forefront of developments (SE, 2005; DH, 2006). This emphasis on convenient access to care, closer to and within the patient's home, highlights the need for flexible and competent community nurses (SG, 2007; DH, 2008). This means community nurses are currently in an unique position to reflect on existing practices and review these for suitability and/or adaptation to meet the changing political agenda.

The Nursing and Midwifery Council (NMC, 2006) makes it quite clear in the standards of proficiency for nurse and midwife prescribers that thorough assessment including risk assessment is vital to the prescribing process. Although not all community nurses prescribe, having the relevant knowledge and skills in relation to assessment is central to delivering safe and effective care. Community nursing assessment practice is therefore worthy of exploration as it provides nurses with an opportunity to reflect on their current assessment skills and knowledge and to identify ways to improve their practice. A starting point is examining what we actually mean by assessment.

DEFINING ASSESSMENT

It is perhaps somewhat surprising that concise contemporary definitions of nursing assessment can be challenging to find in current literature. A broad definition of assessment was given some 10 years ago by Worth (2001) linking the ways in which the needs and requirements of patients/clients drive the subsequent planned care and services. This emphasizes patient need, which is not surprising, and the concept of need is further explored later on in this chapter.Some 10 years earlier Roper *et al.* (1990) were quite specific in relation to patient assessment, highlighting that it included collecting information about the patient, identifying the problems and then determining the priorities. Although this first appears as a superficial approach, far more detail is then provided and it is clear that assessment is an ongoing activity that gathers biographical and health data before considering assessment of the patient's activities of living (Roper *et al.*, 1990). Muncey (2002) grasps the key issue of assessment by the expert nurse as being 'invisible', and explains that it is a cognitive process which is then only articulated once documented in written form. Only then can the visual representation of actual and potential problems and their priority be identified. It is this anticipatory approach that is based on the nurse's underpinning knowledge and skills along with decision-making which focuses on the whole person and their surroundings.

ANALYZING CONCEPTUAL ASPECTS OF ASSESSMENTS

Rushworth (2009) and Wilson and Giddens (2009) state that individual health assessment is undertaken by taking a health history and conducting a physical examination, and this is then followed by a diagnosis and treatment plan. Bickley (2009) agrees and explains comprehensive assessment in relation to a health history and complete physical examination, which includes family, personal and social history as part of the seven components required. In complete contrast, Wright and Leahey (2009) look at family assessment and include physical or spiritual suffering, illness, relationship issues or family crisis as indications for a family assessment. Although a health history described by Bickley (2009), Rushworth (2009), and Wilson and Giddens (2009) is suitable for the context of individual patients presenting with a physical complaint or illness, this is clearly a different context from that of a family with health needs in the community setting that Wright and Leahey (2009) are alluding to. This highlights the complex nature and diversity of community nursing assessment, as it is often the client group along with the type of community nursing service involved that dictates the form of assessment.

Although a health history does include social, family history and lifestyle, the focus of the consultation is usually around the presenting complaint and has a strong physical component. Even though this type of consultation clearly has a place in community nursing, for example in long-term condition management and prescribing, the emphasis can appear medicalized. Indeed the position statement on Advanced Level Nursing (DH, 2010) emphasizes the significance of advanced health needs assessment for nurses working at this level. Advanced physical examination and interpretation of diagnostic tests are recent skills for nurses, and highlight key elements of this advanced level of assessment. Although this advanced stage of nursing is linked to a level of expertise well beyond initial registration and would be undertaken only by those practitioners who had additional education and expertise, the position statement (DH, 2010) does indicate that the assessment takes a holistic perspective. For that reason a wider understanding of holistic assessment along with consideration of the nurse–patient relationship and the models or frameworks that guide us are areas worthy of further consideration (Winder, 2001; Roberts *et al.*, 2005; Maher and Hemming, 2005; NMC, 2006).

ACTIVITY 7.1

Defining terms: holism

From your own perspective note the key components of holism. Now link these ideas to community nursing assessment and write a short definition of 'holistic nursing care'. Continue reading through the chapter and then review your definition against those drawn from the literature in the following section.

HOLISM

Although holism is a term used frequently within nursing literature in relation to health assessment (Roper *et al.*, 1990; Aggleton and Chalmers, 2000; Fox, 2003; RCN 2006; Beckwith and Franklin, 2007), a more detailed analysis of the term is often absent. According to Dossey and Guzzetta (2005: 8), Holistic Nursing Consultants in the USA, 'Holistic nursing is the most complete way to conceptualize and practice professional nursing'. The bio-psycho-social-spiritual concept that Dossey and Guzzetta (2005: 8) describe for patient care necessary to achieve the best results closely resembles the approach supported by Gough (2008), Freeman (2005) and Haworth and Dluhy (2001), which embraces physical, psychological, social, environmental, spiritual and cultural factors that make up an individual as a whole (Haworth and Dluhy, 2001; Freeman, 2005; Gough, 2008). This is a sound perspective for community nurses to start from, as it reflects a social model of health and places the patient in a community setting. This links to Kennedy's (2004) work, which looked at community nursing assessment and reinforced the wider aspects of care that included psychosocial and spiritual features and the impact these factors have on health and wellbeing. Therefore, holistic assessment involves gathering information and data from a patient or client in relation to their physical, psychological, social, environmental, spiritual and cultural wellbeing. The Family Health System (FHS)

(Anderson and Tomlinson, 1992) also embraces a biopsychosocial approach, and the five realms of family life that make up the detail of the assessment plan suggest that environmental, cultural and spiritual wellbeing would be included. It is reassuring then that compatible assessment approaches from the disciplines of community and family nursing co-exist.

Retrieving guidance in the form of a model or framework that assists the practitioner to undertake a holistic assessment however is not straightforward. Two years ago, in an attempt to provide novice prescribers with guidance for assessment, Gough (2008) developed a holistic assessment model based on relevant theoretical perspectives. Although a limitation of this holistic framework is that it has not been formally validated to determine its inter-rater reliability, the content can guide practitioners and help them evaluate the assessment models that they currently use. Developing an assessment tool for a group of patients is not a new phenomenon, although failure to disseminate it through nursing literature perhaps is. Over 10 years ago Matthews and Hegarty (1997) failed to identify a recognized assessment tool for people with a learning disability and as a result designed a checklist to identify the health needs of this group of clients. Called the 'OK Health Check' the assessment checklist was devised to identify recognized health problems and health needs for this specific client group. Although assessment checklists can be deemed as superficial, it was accepted by Matthews and Hegarty (1997) that the tool had to be suitable for untrained carers to use and this may have been the factor that encouraged the development of a checklist rather than a comprehensive assessment tool for qualified nurses. A high level of inter-rater reliability was evidenced in relation to the checklist, and Matthews and Hegarty (1997) intimated their keenness for further development. The FHS (Anderson and Tomlinson, 1992) focuses on the five realms, which are the interactive (such as family relationships), developmental (the lifespan stages), integrity (family values), coping (managing crisis) and health processes (health beliefs and current health issues), making up the five realms of family life. Within the assessment process each of these areas is reviewed along with the construction of a genogram and ecomap, both of which will be explained later in the chapter. This is a very comprehensive holistic approach with all family members considered; however, a limitation in relation to the time required to undertake and document the findings from an FHS in this way needs to be recognized along with the wide-ranging knowledge and skills that the nurse appears to require.

PATIENT-CENTRED CARE

In addition to this understanding of holism, the RCN (2006) stresses that individualized assessment requires the patient or client to be a key partner to inform the management plan. This idea of patients being at the centre of their care was established in the Patients' Charter in 1991 and introduced the concept of the named nurse (Kingsfund, 2009). Principles of patient-centred care are detailed in Box 7.1 and it is clear that these key areas represent an approach to practice, as opposed to a definitive framework.

> **Box 7.1 Principles of patient-centred care**
>
> **Consideration of**
> • the patient's needs and beliefs
> • the patient as an individual
> • the patient's view in decision-making
> • the patient's fears and concerns
> • the patient's family, carers and friends

Furthermore, the principles of patient-centred care link to holistic assessment, recognizing need and shared decision-making. Support for this patient-centred approach is augmented in practice by the growing understanding of the term concordance and the resulting 'informed partnership agreement which is negotiated between the prescriber and the patient' (Beckwith and Franklin, 2007). This partnership agreement is explained in more detail by the Department of Health (2007), which differentiates between concordance and compliance in relation to medicines management by stating:

> Concordance describes a partnership approach to medicine prescribing and taking. It is different from 'compliance', which describes the patient's medicine taking in relation to the prescriber's instructions. Concordance recognises that people make their own decisions about whether or not to take a prescribed treatment and acknowledges that a well-informed patient may decide to decline treatment after learning about the relative benefits and risks.

This partnership approach to assessment practice, which illustrates the sharing of power between patient and professional, had already been recognized by Bryans (2000) as a social and participative process, in which both nurses and patient-client take part. Being able to view patients as individuals with diverse needs while exhibiting a positive interpersonal approach is a cornerstone of patient-centred care.

Notwithstanding, this approach can introduce complex challenges for community nurses as sharing information, providing autonomy for patients, delivering health promotion and responding to any potential issues that may impact on concordance are likely to be time-consuming. At a time where resources are constrained and community nurses need to justify the time spent in patients' homes, the concern is that achieving genuine holistic patient-centred care could be compromised.

ADOPTING NEW ROLES

The context of health assessment, however, can subtly change its focus directly due to nurses adopting new roles in practice. This can be seen when the term 'patient consultation' is introduced into contemporary nursing along with details of consultation models which are finding their way into nursing literature (Hastings, 2006; Young *et al.*, 2009; Harper and Ajao, 2010; Young and Duggan, 2010). The aforementioned authors analyzed the history-taking process in relation to a patient consultation, and it is clear that this reflects advanced skills in comparison to assessment of need by current community nurses. Among other things, these skills include *clarifying the complaint* and *identifying any red flags* (Young *et al.*, 2009; Young and Duggan, 2010), and for those with a prescribing background these terms in relation to risk assessment (NMC, 2006) will no doubt be familiar. Although current consultation models clearly have an assessment component drawn from nursing, along with recognition of interpersonal skills, this does introduce advanced clinical proficiencies that nurses moving into these roles need to develop (Young *et al.*, 2009). Regardless of the type of assessment that nurses in the community are involved in, being able to identify the health needs from both a patient and a nurse perspective is crucial.

EXPLORING THE CONCEPT OF NEED

A key aspect of health assessment links to the concept of need, and it would be difficult to undertake holistic assessment without consideration of need. Health needs can relate to different levels depending on the context, for example helping patients to identify their own health needs takes a different approach from identifying broad health needs within a local community (Coles and Porter, 2008). Bradshaw (1972) identified a taxonomy of need from a sociological perspective that helps to explain individual need and this is outlined in Box 7.2.

Box 7.2 Bradshaw's taxonomy of need

Normative need is explained as the need that the health/social care professional identifies. Although professionals are educated to recognize need, it has to be acknowledged that various professionals may identify different needs from each other. Furthermore health needs can change over time.

Felt need is described as a need identified by the patient or carer. Although the patient or carer will be able to identify some of their own needs, they may not have a grasp of all that they require.

Expressed need is the articulation of a felt need by the patient or carer.

Comparative need is when in certain areas the patients or carers are not receiving the same standard of care that is available elsewhere.

Although this does provide a theoretical perspective of need that can be practically applied by community nurses, it is worth pointing out that there is no acknowledgement of any associated resources, including availability of services. This means that although needs in relation to individuals or families may be identified, an issue arises when the resources are limited and these needs cannot be met. In reality this means that although assessment identifies healthcare needs for an individual, for example referral to a leg ulcer clinic or a nursery placement, any treatment or service provision will need to be justified economically. Furthermore, if the need cannot be met because there is no transport to the leg ulcer clinic or the nursery has no spaces, then alternatives have to be considered. Working within these constraints can be very challenging for the community nursing team and can result in frustration and concerns when trying to deliver evidenced-based practice. As determining need along with an available resource is part of the assessment process, then reviewing assessment frameworks is the next logical step.

DISCUSSION OF ASSESSMENT FRAMEWORKS

A starting point for analysis of existing frameworks is consideration of those currently in place that guide community nursing assessment.

ACTIVITY 7.2

Reflection point

Reflect on the way in which you currently assess a patient/client in practice including the assessment framework or model that guides you. Consider the age and context of the framework/model that you currently use and judge whether:

1. It is fit for purpose

You may wish to consider its strengths and limitations (is it simply a tick list?) and its ease of completion along with any gaps you identify. Gaps in assessment frameworks often result in the practitioner having to add in additional information using free hand.

2. Does it have an evidence base?

Can you clearly identify the literature or research that underpins the tool?

If you are using a Trust/NHS assessment framework then you still need to question the evidence base and identify the literature or research that underpins the tool.

It may be that you are unsure what assessment framework is available to you in practice: this is an important discovery. Practitioners can find themselves using the documentation that their employing organization provides them with and mistakenly believe this to be an assessment tool. Of course in some cases a validated assessment tool will be incorporated into the documentation, and as practitioners you should be able to identify this clearly. In an article on patient documentation by Irving *et al.* (2006), there is an assumption made that nursing records mirror the assessment made. The problem with this is that although the nurse enters the findings from the assessment into the nursing record, there is no guarantee that the documentation is in fact an assessment tool. This is then problematic if it is the documentation that drives the assessmentbecause the focus may not be holistic or, even worse, crucial information may be missed. Furthermore, if the tool only allows the nurse to document 'tasks' then the ethos of holistic assessment, decision-making and anticipatory care, which are the key elements of community nursing practice, is lost.

This link to 'task-orientated' nursing can be identified subtly in the aforementioned study by Irving *et al.* (2006). The study suggested that the objective biomedical information gathered from patients had more of a focus in the nursing notes than the subjective patient perspective, as this was often the least clearly cited. So measurement of physical wellbeing seemed to rate a higher significance than perhaps patients' emotional and psychological health. Certainly this study was undertaken in relation to four acute hospitals focusing on specific individual patients, whereas within a community setting it would be more likely to have family, carers and significant others featuring in assessments. Nevertheless, we cannot assume that community settings guarantee a holistic approach to assessment.

NURSING MODELS

Nursing models were introduced into the UK nurse education and practice in the 1980s. Designed to inform assessment by collating appropriate data (Aggleton and Chalmers, 2000) they were developed to guide nurses to deliver practice in a less chaotic and more organized fashion. Roper *et al.*'s (1990) model for nursing is perhaps the most well known in the UK, which is no surprise as the authors are British. Although the five components of the model include the activities of living and influencing factors, the lifespan, dependence–independence continuum and individuality in living (Roper *et al.*, 1990), it is almost always the activities of living that are evident in assessment frameworks within practice. Unfortunately, if the whole model is not used, the activities of living become a checklist and as a result the information gathered can often become superficial and lack crucial detail. It is perhaps no surprise that current literature which promotes the use of nursing models in contemporary community nursing practice is scarce, and this may reveal a lack of interest from educators and practitioners alike. Not surprisingly, when models of nursing, such as Orem's self-care model and Roy's adaptation model (Aggleton and Chalmers, 2000), are explored for clarity and understanding it becomes evident that the terminology implemented is not always user friendly and the language used is somewhat complicated. Perhaps it is this less than straightforward approach combined with a difficulty in application that has contributed to their decline.

It is likely that a search for the perfect assessment tool for community nursing is not realistic; however, there are various diverse theories and concepts available in the literature to assist nurses to develop holistic approaches for their area of practice.

HOLISTIC ASSESSMENT TOOLS

Finding a generic holistic assessment tool can be problematic, and it was exactly the nature of this problem that resulted in the development of such a tool for novice community practitioner nurse prescribers. The holistic assessment tool created by Gough (2008), which can be viewed in Box 7.3, was developed with a prescribing focus in mind. That said, the tool is arguably useful for gathering information from a range of patients/clients who have an identified health need in a community setting. Drawing on the dimensions of health (adapted from Aggleton and Homans, 1987, and Eweles and Simnett, 1999), the Determinants of Health (Dahlgren and Whitehead, 1991), Bickley's (2009) physical examination and history taking along with the prescribing pyramid (NPC, 1999), which includes the Mnemonic WWHAM used in pharmacies for advising about over-the-counter treatments (Box 7.4), a flexible assessment tool emerged. The tool provides guidance for community nurses to undertake a holistic assessment using free text and avoids completing a tick box checklist. Although every aspect may not be assessed at the first visit the assessment tool allows community nurses to respond to the needs determined by both the patient and nurse whilst implementing a partnership approach.

The flexibility of the assessment tool developed by Gough (2008) promotes the identification of priorities while at the same time providing an opportunity to include additional information at a later date. Although not yet validated, the assessment tool can prompt community nurses to respond to a holistic approach to assessment.

Box 7.3 Holistic assessment tool for community practitioner nurse prescribers (Gough, 2008)

Name and address
DOB
Occupation
(hazards, working
conditions, risks)
Reason for assessment/presenting complaint

Physical health
Onset, duration and severity of condition
Previous history of complaint, treatment and results

Previous medical history
Family history
Current health status and appearance
Medication
Prescription-only medication (POM), Pharmacy medication (P), general sales list (GSL) and other
Herbal/homeopathic
Known allergies (drugs and substances)
Alcohol history (can include family if client a child)
Smoking history (can include family if client a child)
Diet and fluids
Mobility (aids and adaptations)
Dexterity (aids and adaptations)
Visual acuity (aids and adaptations)
Additional physical findings specific to complaint (e.g. bowel habit, oral hygiene, broken skin)
Clinical findings (if examination required)
Additional specific assessment tool required (pain, wound, depression, nutritional assessment tool)

Emotional and psychological health
Emotional effects of condition
Cognitive (ability, disability, memory)
Mental health (anxiety, worry, confusion, depression, dementia)

Social/environmental health
Home occupants
Dependants
Carers (statutory and voluntary)
Living conditions (housing, access, safety)
Financial (needs, allowances, exemptions)
Local amenities (shops, transport, sanitation)

Sexual health
Impact of condition on sexuality and sexual health

Spiritual health
Impact of condition on religion, beliefs, faith and culture
Additional information

Box 7.4 Mnemonic WWHAM

W   Who is it for?

W   What are the symptoms?

H   How long have the symptoms been present?

A   Any action taken so far?

M   Any other Medication

NPC (1991)

FAMILY HEALTH NURSING

Family health nursing takes a distinct approach to assessment and like nursing models has its foundation in North America. As part of family assessment family health nursing uses genograms to gather information about the composition of a family and ecomaps to gather information about the associated relationships. Genograms provide a diagrammatic picture of the generations of a family and include any patterns of health or genetic trends (Rowe Kaakinen and Harmon Hanson, 2005; Rempel *et al.*, 2007). An ecomap details any stressors or external issues that impact on the family and its relationship with the wider community (Rowe Kaakinen and Harmon Hanson, 2005). Compared with individual assessment, family assessment has a focus on all of those who make up the family and for some community nurses this may be a quantum shift in philosophy with implications for the time that is spent with one family in tandem with the number of families that the community nurse has on their caseload. Furthermore, the family assessment described by Anderson and Tomlinson (1992), and illustrated using a case study approach in Anderson (2000), does however introduce a different service of healthcare delivery in the USA compared with that in the UK. Not only that, but it seems that the level and scope of practice do not appear to be comparable with the UK, where community nurses are expected to exercise high levels of clinical decision-making and therefore autonomy.

Despite these service issues it is clear that this kind of data is very important when supporting families in the community, and ecomaps and genograms as part of a holistic assessment could be integrated by most community nursing specialities. This would capture this unique perspective in relation to family assessment and assist the community nurse with decision-making and planning care or interventions. Understandably, before community nurses incorporated these additional aspects into their existing assessment, consideration would need to be given to education and practice for nurses, not only to explain the concept and theory behind these tools before their use in practice but to set them in context. This means that depending on the context of the assessment, the use of ecomaps and genograms may or may not be appropriate so consideration needs to be given to the focus of the assessment. For example, if a client presents with an acute situation that requires a clinical intervention then gathering information to develop a genogram will not be a priority at that time. However, if a community nurse is going to be involved with a client and family over a period of time, then clearly genograms and ecomaps are valuable tools in gathering information and planning interventions. Focusing on a family and a community setting is likely to involve several health and social care professionals so it is perhaps no surprise that policy drivers to introduce a shared assessment process have already emerged.

SHARED ASSESSMENT

This approach to assessing adults in the community was adopted by all four UK countries to help standardize health and social care delivery and avoid duplication of services (Miller and Cameron, 2011). Driven from a policy agenda (DH, 2000; SE, 2000; Department of Health, Social Services and Public Safety, 2001; Welsh Assembly, 2001) and termed single assessment in England, single shared assessment in Scotland, unified assessment in Wales and single assessment tool in Northern Ireland, only Northern Ireland had a developed assessment tool to guide practice. This meant for the remaining three countries that although guidance was available, local areas were left to agree the assessment tool that was to be implemented. A literature review by Miller and Cameron (2011) also highlighted variations in the type of assessment adopted in relation to gathering information, and this ranged from being able to complete free text to a tick box approach. It would therefore appear that it is the documentation for shared assessment by health and social care that drives the assessment in place of an assessment tool, although this does not negate the assessment skills that practitioners have in the community setting. This lack of standardization however does raise a concern and links to issues around comparative need and fairness discussed earlier. Although Miller and Cameron

(2011) did identify some positive aspects of shared assessment in relation to joint working and the sharing of information, they concluded that identifying the outcomes of shared assessment was the way forward.

Holistic assessment tools often require to be supplemented by additional specific assessment tools, for example for pain assessment, assessing postnatal depression, nutrition or assessing spiritual needs.

ACTIVITY 7.3

Reflection point
Now consider any additional specific areas of assessment (pain, wound, memory, mental state, nutrition, etc.) that you might want to undertake with your client group. What evidence-based tools or frameworks are available to you in your area? Now consider the ways in which you could search, retrieve and disseminate these with neighbouring community nurses.

Not surprisingly assessment practice does not stand independently and decision-making is a close relation that needs to be embraced in tandem alongside it. Decision-making is part of the crucial cognitive process when assessment is being undertaken and ties together the evidence base that should underpin community nursing assessment practice.

CRITICAL REFLECTION ON DECISION-MAKING

It is clear therefore that assessment cannot exist in a vacuum without decision-making processes with which to move the episode of care along.

ACTIVITY 7.4

Reflection point
Reflect on your current assessment practice and determine what currently guides your decision-making. If you are unable to answer this then please do not panic as help is at hand in the following section.

If you can identify a guide to your decision-making practice, now consider whether it has an evidence base.

Can you clearly identify the literature or research that underpins this guide?

If not then this is something that you can investigate within your local Trust/ NHS organization.

Sometimes it can be difficult to actually unpick what we mean when thinking about what guides decision-making, but what is clear is that for community nurses, nursing care requires to be evidenced based and not as a result of a whim or, worse, a comment like 'we always do it like this here'. As accountable practitioners a rationale needs to be provided for our actions and decisions (NMC, 2008) and having a guide to support our decision-making and to reflect with afterwards helps us to learn from experience.

CONTEXT OF DECISION-MAKING

As already mentioned, within community nursing there is a wide variety of contexts of practice in relation to the patient group and the discipline involved, for example young children and the potential input from health visitors/public health nurses or community children's nurses, those with mental health conditions and likely input from community mental health nurses and finally unwell older adults receiving care from district nurses and practice nurses. These contexts are important as they determine the skills and knowledge required to deliver care and are highlighted specifically in relation to decision-making and healthcare by Croskerry (2009). This article highlights two main systems of decision-making. The first is *system one*, the intuitive route, which relies on a reflexive approach that expends little effort and does not depend on evidence to underpin the decision. Although this will be familiar to community nurses, the problem is that it can be unreliable and errors are frequent, so relying on this approach is unlikely to provide quality patient care and in the extreme could be fatal. Errors in decision-making are explained as slips, lapses and mistakes (Thomson and Dowding, 2002). Furthermore, mistakes take place when the practitioner's thinking is faulty (Thomson and Dowding, 2002); for example, the diagnosis of a red painful wound as infected when it is actually inflamed.

System two described by Croskerry (2009) is the analytical route, which relies on a rule-based approach that requires significant effort and has a scientific base. The problem with this analytical approach is that although it is a more reliable system of decision-making, there is an associated cost and time issue that cannot be ignored. Therefore, a balance between both systems needs to be considered. The case study illustrates this from a community nursing practice perspective.

CASE STUDY

Mrs Grant is aged 84 years and is unknown to you. She has requested that you visit as she would like some help and advice in relation to a problem with constipation.

Intuitive approach – fast, reflexive with minimal effort

Your experience with patients in this age group links constipation to medication side-effects, reduced fibre in the diet along with a lack of fluids and low mobility. This intuitive approach relies on the context to guide the decision and in this case it's the gender, age and assumed comorbidity of the patient.

Analytical approach – slower, deliberate with considerable effort

Your experience with patients in this age group links constipation to medication side-effects, reduced fibre in the diet along with a lack of fluids and low mobility. However, you are aware that a change in bowel habit and any bleeding could indicate bowel disease or cancer. This knowledge combined with the use of the Bristol Stool Chart and a history of the complaint will identify a normal bowel pattern and stool consistency.

It is not Mrs Grant who has constipation as you first thought, and it turns out that Mrs Grant would like some help and advice about her husband as she is his main carer. Mr Grant has multiple sclerosis and he has had several recent falls. As a result he has stopped the osmotic laxative he had been taking for several months as his bowel movements are loose and he needs to rush to the toilet fairly frequently. He has been soiling underwear and sheets frequently, which has been upsetting for them both, and now his normal bowel pattern has ceased. Mr Grant now feels very uncomfortable and nauseous. This analytical approach extracts any irrelevant information (in this case the patient with constipation is not Mrs Grant), does not focus on the specific context and uses guidelines to support clinical practice.

While repeated specific experiences may convert analytical decisions into intuitive ones, a raised awareness of the context of situations, although helping us to make sense of the situation, can also provide a distraction from the reality and lead us to assumptions that are not accurate. Earlier work by Croskerry (2002) in relation to pattern recognition explains a situation whereby a patient presenting with particular visual aspects of a complaint and their appearance can trigger a bias in the decision-making. Furthermore, any subsequent data gathered from the patient can be used to confirm the initial diagnosis, even when it is not accurate. For example, a patient presenting with a painful mouth with evidence of an ulcer and white plaques on their tongue who confirms that they have just completed a course of antibiotics may result in a bias towards oral thrush when the ulcer may actually be the beginnings of oral cancer. Although this article by Croskerry (2002) is aimed at medics and in particular those who work in emergency medicine, it can illustrate how a failed approach to decision-making can occur, a fundamental message that community nurses need to be aware of.

DECISION-MAKING FRAMEWORKS

Providing a rationale for decisions often requires a reflective approach and in 1996 Bryans and McIntosh undertook this by analyzing decision-making in relation to community nursing assessment practice. Although Bryans and McIntosh (1996) do not articulate the intuitive and analytical approaches that are described above, they do introduce a seven-stage framework and the first two stages of the framework link to decision-making prior to meeting the patient. These first two stages (Carroll and Johnston, 1990) of the decision-making framework are problem recognition and formulation which are explained as 'pre-decisional activity' (Bryans and McIntosh, 1996: 25). Just like the 'context' discussed above these first two stages are when the community nurse forms ideas about a new referral, for example, and what the subsequent assessment will involve. If it is a familiar situation then there is a risk that assumptions and judgements may be made about their patient, such as their address if the referral is for a family with allergy problems in an affluent area, or the patient's age if very elderly or indeed if the family name is well known to most of the local health and social care agencies.

The Carroll and Johnston (1990) decision-making framework moves onto subsequent stages that include stages 3 (alternative generation), 4 (information search) and 5 (judgement or choice). These stages are explained as those where the community nurse undertaking the assessment begins to think the problem through and weighs up 'the pros and cons' of the choices available. What must be remembered is that mistakes could still be made here if the practitioner has gaps in their knowledge base. Thomson and Dowding (2002) point to evidence-based guidelines to minimize this risk. Furthermore, pattern recognition discussed earlier could also result in missed problem recognition. The penultimate stage is stage 6 which actions the decision and stage 7 is about feedback when the community nurse evaluates the situation following intervention, a final stage essential for community nursing practice. Carroll and Johnston's decision-making framework was originally published in 1990 and was included in Bryans and McIntosh's (1996) research work 6 years later. Arguably its relevance for community nurses is still apparent, as it has been contextualized specifically for community nurses and can be used to provide a rationale for any actions taken within community nursing care. In other words by using this framework reflectively, decision-making in relation to patient care can be reviewed and the steps taken to reach a transparent decision are made.

SHARED DECISION-MAKING

The competency framework for shared decision-making (NPC, 2007) is very detailed and describes behaviours that will guide a prescriber when building a relationship with the client/patient. Although designed for prescribing, many of the components have a generalized approach, with only a few aspects relating specifically to medicines. This means this framework is ideal for community nurses to consider as a guide to patient-centred decision-making.

The competency framework (NPC, 2007) provides eight areas of practice that include interpersonal skills such as *listening* and *communicating* along with consideration of the practitioner's *knowledge*. The context of the assessment, although advocating a patient-centred approach (patients *understanding* and *deciding*) throughout, is also well thought out. *Exploring* treatment options and the patient's views are then followed by a *monitoring* aspect; however, unlike the Carroll and Johnston (1990) framework this does not include review. Having said that the competency framework is meticulous in its approach and although at first it appears to be complex, closer examination reveals that it is actually in the final part of the framework, 'sharing a decision', that the focus on decision-making is revealed. For nurses moving into the delivery of care previously undertaken by medical staff, clearly an additional vigorous approach to clinical decision-making would need to be considered. Certainly the strategies advocated by Croskerry (2002) would be an ideal starting point.

CONCLUSION

So it would seem that in order to deliver effective care to patients in the community, assessment needs to be placed under scrutiny. Determining existing assessment strategies and underpinning theory that supports assessment in practice is a starting point. Holistic assessment in community nursing practice involves a person-centred approach where information is gathered in relation to the individual's physical, psychological, social, environmental, spiritual and cultural wellbeing using recognized evidenced-based frameworks. Family and carers are included in the assessment where appropriate, and, depending on the needs prioritized, the focus of the assessment can move along a spectrum from concentrating on a physical assessment utilizing advanced clinical skills with one individual, to focusing on a broad family assessment where developing ecomaps and genograms along with a spiritual assessment may be beneficial. It is this flexible approach practised by a body of community nurses that is a real strength.

Undertaking robust evidenced-based assessments that have clinical decision-making embedded in the process, a clear understanding of accountability and the essential underpinning knowledge and skills in relation to delivering patient care will facilitate community nurses to deliver the high-quality care that most patients expect and deserve. By revisiting theories of assessment, including assessment tools and decision-making frameworks, current and future community nurses will be able to provide a clear rationale for their practice and take responsibility for implementing any improvements within their clinical area.

REFERENCES

Aggleton P and Chalmers H (2000) *Nursing Models and Nursing Practice*, 2nd edn. London: Macmillan Press Limited.

Aggleton P and Homans H (1987) *Educating about AIDs.* Bristol: NHS Training Authority. cited in Naidoo J and Wills J (2000) *Health Promotion: Foundations for Practice*, 2nd edn. Edinburgh: Harcourt Publishers.

Anderson KH (2000) The family health system approach to family systems nursing. *Journal of Family Nursing* 6:103–19.

Anderson KH and Tomlinson PS (1992) The Family Health System as an emerging paradigmatic view for nursing. *Journal of Nursing Scholarship* 24:57–63.

Beckwith S and Franklin P (2007) *Oxford Handbook of Nurse Prescribing.* Oxford: Oxford University Press.

Bickley LS (2009) *Bates' Pocket Guide to Physical Examination and History Taking*, 10th edn. Philadelphia, PA: Lippincott Williams & Wilkins.

Bradshaw J (1972) The concept of social need. *New Society* March:640–3.

Bryans A (2000) Providing new insight into community nursing know-how through qualitative analysis of multiple data sets of simulation data. *Primary Health Care Research and Development* 1:79–89.

Bryans A and McIntosh J (1996) Decision making in community nursing: an analysis of the stages of decision making as they relate to community nursing assessment practice. *Journal of Advanced Nursing* 24:24–30.

Carroll JS and Johnson EJ (1990) Decision research: a field guide. In Bryans A and McIntosh J (1996) Decision making in community nursing: an analysis of the stages of decision making as they relate to community nursing assessment practice. *Journal of Advanced Nursing* 24: 24–30.

Coles L and Porter E (2008) *Public Health Skills: A Practical Guide for Nurses and Public Health Practitioners*. Oxford: Blackwell Publishing Ltd.

Croskerry P (2002) Achieving quality in clinical decision making; cognitive strategies and detection of bias. *Academic Emergency Medicine* 9:1184–204.

Croskerry P (2009) Context is everything or How could I have been that stupid? *Healthcare Quarterly* 12(special issue):171–7.

Dahlgren G and Whitehead M (1991) *Policies and Strategies to Promote Social Equity in Health*. Stockholm: Institute for Future Studies.

Department of Health (DH) (2000) *The NHS Plan: A Plan for Investment, A Plan for Reform*. London: Department of Health.

DH (2006) *Our Health, Our Care, Our Say: A New Direction for Community Services*. London: Department of Health.

DH (2007) *Management of Medicines – A Resource to Support Implementation of the Wider Aspects of Medicines Management for the National Service Frameworks for Diabetes, Renal Services and Long-Term Conditions*. London: Department of Health.

DH (2008) *A High Quality Workforce: NHS Next Stage Review*. London: Department of Health.

DH (2010) *Advanced Level Nursing: A Position Statement*. London: Department of Health.

Department of Health, Social Services and Public Safety (2001) *People First: Community Care in Northern Ireland*. Belfast: Department of Health, Social Services and Public Safety.

Ewles L and Simnett I (1999) *Promoting Health: A Practical Guide to Health Education*, 4th edn. Edinburgh: Harcourt Publishers, cited in Naidoo J and Wills J (2000) *Health Promotion Foundations for Practice* Edinburgh: Harcourt Publishers Limited.

Dossey BM and Guzzetta CE (2005) Holistic nursing practice. In Dossey BM, Keegan L and Guzzetta CE (eds) *Holistic Nursing: A Handbook for Practice*, 4th edn. Boston: Jones and Bartlett Publishers, pp. 5–40.

Fox C (2003) The holistic assessment of a patient with leg ulceration. *British Journal of Community Nursing Wound Care* March:26–30.

Freeman J (2005) Towards a definition of holism. *British Journal of General Practice* February:154–5.

Gough H (2008) Plugging the gaps and getting assessment right: a new holistic assessment framework for the community practitioner nurse prescriber. *Care* 2:24–40. ww.gcu.ac.uk/care.

Harper C and Ajao A (2010) Pendleton's consultation model: assessing a patient. *British Journal of Community Nursing* 15:38–43.

Hastings A (2006) Assessing and improving the consultation skills of nurses. *Nurse Prescribing* 4:418–22.

Haworth S and Dluhy N (2001) Holistic symptom management: modelling the interactive phase. *Journal of Advanced Nursing* 36:302–10.

Irving K, Treacy M, Scott A, *et al.* (2006) Discursive practices in the documentation of patient assessment. *Journal of Advanced Nursing* 51:151–9.

Kennedy CM (2004) A typology of knowledge for district nursing practice. *Journal of Advanced Nursing* 45:401–9.

King's Fund (2009) Patient Centred Care. (Accessed 12 November 2010) www.kingsfund.org.uk/topics/patientcentred_care/#keypoints.

Maher D and Hemming L (2005) Understanding patient and family: holistic assessment in palliative care. British *Journal of Community Nursing* 10:318–22.

Matthews D and Hegarty J (1997) The OK health check: a health assessment checklist for people with learning disabilities. *British Journal of Learning Disabilities* 25:138–43.

Miller E and Cameron K (2011) Challenges and benefits in implementing shared interagency assessment across the UK: a literature review. *Journal of Interprofessional Care* 25:39–45.

Muncey T (2002) .In Muncey T and Parker A (eds) *Chronic Disease Management: A Practical Guide.* Basingstoke: Palgrave.

National Prescribing Centre (NPC) (1991) Signposts for prescribing nurses – general principles of good prescribing. *Nurse Prescribing Bulletin* 1:1–4.

NPC Plus (2007) *A competency framework for shared decision making with patients.* Keele: National Prescribing Centre Plus.

Nursing and Midwifery Council (NMC) (2008) *The Code.* London: Nursing and Midwifery Council.

NMC (2006) *Standards of Proficiency for Nurse and Midwife Prescribers.* London:Nursing and Midwifery Council.

Rempel GR, Neufeld A and Kushner KE (2007) Interactive use of Genograms and ecomaps in family caregiving research. *Journal of Family Nursing* 13:403–19.

Roberts D, Taylor S, Bodell W, *et al.* (2005) Development of a holistic admission assessment: an integrated care pathway for the hospice setting. *International Journal of Palliative Nursing* 11:322–32.

Roper N, Logan WW and Tierney A (1990) *The Elements of Nursing: A Model of Nursing Based on a Model of Living*, 3rd edn. Edinburgh: Churchill Livingstone.

Rowe Kaakinen J and Harmon Hanson SM (2005) Family nursing assessment and intervention. In Harmon Hanson SM, Gedaly-Duff V and Rowe Kaakinen J (2005) *Family Health Care Nursing: Theory, Practice and Research*, 3rd edn. Philadelphia, PA: FA Davis, pp. 215–42.

Royal College of Nursing (2006) *Caring in Partnership: Older People and Nursing Staff Working towards the Future.* London: Royal College of Nursing.

Rushworth H (2009) *Assessment Made Incredibly Easy.* Philadelphia, PA: Lippincott Williams, Wilkins.

Scottish Executive (2000) *Report of the Joint Future Group.* Edinburgh: Scottish Executive.

Scottish Executive (2005) *Building a Health Service Fit for the Future: A National Framework for Service Change in the NHS in Scotland.* Edinburgh: Scottish Executive.

Scottish Government (2007) *Better Health, Better Care: Planning Tomorrow's Workforce Today.* Edinburgh: Scottish Government.

Thomson C and Dowding D (2002) *Clinical Decision Making and Judgement in Nursing.* Edinburgh: Churchill Livingstone.

Welsh Assembly (2001) *National Service Framework for Older People.* Cardiff: Welsh Assembly.

Wilson SF and Giddens JF (2009) *Health Assessment for Nursing Practice*, 4th edn. St Louis, MO: Mosby Elsevier.

Winder A (2001) Devising an effective general continence assessment tool. *British Journal of Nursing* 10:93–5947.

Worth A (2001) Assessment of the needs of older people by district nurses and social workers: a changing culture. *Journal of Interprofessional Care* 15:257–66.

Wright LM and Leahey M (2009) *Nurses and Families: A Guide to Family Assessment and Intervention*, 5th edn. Philadelphia, PA: FA Davis Company.

Young K and Duggan L (2010) Consulting with patients: the structure of history taking. *Journal of Community Nursing* 24:30–2.

Young K, Duggan L and Franklin P (2009) Effective consulting and history-taking skills for prescribing practice. *Journal of Nursing* 18:1056–61.

FURTHER READING

Rempel GR, Neufeld A and Kushner KE (2007) Interactive use of Genograms and ecomaps in family caregiving research. *Journal of Family Nursing* 13:403–19.

Carers: the keystone of communities and families

Fiona Baguley

LEARNING OUTCOMES

- Discuss the role of carers in the community setting
- Explore some of the difficulties and rewards of caring in the community setting
- Critically appraise carer assessment tools and their use
- Reflect on the support needs of carers

INTRODUCTION

Carers are now acknowledged as the 'bedrock' of community care (McNamara, 2010), but there still exists some confusion around who we are referring to when we talk about carers. In this chapter the definition of 'carer' in the UK will be examined; the role they carry out; the contribution they make to society; relevant issues they have to face; and the role nurses have to identify, assess and support them.

WHO IS A CARER?

Generally in the UK a carer is someone who provides a substantial amount of unpaid care, on a regular basis, to an adult or child who may not be able to manage daily activities because of frailty, illness or disability. Others who provide care, for example care workers who work for social services or private agencies that provide personal care, are often mistakenly referred to as carers. These people are employed to provide care and receive payment for doing so.

Anyone might become a carer during their lifespan, sometimes caring for several people at once, or perhaps fulfilling the carer role on more than one occasion, for example a mother who then cares for her mother, then her father-in-law. Carers can be family members, perhaps juggle several roles at once, have learning disabilities or be physically frail themselves. Carers can be under 16 years of age, a refugee or perhaps a travelling gypsy. Those who need care are also diverse in need and ability. In order to be legally recognized as a carer a person must provide a substantial amount of care on a regular basis for either an adult or a child, when that adult or child receives, or is eligible to receive, a qualifying disability benefit. Family members caring for children in a range of circumstances will not come under the legal definition of a carer unless the child in question has a disability or is affected by disability.

For several reasons carers are often difficult to identify. They might not or are unwilling to recognize that they are carrying out that role for many complex reasons. This can result in them receiving little or no support from any other agencies or professionals. Appropriate and uniform recognition, definition and use of the term 'carer' is important in enabling the identification of carers throughout the country, publicizing the support needed for those carers and directing appropriate financial provision to them.

THE IMPACT OF POPULATION CHANGE

According to the 2001 Census (Carers UK, 2006), approximately 10% of the population are carers in the UK and Northern Ireland. It is projected that 174 995 people under 18 years of age in the UK and Northern Ireland are carers, just over 13 000 of whom provide more than 50 hours of care a week. It is anticipated that by 2031 the working age population in the UK will have reduced from five to three people for every person over the age of 65. These demographic predictions have implications for the availability of carers and the future of care in the community setting, which will impact on the role and responsibilities of healthcare practitioners (Carers UK, 2006).

The financial value of the care provided by carers in the UK is estimated at £87 billion per year (Carers UK, 2007). The need for carers to take on this responsibility will continue to increase as the population ages and more people live with long-term conditions. The UK-wide Health Service focus on preventative, anticipatory care will only be possible if carers become equal partners in care delivery. The potential cost to health and social services if this informal care situation breaks down is highly significant for future economic sustainability of society (Jarvis, 2011).

Nurses in the community setting often work in partnership with carers and are invaluable in identifying, supporting and assessing carer needs in a professional and accountable manner.

ACTIVITY 8.1

Reflection point
Consider the role of a carer you have known, either in the clinical setting or personally.

- What support has that carer received?
- Did they identify themselves as a carer?
- What other life commitments did that carer have to manage?
- Do you agree with the definition of formal/informal carer?

THE IMPACT OF CARING

Age

Carers of older people and those with long-term conditions in the community are often spouses and older themselves. Rees *et al.* (2001) postulate that it is this very group who cope least well with the responsibility of caring, physically and emotionally, for a dependent person. A lack of support, education, ability or willingness can often result in carer depression, illness, exhaustion and mortality. In the UK carers can feel isolated, particularly partner carers, who might live alone with their dependent person and in poverty, or carers who live in a rural situation. Sometimes carers exhibit reluctance to admit that they are having difficulty coping because they are unaware of the help and support that can be offered to assist the home situation (Rees *et al.*, 2001). The effective identification of carers and appropriate assessments and interventions can ease the role of caring for those who are struggling and prevent other carers becoming isolated and burnt out, thus maintaining the quality of the carer's life and sustaining the carer relationship and quality of life for the dependent person.

Financial assistance

The main financial assistance for carers is the Carer's Allowance (or Invalid Carer Allowance in Northern Ireland). Despite one in 10 carers being eligible to receive the Carer's Allowance, £840 million goes unclaimed each year in the UK. There are strict criteria the carer has to meet to be allocated this allowance, and it is not available to carers under the age of 16. Other benefits they might receive if not receiving the Carer's Allowance are Incapacity Benefit, State Pension or other allowances, depending on their circumstances. However, it is widely acknowledged by Carers UK that many carers who are on benefits find it very difficult to manage. There are additional costs incurred by caring for a disabled person, together with the inadequacy of benefits and the cost of services.

Financial impact

The financial cost of caring can be increased by simple daily life, for example increased laundry bills, higher heating costs and transportation costs. Carers in poverty have to make drastic compromises in their diet, use of fuel and accumulation of debt in order to survive at a basic level, all of which can have an impact on the carer's health.

For many carers it is the idea of having to meet set criteria in order to be eligible for and have access to the help they need that is one of the most difficult aspects of the caring role to cope with.

Carer health and Work

For those carers who are unwell themselves, it is not uncommon for them to dismiss their own health and wellbeing in order to fulfil their role as carer. Yet the health and ability of the carer to cope are essential to enable the dependent person to stay at home and receive the assistance they need.

In the UK, according to the 2001 Census (Carers UK, 2006), eight out of 10 carers are of working age, the majority of whom have no income coming into the home except benefits. Four hundred thousand carers juggle full-time work, while also providing over 20 hours of care per week. Working carers have been found to compromise their career prospects, and according to the 2001 Census (Carers UK, 2006) retire earlier, incurring financial loss.

Young carers

Young carers are children and young people under the age of 18 who provide, or intend to provide, care, assistance or support to another family member who is disabled, physically or mentally ill, or has a substance misuse problem. They carry out, often on a regular basis, significant or substantial caring tasks, taking on a level of responsibility that is inappropriate to their age or development. Young carers who care for a dependent person for many hours per week often for many years are especially vulnerable to the negative impact of caring physically and psychologically (Banks *et al.*, 2002).

Impact on young carers

The young carer populations are more predisposed to having problems at school with attendance, engaging in work and in attaining qualifications. They are often isolated from their peer group or bullied. Young carers feel that their difficulties are not understood and feel unsupported by health, social and education professionals. They can experience feelings of guilt and resentment because of the conflict between the needs of the person they are caring for and their own lifestyle, emotional and recreational needs. This all accumulates, and problems often occur when they move into adulthood, finding employment, living independently and establishing relationships (Banks *et al.*, 2002).

The difficulties that young carers can experience can be expressed through disruptive or antisocial behaviour, drug taking, depression, ill health and so forth. Although it cannot be said that young people should not be in a caring role at all, because each situation is unique, the community health practitioner does have an important role in the identification, assessment and support of young carers, together with social services, educational services and voluntary services. The difficulty is identifying young carers, resulting in appropriate support from statutory services not being given.

Epidemiology and national policies

It has been predicted that by 2021 the number of people aged over 75 years in the UK will have increased by 75% and the percentage of young people will have fallen by 20%. People will be living longer and also living with long-term conditions for a significant part of their lives (DH, 2008). The need for carers will increase and the situation now is not unusual where two older people live together, one caring for the other, but neither with good health.

It is in response to these changes that the UK governments wish to increase the relationship between primary healthcare, social services, charities and the acute sector. There will be a continuing emphasis on the development of the role of primary care, health promotion and sustaining people at home.

Each country in the UK and Northern Ireland has produced its own carer strategies and policies (see Further reading) and to a certain extent Scotland does have an alternative system when financing personal care provision to a disabled/dependent person. However, the aims and desires of all UK countries are broadly the same, as are the needs of carers. Whether a carer fulfils the criteria to receive benefits or not, the focus for health practitioners is to improve the effective identification of carers, increase the uptake and quality of carer assessment and provide information and advice. Carers, health, wellbeing and support can be enhanced by assisting them to contact voluntary agencies, promoting short breaks (previously called respite) and providing education with skills such as moving and handling. Health and social professionals working closer together with other appropriate local services can provide and participate in partnership training. GPs are being encouraged to advocate regular health checks for carers between the ages of 40 and 65 years. This is an appropriate opportunity for the community nurse to assess how they are coping with the role of caring.

The changing face of carer empowerment

Carers' rights and recognition Europe-wide have increased greatly in the last 10 years, and in the UK the aim is to develop in the next 5 a Carers Rights Charter that will promote an environment in which carers can have a life apart from caring. There has been an increase in carer information services and carer support groups, and in some respects the voice of carers is becoming louder. The most important action cited by carers that would improve their quality of life is to gain greater recognition and respect as key partners and providers of care, perhaps through the development of a rights-based policy framework to support carers (Carers UK, 2006, 2007).

ACTIVITY 8.2

Reflection point
Identify and reflect on the rewards of carrying out the role of carer and the costs, considering emotional, physical and financial aspects.

SUPPORTIVE ASSESSMENT OF CARERS

Nursing assessment

In community nursing there is generally a good understanding of the importance of carrying out health needs assessments as discussed in Chapter 1. The assessment of need can be carried out for individuals, families, communities and carers, depending on the situation the community practitioner encounters. Much of the emphasis on nursing assessment has traditionally been on the patient/individual rather than the carer, although some assessment tools do include the carer within them.

Rationale for carer assessment

Carers are often asked to make proxy decisions on behalf of patients, and their own interests and perceptions of their situation and choices available can influence these judgements. This is important for the healthcare practitioner to be aware of in order to protect and be an advocate for the dependent person. A specific carer assessment will often help healthcare professionals understand carers' experiences and enable them to give the support that carers need to fulfil the role or work in partnership with others if needed (Dahlberg *et al.*, 2007).

The 2004 Carers (Equal Opportunities) Act emphasizes the responsibility health and social care professionals have to work together to endorse and protect the health of carers. Over the last 10 years researchers and practitioners have developed tools for assessing people identified as carers, recognizing them and promoting the recognition of them in their role and acknowledging their value in the success of the care situation. The effective and sensitive use of such tools has had positive results for both the carers and the dependent person (Guberman, 2003). Effective carer assessment at an appropriate time promotes the improvement of interventions and the effectiveness of healthcare staff in their professional capacity. The assessment tool format often allows the carer to voice simple issues, which, if addressed, improve care and results for the dependent person. However, carer assessment tools are still underused and there remains a policy-to-practice gap (Guberman, 2003).

The sensitivity of the healthcare professional when carrying out an assessment of the carer is vital for the success of the tool. Some carers might think that because they are being assessed their ability or suitability to provide care is under question, causing anxiety. It would be helpful if the carer assessment was viewed by all as a carers' support tool.

Single shared assessment

All people over the age of 16 who meet the definition of carer in their local area are entitled to an assessment by Social Services, or a Single Shared Assessment by Social Services and the National Health Service together (DH, 2000; Department of Health, Social Services and Public Safety, 2001; SE, 2000; Welsh Assembly, 2001). These tools are used by social services and healthcare workers to assess the carer's experience, their ability or willingness to cope and their quality of life.

The development of carer assessment tools

In recognition of the fact that all European countries face similar changes in their epidemiology, resulting in an increase in their dependent population, there has been a Europe-wide desire for some time to develop a Carers Assessment Tool to be used by health practitioners (Guberman *et al.*, 2003).

COPE (Carers of Older People in Europe) was a European-funded project that led to the development of the COPE Index, a first-stage assessment tool, developed and tried in 1998–2001. COPE was a project to promote a uniform assessment of family carer need. It was a simple but holistic tool, focusing on the positive and negative aspects of caring and the needs of the carer (Nolan and Philip, 1999). As a first-stage tool the COPE Index is a concise assessment tool and identifies to the health professional carers who might require a more comprehensive second-stage assessment. There is a selection of second-stage tools being used and developed, examples of which are CADI (Carers Assessment of Difficulties Index), CAMI (Carers Assessment of Managing Index) and CASI (Carers Assessment of Satisfactions Index). These tools have been used successfully in several European countries and have obtained favourable results from carers and practitioners (McKee, 2009).

The Carers Outcome Agreement Assessment Tool (COAT) was developed between 2003 and 2005 in recognition of the global significance of the role of carers and the sensitive priority that must be given to their need and ability to fulfil their role (Hanson *et al.*, 2008). It successfully gave a voice to carers and is a model that enables an honest reflection of the carer's personal, daily situation. The development of COAT has been successful in enabling a holistic perspective to be gained by the professional, but also enabled problems to be identified, negotiated and a management plan developed. It is a step closer to a partnership agreement between carer and assessor and service provider.

Practitioner approach

Something to note is that the health professional carrying out the assessment should not assume that the carer wants to continue in the caring role. Sometimes a carer can think that if they do not care for their dependent person it will be assumed that they also do not care about the dependent person, resulting in them taking on a responsibility they are not able or willing to carry out, to the detriment of all concerned. Any assessment or support tool will require sensitivity and communication skill from the professional, enabling a relationship of trust and honesty to develop. The development of a trusting relationship and support building takes time, investment and effort, both at a higher and at a local level.

ACTIVITY 8.3

- What theory currently underpins your assessment of a carer's needs?
- Review two carer assessment tools from your reading, then compare and contrast them in terms of their strengths and weaknesses.

COPING WITH DIFFICULT BEHAVIOURS

Recognizing difficult behaviours

The King's Fund (2008) stipulates that future changes in an ever-changing community healthcare environment will fail if they neglect the needs of carers.

One of the issues of care-giving that can be ignored or hidden is that of carers experiencing difficult behaviours on a frequent and regular basis, leading to carer anxiety, grief and a breakdown in the caring relationship.

Definition of difficult behaviours

The definition of difficult behaviours is not clear–it can be as simple as the dependent person refusing to eat after requesting something specific for lunch, or it can be violence, spitting, deliberate defecation and so forth.

Impact on carers

Difficult behaviour that is repeated in the home environment is a stress that may well contribute to the challenge of caring. If one person becomes more dependent on the other and the balance of the close relationship, such as a partner or spousal relationship, changes, the carer's patience and care satisfaction can be lowered when they are on the receiving end of 'troublesome behaviours'.

Carers sometimes do not identify themselves as being on the receiving end of abusive behaviour because of the perceived lack of intention to harm by the perpetrator, e.g. in dementia/mental illness/frustration (Mowlam, 2007). In their study looking at the mistreatment of older, partnered, female carers, Zink *et al.* (2006) identified that mistreatment of a carer often takes place in relationships when change occurs, e.g. the spouse becomes a carer and the relationship balance is altered. In relationships where historically there has been evidence of maltreatment in a physical or sexual manner from the now dependent person, the abusive behaviour continues, but often changes in nature. Also, as spousal carers age they may actually become more psychologically vulnerable than before.

CARER SUPPORT

Access to help

Generational beliefs about their role as a spouse, the confusion between caring for and caring about their partner, shame and the fear of change can stop carers who are exposed to repeated difficult behaviours from seeking the help and support they need. Rees *et al.* (2001) state that when they analyzed the literature on carer assessment, the quality of life of the carer tended to be 'worse than that of the patient'.

For the healthcare practitioner, assessing a situation and establishing the balance between the carer getting the support they need and being able to care for the dependent person if they want to is essential. Buhr *et al.* (2006) identified that it is the carer's life satisfaction and quality of health in the year prior to the dependent person being admitted to a residential placement that predicts the admission of the dependent person into institutional care. Any extra pressure on the carer or perceived extra pressure by the carer may eventually lead to the breakdown of the care situation. This is a particularly important issue when the carer is hidden and no-one has any insight into the carer's needs and the treatment the disabled person is receiving. It is essential for community practitioner understanding to verify different groups of carers and carer experiences if they are to offer the support that carers need to fulfil the role they have in today's society. It is important to identify the 'hidden carers': those carers who are in the majority, who receive no help, no support, are not aware what help they are entitled to and do not know how to access assistance. In some areas of the UK, this is being done through setting up a 'carers point' in the general hospital, where carers can go to identify themselves, get advice and information. GP case notes are also highlighting carers more clearly in the surgery, while the acute sector admission and assessment process now notes if someone is a carer, or depends on a carer.

Interprofessional working

It is important for community practitioners to have effective working relationships and regular communication with the multidisciplinary team. Interprofessional appreciation of what each can offer and what they can offer together will effectively use resources and highlight more unidentified carers.

Dealing with change

In their research into the experiences of spousal carers where the dependent person has multiple sclerosis, Cheung and Hocking (2004) discussed the chronic loss that the carer experiences due to the relationship changes that take place, without the physical loss of the spouse. Also taken into consideration is the loss of self in the care situation. Carers often feel a loss of identity and status. Carers often identified themselves as having little recognition or understanding within society. The inability to continue their career is also something that can be difficult to cope with, even if the choice was made willingly (Cheung and Hocking, 2004).

The change in relationship between carer and cared for is one of the most complex areas for the nurse to offer support with. Often there has been some role reversal, e.g. child caring for parent, and each home circumstance has to be assessed independently. Some carers will be reluctant to perform personal tasks, while others feel quite comfortable with the role. For some carers, the change in roles and relationships as one person becomes more dependent on another is identified as being the natural progression of that relationship, whereas for others it identifies the end of the relationship that was.

Ethnicity

Those carers among ethnic minority populations in the UK and Northern Ireland have traditionally been less likely to access health practitioners or social services. It has been argued that it is those populations who cope best with the caring role, identifying it as a natural and expected turn of events, especially in marital or parental relationships. This positive perspective helps to balance out feelings of carer strain, isolation and fear. For many carers, whatever their relationship or background, the role of carer can be viewed as one that gives satisfaction and fulfilment. It can be perceived as being virtuous in nature. There is some evidence to suggest that those who cope less well with the caring role and find it more difficult to adapt to are white, well-educated women (Lawrence, 2008). However, as a healthcare professional it is worth being aware that perhaps it is the white, well-educated women who are able to voice their needs and difficulties more and access services in order to get support, whereas others who seem to cope are less aware of or able to ask for help and have a greater sense of duty. For those adult children who now care for parents, there might be a desire to give back the care and support shown to them as they were growing up.

Lifestyle

For all carers the unpredictable nature of the role means that they focus on coping with the daily activities of caring and have little emotional or mental capacity to plan for the future, e.g. plan a holiday. Most carers who live with the person they are caring for find the constant need to be present and vigilant the most mentally taxing aspect of the role.

Carer perspectives

It can be difficult for a carer to stand back mentally and gain an overview of what plans if put into place could give some balance to their life and identity, such as a short break, day care or carers' support groups. The health professional can be invaluable in providing advice, objectivity, empathy and direction.

Some carers look after a dependent person because they see residential and nursing home care as a last resort and one that is negative (Bolan and Sims, 1996). However, the use of respite care and other services can positively enhance the carer's experience and enable the care situation at home to continue for longer, perhaps avoiding a crisis.

Perceptions of whether caring is predominantly a burden or has some reward are closely tied up with cultural background, as has already been mentioned, and also religious beliefs and life expectations. Carer empowerment through education, support and recognition is a significant aspect of the community practitioner's role.

Agencies

A voluntary agency, usually a charity or grant-funded body, meets a particular need. The Princess Royal Trust for Carers would be an example of a voluntary agency.

The aim of voluntary and charitable agencies in relation to carers is to make a practical and positive difference through the provision of information, care relief, a listening ear, group support, respite care and practical support to all who need it. These agencies have the carer and the dependent person at the centre of their philosophy and are often run by carers themselves or their representatives. This gives a significant and informed insight into the needs of carers.

Voluntary and charitable organizations are ideally placed to empower carers. However, as their role increases the skills that they need, such as moving and handling training, education, definition of role and responsibilities, will be called into question. One of the overall benefits of the voluntary agencies is that in the past they have been less bureaucratic and able to respond to need quickly.

A statutory agency (or in Scotland Public Body) is one provided under law and is usually the responsibility of a Local Authority or Central Government department. Examples are various health and social care organizations. These agencies (voluntary, charitable, statutory and public) work slightly differently from country to country and between localities. However, it remains important, especially in the ever-changing face of healthcare provision, that agencies work together for the common good. They need to share information, communicate effectively and be aware of the others' roles and responsibilities.

ACTIVITY 8.4

Jean and Sid have been married for 18 years and have two children, a girl aged 10 and a boy aged 14. Sid was a successful businessman until recently, when the business was sold because he was unable to manage it. Sid was diagnosed 13 years ago with multiple sclerosis. He mobilizes using an electric wheelchair and requires assistance from his wife to maintain personal hygiene, to dress and for emotional support. He has recently become emotionally labile, which Jean says has had an impact on the children.

The district nurse has been called in to discuss intermittent catheterization with Sid. She has not met the family before because Jean has tried to protect the home environment from medical and healthcare personnel.

Jean does not recognize herself as a carer because she thinks that in doing so it will confirm her husband's frailty, while also confirming to her that he is deteriorating.

* What assessments need to be carried out in this home?
* What support could you envisage introducing to this family?
* What other agencies in your area could be involved if appropriate?
* What skills would the district nurse need to apply in this situation?

CONCLUSION

In this chapter some aspects of carrying out the role of carer have been investigated. The future of caring in the community, with an ageing population and more people living with long-term conditions, mental health issues or drug abuse, is being taken seriously by government and service providers throughout Europe. The important issues of carer identification, assessment, education and partnership recognition have been acknowledged. The role of assessment and support by an educated, skilled and multiprofessional health and social care team is valued as the keystone of the carer's ability to cope. Governments are also funding and championing charities and voluntary organizations which are essential providers of relief for carers. Although the picture can seem daunting, there are constant changes taking place in the world of telehealth and ecare that could make the responsibility of caring lighter and enable people, although physically isolated, to access support and maintain communication with the world around (King's Fund, 2008).

ACKNOWLEDGEMENTS

Many thanks to the staff of the Voluntary Service Aberdeen Carers Centre, Aberdeen who are part of the Princess Royal Trust for Carers network, for their time and support.

REFERENCES

Banks P, Cogan N and Riddell S (2002) Does the covert nature of caring prohibit the development of effective services for young carers? *British Journal of Guidance and Counselling* 30:3.

Bolan DL and Sims SL (1996) Family care giving at home as a solitary journey. *Journal of Nursing Scholarship* 28:55–8.

Buhr GT, Kuchibhatla M and Clipp EC (2006) Caregivers' reasons for nursing home placement: clues for improving discussions with families prior to the transition. *Gerontologist* 46:52–61.

Carers UK (2006) *More than a Job: Working Carers: Evidence from the 2001 Census.* London: Carers UK.

Carers UK (2007)*Valuing Carers – Calculating the Value of Unpaid Care.* London: Carers UK.

Cheung J and Hocking P (2004) Caring as a worrying experience of spousal carers. *Journal of Advanced Nursing* 47:475–82.

Department of Health (DH) (2000) *The NHS Plan: A Plan for Investment a Plan for Reform.* London: Department of Health.

DH (2008) *Carers at the Heart of 21st Century Families and Communities: A Caring System on Your Side, A Life of Your Own.* London: Department of Health publications.

Department of Health, Social Services and Public Safety (2001) *People First: Community Care in Northern Ireland.* Belfast: Department of Health, Social Services and Public Safety.

Dahlberg L, Demack S and Bambra C(2007) Age and gender of informal carers: a population-based study in the UK. *Health and Social Care in the Community* 15:439–45.

Gubernam N, Nicholas E, Nolan M, *et al.* (2003) Impacts on practitioners of using research-based carer assessment tools: experiences from the UK, Canada and Sweden, with insights from Australia. *Health and Social Care in the Community* 11:345–55.

Hanson E, Magnusson L and Nolan J (2008) Swedish experiences of a negotiated approach to carer assessment: the Carers Outcome Agreement Tool. *Journal of Research in Nursing* 13:391–40.

Jarvis A (2011) Working with carers in the next decade: the challenges. *British Journal of Community Nursing*15:125–8.

King's Fund (2008) *Telecare: Researching the Impact on Carers and Care Workers.* www.wsdactionnetwork.org.uk/news/features/telecare.html.

Lawrence V, Murray J, Samsi K and Banerjee S (2008) Attitudes and support needs of Black Caribbean, South Asian and White British carers of people with dementia in the UK. *The British Journal of Psychiatry* 193:240–6.

McKee K, Spazzafumo L, Nolan M, *et al.*(2009) Components of the difficulties, satisfactions and management strategies of carers of older people: a principal component analysis of CADI-CASI-CAMI. *Ageing and Mental Health* 13:255–64.

McNamara B and Rosenwax L (2010) Which carers of family members at the end of life need more support from health services and why? *Social Science and Medicine* 70:1035–41.

Mowlam A, Tennant R, Dixon J and McCreadie C (2007) UK Study of abuse and neglect of older people: qualitative findings. *National Centre of Social Research and Kings College London.* 8–80.

Nolan M and Philip I (1999) COPE: towards a comprehensive assessment of caregiver need. *British Journal of Nursing* 8:20.

Rees J, O'Boyle C and MacDonagh R (2001) Quality of life: impact of chronic illness on the partner. *Journal of the Royal Society of Medicine* 94:563–6.

Scottish Executive (SE) (2000) *Report of the Joint Future Group.* Edinburgh: Scottish Executive.

Welsh Assembly (2001) *National Service Framework for Older People.* Cardiff: Welsh Assembly.

Zink T, Jacobson J and Regan S (2006) Older women's descriptions and understandings of their abusers. *Violence Against Women* 12:851.

FURTHER READING

Carers' Strategy for Wales – Action Plan. 2007. http://wales.gov.uk/topics/olderpeople/publications/carersactionplan2007?lang=en.

Department of Health (1998) *'They look after their own, don't they?' Inspection of community care services for black and ethnic minority older people.* London: The Department of Health publications.

Mutch K (2010) In sickness and in health: experience of caring for a spouse with MS. *British Journal of Nursing* 19:214–19.

Obadina S (2012) Parental mental illness: effects on young carers. *British Journal of School Nursing* 3:135–9.

Rees J, O'Boyle C and MacDonagh R (2001) Quality of life: impact of chronic illness on the partner. *Journal of the Royal Society of Medicine* 94:563–6.

The Scottish Government (2010) *Carers Strategy.* www.scotland.gov.uk.

FURTHER RESOURCES

www.carersuk.org

www.ageuk.org.uk

www.carersinformatiobn.org.uk

www.diabetes.org.uk

www.mssociety.org.uk

http://alzheimers.org.uk/site/index.php

www.youngcarers.net

www.barnardos.org.uk/what_we_do/our_projects/young_carers.htm

www.macmillan.org.uk/Cancerinformation/Ifsomeoneelsehascancer/CringForSomeone.aspx

Spirituality: a neglected aspect of care

Ann Clarridge

LEARNING OUTCOMES

- Critically discuss the concept of 'spirituality' and spiritual care within nursing
- Describe the principles underpinning spiritual assessment and appraise the associated tools and interventions available
- Explore the concept of 'self-awareness'
- Critically discuss how, as a community nurse, developing self-awareness can enhance the spiritual assessment of patients/clients

INTRODUCTION

This chapter is concerned with the concept of spirituality in the care provided by nursing professionals. Reference is made to some of the relevant research and literary reviews which offer a useful context for this complex subject area. Some definitions of spirituality are outlined and the place of spirituality within community nursing is considered. The consequent implications in terms of spiritual assessment and possible interventions are discussed. The need for self-awareness and its development in nurses is explored. Finally, the competence of nurses to deal with the spiritual aspects of care is considered together with the importance of observational skills and communication, essential tools in the repertoire of all nursing professionals.

LITERATURE REVIEW AND RESEARCH

There is a growing interest surrounding the place of spiritual care in nursing, and this is supported by a plethora of literature. Some of this research is considered here.

MacKinlay and Hudson undertook a review of the extensive literature for the year 2006. On the basis of the key words ageing, chronic illness, frailty, nursing research, older people, nursing and spirituality a total of 41 articles were selected. Seven main themes on spirituality and ageing emerged that highlighted issues relevant to spiritual care and to practice in nursing older people. The themes were spirituality concept development and models, spirituality and chronic illness, promoting spiritual health and wellbeing, spirituality and dying, cross-cultural and multifaith issues, spiritual assessment and ethics (MacKinlay and Hudson, 2008: 143).

Ross (2006) undertook a thorough and comprehensive review of research on spiritual care in nursing between 1983 and 2005 using the key words of ethics, spirituality, spiritual care and spiritual research. The results of the original search using the key words drew a response of 1420 papers. Following a process of sorting and selection that included the discarding of book chapters, videos and editorials, 45 original research papers were included for the review. These 45 original papers were categorized under five main headings: nurses; patients/clients/carers; nurses and clients/carers; nurse education; and instrument development. Using a template created especially for the purpose, which included information regarding the design and the focus of the study, all 45 papers were reviewed. A summary of the findings and a critique were also undertaken.

The results of this review provided insight into how nurses, clients and their carers perceive spirituality and spiritual care with relevance to clinical practice. It would seem that nurses identify spiritual needs not only from specific religious requests made by clients but also from their non-verbal cues such as anxiety, depression and being withdrawn (Ross, 2006). Some nurses did not always respond to those needs because of feelings of inadequacy and lack of preparation. The nurses who reported feeling confident to meet spiritual needs were those who were aware of their own spirituality, beliefs and values. Most nurses, however, were happy to listen to clients or simply be present with a client. Clients who expressed particular needs were often referred to another experienced professional, for example a chaplain or appropriate religious leader dependent upon the client's preference (Ross, 2006). The overall conclusions to be drawn from this extensive review point to the need for further, systematic and coordinated research, particularly in the area of preparation of nurses in the assessment and provision of spiritual care. The overriding problems that emerge are how, what, where and when spiritual care should be taught and who should teach it.

ACTIVITY 9.1

Reflection point
Consider the following questions:
- What is your experience of being taught about spiritual care?
- Would you have found it helpful if spirituality had been included in your education and training?
- What knowledge and skills would be helpful to enable you to explore a patient's spiritual needs with confidence?

DEFINING SPIRITUALITY

The concept of spiritual care is equivocal. There is a need to define spirituality and consider how it relates to nursing care.

The terms spiritual and religious are often used to mean the same thing, and although there is an overlap between the two, not everyone would agree that an individual needs to be religious in order to be spiritual or vice versa (Clarke, 2009). Koenig *et al.* (2001) mark very distinct differences and define religion as 'an organised system of beliefs, practices, rituals and symbols' and spirituality as the personal quest for understanding answers to ultimate questions about life, about meaning, and about relationship to the sacred or transcendent which may or may not lead to or arise from the development of religious rituals and the formation of community.

(Koenig et al., 2001, cited in MacKinlay, 2008: 140)

Thus it could be argued 'that the practice of religion is a way that humans relate to the sacred, to otherness' and that all humans have a spiritual dimension but not all humans practise religion (MacKinlay, 2008: 140).

'Spiritual but not religious' is a phrase used by many people to express the belief that real spirituality is the concern of the individual (Sulmasy, 2009). Those who hold this view will affirm that their individual experience is one thing and institutionalized religion is another (Jamison, 2006: 142). On one side classical religion, including all the main world religions each with its own specific doctrine, rituals and beliefs, 'offers us an educative process that helps us to see the whole of life in a different way' (Jamison, 2006: 146). On the other side, modern spirituality might well be defined as 'psychological well-being combined with the moral golden rule – do unto others as you would have them do unto you' (Jamison, 2006: 143). Chochinov (2006a) suggests that spirituality is to 'invoke a sense of searching or yearning for significance or meaning in life' (Chochinov, 2006b: 88).

Spirituality outside religion often signifies a believer whose *faith* is personal, more open to new ideas and numerous influences than the *dogmatic* faith of mature religions. Such believers tend to regard spirituality not as a religion but as the active and vital connection to a force, power or energy, or a sense of the deep *self*. It can also signify the personal nature of the relationship or connection with the god(s) or *belief system*(s) of a believer as opposed to the general relationship with a *deity* and the rites of group worship shared by members of a given faith. Those who claim that they are spiritual but not religious often believe in the existence of many 'spiritual paths' and would refute that there is an *objectively* definable best path to follow. They often emphasize the importance of finding one's individual path to the divine and may or may not believe in the supernatural. Where there is such a belief and a relationship with supernatural beings represents the foundation of happiness then that will form the basis of spiritual practice. Where there is no such belief, a different form of practice provides the way to manage thoughts and emotions which otherwise would prevent happiness (Sulmasy, 2009).

Definitions of spirituality are constantly evolving so it would seem appropriate, therefore, in the context of this chapter to accept Chochinov's (2006a) simple definition without necessarily invoking religion. Thus spirituality may be understood to be that search for inner peace and the foundation of happiness which requires some form of spiritual practice but which is essential for the promotion of personal wellbeing. Chochinov identifies a client who speaks of loss of hope, feelings of being a burden to others, loss of dignity or loss of the will to live as being one who is experiencing spiritual distress. Many techniques and practices have been explored and developed in religious contexts, such as meditation or contemplative reading, and are immensely valuable in themselves as skills for managing aspects of the inner life.

Reflection point
Consider the following questions:
• What does spirituality mean to me? How would I define it for myself?
• What does it mean when an individual is said to be 'spiritual'?

Spirituality and community nursing

Spirituality and all its associated vocabulary are terms much in vogue: they sound significant, with a touch of mystery. As with all jargon, however, it provides us with a language that enables us to think and talk about issues and concepts which are otherwise difficult to articulate. Individual spirituality as an important element in nursing practice is now being generally and officially recognized (Editorial (2006), Department of Health 2006, 2007). The importance of addressing a person's spiritual needs with an emphasis on competence in spiritual care is placed firmly within the professional regulatory body in the Code of Standards, Conduct, Performance and Ethics for Nurses and Midwives (NMC, 2008). Health boards and government policies also support the importance of meeting the spiritual needs of patients. The International Council of Nurses (ICN) specifies 'an environment in which the human rights, values, customs and spiritual beliefs of the individual, family and community are respected' (ICN Code of Ethics, 2000: 5). The Department of Health (2002) in its guidelines for Chaplaincy and Spiritual Care in the NHS in Scotland includes an aim 'to develop and implement spiritual care policies' which are appropriate to our 'increasingly multi-cultural society' (MacLaren, 2004: 457). 'Spiritual nursing can be an opportunity for nurses to enquire into that which is fundamental about the human condition and to give truly whole person care in a multi-faith society' (MacLaren, 2004: 461).

Community nurses need a definition of the context for the care they provide. The term 'community' frequently describes a wide range of patterns of relationships but generally includes two important characteristics. The first describes those who share values and a sense of purpose and who encourage and support each other in the challenges of daily life. 'The giving and receiving of love is an important element for this community of people' and such a community might be the local church, neighbours or family (Runcorn, 2006: 55). The second describes shared work, special circumstances or interests.

It would seem at first glance that community nursing could be defined through shared work and special circumstances. However, a closer look at what actually underpins nursing–*The Code of Conduct, Standards and Ethics for Nurses and Midwives* (NMC, 2008), for example–suggests that community nursing may well be identified by the first characteristic – the shared values and sense of purpose. So, in effect, both descriptions could be said to apply to the work of the community nurse.

Nurses who work within the context of a community as opposed to an institution fulfil a very specific role. They care for individuals and families with a variety of conditions in their own homes or in homely settings. They are involved with people from different ethnic backgrounds, with those who have and with those who do not have an expressed religious faith. In every case the nurse needs to be aware of the spiritual dimension of each individual no matter how it finds expression. In 1964 Jean Vanier established a community where people with various physical and learning difficulties could live as equals with able-bodied people. He asserted that 'the fundamental right of each person includes amongst the right to life and care, the right to a spiritual life' (L'Arche Charter, in Runcorn, 2006: 55).

Community nurses find themselves in the role of 'key players', able to recognize and meet the spiritual needs of clients and their families (McSherry and Ross, 2010). They would argue that holistic care of the individual and not just physical need has always been their concern. Indeed their claim is justly supported by the plethora of nursing models of care. A holistic approach to care reflects the underlying principles and philosophy that all nurses draw upon to shape the way in which they act and carry out their nursing practice. Although conceptual models of nursing differ quite considerably because nurses have different ideas about what nursing means for them, fundamental to most models is the person or the individual. Each model has something to say about this key element, especially in the assessment for proposed care. It is here, within this area of the model, that the spiritual needs of the patient can be addressed (Smith, 2004).

Research undertaken by Perry (2005) identified four areas that were of importance to nurses: 'affirming the value of the person, defending dignity, enabling hope and helping patients find meaning' (Perry 2005, in McSherry and Ross, 2010: 155). Neuman (1995) and Roper et al. (2000) revised their nursing theories to include spirituality, thus seeking to provide true holistic care (Smith, 2004).

In times of illness or loss of independence patients will frequently raise fundamental questions concerning the meaning or purpose of life wherever they may be on the spectrum of religious belief. It is the experience of community nurses that at such times patients turn to those who are caring for them for answers, help and support.

Research literature suggests that nurses need to be aware of their own beliefs and values in order to best meet the spiritual care needs of patients. They need to be clear about how they express their beliefs in their own lives, whether through doctrine, ritual or membership of a religious community. Such clarity is essential if they are to remain objective when assessing, planning and delivering holistic patient care, including spiritual support, without influence or indoctrination, however unwitting. Nurses would then be in a position to demonstrate an interest in and a willingness to discuss issues of a spiritual nature with patients without the necessity of a wide-ranging knowledge of the doctrines, rituals and practices of the many religions. A review of research established that the level and amount of spiritual care given by a nurse were related to the amount of time available for listening and the possession of spiritual awareness, sensitivity and communication skills of the nurse (Ross, 2006).

ACTIVITY 9.3

Refelction and action point

To explore your spiritual beliefs and feelings about other people's beliefs. (Adapted from Burnard, 1992: 16,17)
Write a short passage that sums up what you believe in.
Some helpful questions:
- Do you believe in God, and if so what does your concept of God involve?
- If you do not believe in God, what do you think about people who do?
- What do you consider to be the purpose of your life?
- How did you develop your beliefs and where have they come from?
- How might you respond if colleagues said (a) they did not believe in God, (b) tried to convince you of their belief?
- How might you respond if a patient were to tell you that life is meaningless or hopeless?
- You might like to discuss what you have written or discuss the questions with a friend.
- Share your thoughts and ideas and note the degree to which you agree or disagree with each other.
- Consider what it might be like to take the opposite approach to the one that you hold and what that might mean to you.

Spiritual assessment and intervention

The importance of assessment in the approach to client care is paramount, with the inclusion of the spiritual needs of the client as an integral element of a holistic approach. There are a number of guidelines and strategies within the discipline of social work and family therapy for assessing spiritual needs of families (Frame, 2000; Hodge, 2001). In the past there have been fewer within nursing literature but the situation is changing. Most health and nursing care assessments include a question regarding religious affiliation (Orem, 1980; Peplau, 1988). In recognition of the importance of a patient's spirituality, the number of published guidelines and models in the nursing and spirituality literature is now increasing (Narayanasamy, 2006a; McSherry, 2006; Koenig 2007).

Tanyi (2006) suggests that when assessing the needs of clients and their families, there are three major goals to spiritual assessment:

> to support and enhance families' spiritual well-being and development; to discern spiritual distress and its effect on overall family health; and to ascertain ways to incorporate family spirituality when providing care.
>
> *(Tanyi, 2006: 289)*

However, the nurse must feel comfortable and have already established a relationship of trust with the client before being able to undertake a thorough spiritual assessment and plan appropriate care. Tanyi (2006: 289–90) provides a series of questions and spiritual interventions that can be adapted and used as a guide by nurses to undertake a spiritual assessment and to plan patient care (Box 9.1).

Box 9.1 Guideline questions for spiritual assessment

Strengths
* What has helped you in the past to deal with crisis?
* What gives you strength?
* What do you do to rebuild your strength?

Meaning and purpose
* In your daily life, what gives you meaning?
* What gives you peace, joy and satisfaction?

Relationships
* Who is the most important person in your life?
* To whom do you turn when you need help?

Beliefs
* Do you have a relationship with God/deity, universe, or other?
* If yes, how would you describe it and what does it mean to your health?
* Do you practise rituals such as prayer, worship or meditation?

Personal spirituality and preference for spiritual care
* How do you express/describe your spirituality?
* Do you consider anyone as your spiritual leader and if necessary can this person be contacted?

These questions are provided as a general guide and can be adapted for use according to the individual and the nurse's preference. (See Further reading for a full text of the guidelines to spiritual assessment and interventions for families.)

Sources: Tanyi (2006), McSherry and Ross (2010)

McSherry (2006: 905) offers a model that includes a number of components ('the principal components model') and suggests that familiarity with it is likely to give nurses the confidence to tackle some of the difficulties inherent in undertaking spiritual care. For example, it is recognized that when assessing a client's spiritual needs the nurse must develop a relationship of trust which takes time – the very commodity not always available to busy nurses. If sufficient resources are to be made available to enable nurses to support clients appropriately, it is necessary for the medical practice or other directing 'organization' to recognize the value of the relationship and to credit as worthwhile the time spent in listening (McSherry, 2006).

The patient's spiritual history is a critical element in the background information that needs to be taken into account when planning nursing care. It ensures an understanding and recognition of the patient's own beliefs and value systems. In particular, religious beliefs and practices are clarified, so that any intervention by the professional is appropriate. By identifying individual spiritual needs the patient is given a clear message of the respect that will be shown in the delivery of the proposed care. Furthermore, significant information may be gathered that sheds light upon the motivation underpinning the patient's behaviour. Such information can provide a useful resource when identifying the patient's support network, with the added potential of identifying the patient's ability to comply with care. Additionally, the information provides a baseline from which the situation can be monitored (Koenig, 2007).

Koenig (2007) suggests a number of criteria to be considered when choosing an appropriate model. Perhaps the most important is that questions should be open and brief, focused upon the beliefs and value systems of the patients and not of the nurses. Hodge (2001) identified this as an important aspect of assessment recognizing the value of 'personal and environmental strengths being central to the helping process' (Hodge, 2001: 204). Based upon this premise, Koenig (2007: 44) offers a single question: 'Do you have any spiritual needs or concerns related to your health?' This simple question acknowledges to the patient that this is an area of importance for the professional. At this point, however, one might take issue with Koenig. An individual who is in need of care from a nursing professional almost certainly will have spiritual concerns related to health without necessarily being able to articulate them in such terms in response to a blunt question. By listening to what is said and by hearing what is left unsaid, it is for the professional to tease out the spiritual concerns of the patient.

The use of a mnemonic can provide the nurse with a helpful tool when making an assessment based on a series of questions that explores 'spiritual and religious themes' within an 'empathic dialogue' (Hodge, 2001: 205). The following examples FICAA (adapted by Koenig (2007: 44) and HOPE (Puchalski, in McSherry and Ross, 2010: 87) when suited to the linguistic register of the patient could prove to be useful as a mental blueprint.

F-Faith	What is your faith tradition?
I-Important	How important is your faith to you?
C-Church	What is your church or community of faith?
A-Apply	How do your religious and spiritual beliefs apply to your health?
A-Address	How might we address your spiritual needs?
H-Hope	What are your sources of hope, strength, meaning, peace?
O-Organized religion	What role does organized religion have for you?
P-Personal	What is your personal spirituality and does it involve any specific practices?
E-Effects	Does your spirituality affect your decisions regarding medical care?

A more appropriate alternative to taking a spiritual history might be the use of a diagrammatic representation (Hodge, 2001). Genograms and maps as used within the field of family therapy are designed to show psychological and emotional relationships within the family. A genogram can provide a picture of family structure and offers a useful way to organize information (Carter and McGoldrick, 1980). Genograms are also discussed in Chapter 7. Inviting a patient to draw a spiritual genogram or a spiritual map may have a greater appeal than responding to a series of questions. In this way patients can be encouraged to draw a time-line or tree plotting significant spiritual experiences, history, books and events that have added to their spiritual history and development.

Building upon their earlier work in this field, McSherry and Ross (2010) have devised a model for 'actioning spiritual care using a systematic approach' (McSherry and Ross, 2010: 164). See Further reading for the 'model for actioning spiritual care'.

ACTIVITY 9.4

Action point
Try using the mnemonic FICCA or HOPE with a friend or colleague.

Draw a spiritual genogram, map or tree for yourself detailing your spiritual history and development. Include the significant people, books and experiences that have influenced that development. You may find the following website a useful resource for this activity: www.sociology.org.uk/as4fm3a.doc.

Self-awareness

Who we are, what we are like and what other people think of us are all questions that relate to our 'self'. We are made up of many parts, 'our bodies, out thoughts, our feelings, our perceptions of ourselves, our beliefs and our actions' (Burnard 1992: 6). The more we come to know our 'self' – that is, the greater our self-awareness – the more integrated we become as people and the more able we are to offer effective spiritual care.

Reflection is a commonly used term in the education of nursing and provides a useful way to learn about oneself. Much has been written on the subject that is particularly valuable in the development of self-awareness when applied to the richness of experience in nursing practice. Nurses are able to observe the effect they have on patients and the impact of treatment and care. A vital tool in the nurse's repertoire must be the ability to keep feelings and thoughts from private life separate from the issues of the work place. Although personal experiences can enrich and enhance a nurse's empathy for a patient's situation they should not impinge on decisions taken relating to assessment or care. Rather they should inform and guide responses to situations in practice, especially when approaching a sensitive area such as undertaking a spiritual assessment.

Becoming self-aware, according to Rungapadiachy (1999), is essential to effectiveness and comprises three interrelated perspectives: thinking, feeling and acting. If nurses are to be effective practitioners they need to include patients' spiritual needs when addressing all other aspects of patient care. Therefore, it is essential that they are clear about their own spiritual beliefs and are able to avoid the pitfall of assuming that everyone else thinks about things spiritual in the same way that they do. Nurses who have little understanding of their own spirituality and feel uncomfortable discussing such issues are more likely to avoid conversations concerning a client's spiritual needs, whereas those who are secure in their beliefs are less likely to be uneasy when faced with a patient expressing anxieties about the meaning of life and the loss of a sense of purpose (Burnard, 1992). In a professional situation a nurse has a duty of care to the patient but it does not include trying to influence or change the beliefs and values of the patient (Burnard, 1992). Spirituality is a very personal matter: individuals reach their own understanding of what it means for them in the context of their own lives. However, nurses are in a privileged position and those who have considered their own beliefs and values are more able to help others to think and talk through theirs (Burnard, 1992). Such self-knowledge gives the nurse the opportunity to be prepared and plan ahead for those situations where clients need to express their fundamental concerns in the face of a crisis of illness. It enables the nurse to develop the necessary coping skills rather than evasive strategies when providing care for clients and their families.

Effective communication with clients is crucial and most nurses would state that they feel very skilled in this area. Furthermore, when challenged most nurses would be able to give examples of how and when they had been successful in communicating with a patient. They might also be able to state with honesty that they had blocked a conversation with a client when they felt the level of disclosure by the client was entering an area in which they were not comfortable. When confronted by a client who might wish to express anger or fear concerning their current situation or to question the ultimate meaning of life, the nurse with a well-founded knowledge of self would be better equipped to respond to the client's needs (Koenig *et al.*, 2001).

Self-awareness is not a state that can be attained completely (Burnard, 1988) but is rather an ongoing journey of enlightenment. Narayanasamy (2006b) undertook an empirical study relating to the impact of spirituality and culture on nurse education. The resulting model incorporates 'communication – verbal and non verbal; cultural negotiation – being sensitive to and aware of aspects of other people's culture and an understanding of clients' views; establishing respect and rapport and enabling clients to feel culturally "safe"' (Narayanasamy, 2006a: 841). An adaptation of the original model by Ellis and Narayanasamy (2009) offers a valuable approach to the consideration of a nurse's own self-awareness and spirituality in a way that is helpful and open to adaptation (Box 9.2). Thus may a nurse be encouraged to greater confidence when undertaking and identifying a patient's spiritual needs.

Box 9.2 Guideline questions for self-awareness and spiritual nursing

Strengths
What are my personal beliefs, values, prejudices, assumptions and feelings?
Am I aware how these might influence the way in which I care for a patient?

Beliefs
What is the extent of my knowledge and understanding of the rituals and practices of different religious or non-religious beliefs and is it important that I know?

Relationship
Am I enabling a patient to express their spiritual beliefs?
Am I providing a supportive and trusting relationship within 'outside' constraints?
Do I involve other professionals when appropriate to meet the spiritual needs of the patient?

Meaning and purpose
Do I enable a patient to find meaning and purpose in their illness?
What is my response to a patient who speaks of fear of the unknown, loneliness or hopelessness?
These questions are provided as a general guide and can be adapted for use according to individual preference.

Source: Adapted from Ellis and Narayanasamy (2009)

If we wish to become more self-aware and therefore more effective practitioners, Rungapadiachy (1999) suggests that there are three layers of self-awareness that we should consider. The first layer is superficial and related to acknowledgement and awareness of our age and our gender. The next layer is more in-depth and is related to those elements of which we need to be aware if we are to be effective, such as our appearance and attitudes and how they affect our behaviour. The third layer is the deepest and represents those issues that are known only to ourselves, our deepest secrets and thoughts.

A way to explore these layers is by means of the Johari window (Luft, 1969, in Smith 2007: 50). The 'window' comprises four areas of the 'self': open, blind, hidden and unknown. The 'open' area covers what is known to me and to others: feelings, attitudes and behaviours, likes and dislikes. In the 'blind' area is what is not known to me but might be revealed by others: mannerisms or habits of which I am not aware. The 'hidden' area is concerned with those things which I know about myself but would not wish to disclose to others. In the 'unknown' area there are those aspects of the self which are within my deepest self and not brought to the surface except when unexpectedly triggered by a word or circumstance: for example, a sudden irrational anger felt following a comment made by another (Smith, 2007: 50) (Table 9.1).

Table 9.1 Johari window

	Known to Self	Not Known to Self
Known to others	Open area	Blind area
	Example: This is what I know about myself and what others know of me, for example – I am a nurse and hard working	Example: My friends may have a view of me of which I am unaware. I can uncover these views if others tell me about them. This will increase my 'open' area. For example – my friends may think I do not actively listen to them and I am unaware of this fact.
Not known to others	Hidden area	Unknown area
	Example: This is what I know about myself but hide from others. As I disclose more about myself, within a safe environment, my 'open' area will become larger and I may learn more about myself in the process. For example – I am finding my work very tiring.	Example: This is the area that is unknown to one and to others. As we tell others more about ourselves and receive feedback this area will decrease in size. We will become more self-aware.

Adapted from Luft (1969) in Smith (2007).

ACTIVITY 9.5

Action point

Draw a Johari window and fill in each of the quadrants.

You might wish to discuss your observations with a friend or colleague, particularly noting how your view of yourself differs from that of your friend/colleague, recognising that your own view may be the one that you think you should have rather than the one that is truly you.

Make notes on what you have learned about yourself and how this is relevant for practice.

Nursing competence and spiritual care

In an extensive study undertaken by Van Leeuwen *et al.* (2006: 878) a patient noted that it was not possible 'to expect a nurse to be an all-rounder' and questioned 'whether a nurse should be an expert in psychology and religion as well as health care'.

The data for the study were collected from focus group interviews with patients, nurses and hospital chaplains. Certain limitations were acknowledged by the team in that many of the participants were interested in the topic and so were very willing to join the study. In addition the participants were not culturally or religiously diverse so could not be said to reflect a representative cross-section of the population. However, within these limitations some interesting factors emerged that have particular relevance to spirituality and spiritual care.

Patients in general required a nurse who could provide good professional skills in physical care. There was also an expectation that the nurse would 'be there' for patients, would have time for them, be sensitive to their needs and would enable them to express emotions. It is interesting to note that in relation to conversations between nurses and patients these frequently started spontaneously and were often initiated by the patients. Of equal importance to these conversations was whether or not the patients and the nurses 'shared the same ideology' and the same 'religious language'. When asked about actions taken in the area of spiritual care, nurses emphasized how important it was that they did not breach the boundary of an individual's personal limits, their own or the patient's. Praying with a patient was found to be acceptable but only at the patient's request and if the nurse felt able to do so. It must be emphasized that nurses should not initiate a process that they cannot then follow through (Van Leeuwen *et al.*, 2006).

It has been established that the goal of spiritual care in nursing is to help patients find meaning and purpose during times of illness. Unfortunately, spiritual care cannot be administered like a dose of medicine but depends on the quality and success of the relationship between the client and the professional. It is for the nurse a privileged situation to be able to support another in a time of distress (MacKinlay and Hudson, 2008: 21).

It has already been concluded that for nurses to deliver spiritual care in a professional manner they must be competent (Stern and James, 2006). The literature and research on the provision of competencies through education and practice is limited (Baldacchino, 2006: 885). The nurse who wishes to deliver professional spiritual care is required to exhibit the four nursing competencies identified by Baldacchino (2006):

> … role of the nurse as a professional and as an individual person; delivery of spiritual care by the nursing process; communication with patients, the inter-disciplinary team and clinical/educational organizations; and safeguarding ethical issues in care.
>
> *(Baldacchino, 2006: 889)*

To assist in the difficult task of delivering spiritual care there is a need to explore Baldacchino's identified competencies in a little more detail, taking first the role of the nurse as a professional and as an individual. Baldacchino's study was undertaken with nurses whose patients had had a myocardial infarction. Some nurses reported that they were prepared and felt competent in their knowledge, both physiological and medical, but did not feel confident or competent to deal with the spiritual aspect of their patients' care. As a result they were more inclined to leave that aspect to the chaplain, especially when a patient had expressed anxieties about life and the life-threatening nature of the illness. Those nurses who considered themselves to be well developed in terms of both their clinical and their life experiences stated that they felt competent in undertaking spiritual care. However, they also indicated that the support of the chaplain was important to them as well as their professional support. On the basis of these findings, there is clearly a need to include in their training an opportunity for nurses to develop their skills to meet the spiritual needs of their patients. MacKinlay (2010: 20) confirms this need when referring to the required sensitivity of nurses when providing spiritual care 'with all its variations according to culture and religion'.

The second competency refers to the delivery of spiritual care by the nursing process.

The use of a structured approach to care has long been advocated within the nursing profession. Certainly the processes of physiological and medical assessment, planning, implementation and evaluation are relatively straightforward. However, it is more problematic to apply a structured approach when a patient who may be experiencing spiritual distress speaks of fear of the unknown, loneliness or hopelessness. In the study undertaken by Baldacchino (2006) it was found that it was difficult to evaluate the effectiveness of any spiritual care given because patients did not necessarily give feedback to nurses regarding their state of wellbeing. What is possible to evaluate is whether or not nurses were able to spend time developing a trusting relationship with patients listening to their expressed anxieties in a private environment. Here the issues depend upon the communication skills of the nurses and their ability to facilitate strategies or rituals for coping with spiritual dilemmas.

The remaining competencies refer to the involvement of other professionals and the relevant ethical issues of care. The involvement of other professionals, religious or not, at the right time and in the right manner is another sensitive issue (Baldacchino, 2006). A number of nurses in the study reported that they felt it was the role of chaplains to undertake the spiritual dimension of patient care since they did not feel themselves to be sufficiently well prepared. A further difficulty that was reported was how to document a patient's spiritual concerns without breaking the trust and confidentiality that build between a patient and a nurse: a fundamental issue within the *Code of Conduct, Standards and Ethics for Nurses and Midwives* (NMC, 2008). This then becomes an issue of ethics and presents the problem of how much should a nurse 'hand over' to other professionals where the spiritual status of the patient is concerned.

CONCLUSION

The place of spirituality in nursing care is now an acknowledged fact. It is recognized as an important element of the holistic care of patients, whether as inpatients in hospital or out in the community in their own homes. More information is needed to identify relevant assessments and how they may be carried out appropriately. It is clear that there is a need for more training for nurses to enhance their confidence and competence to deliver spiritual care. Further research is needed to clarify how such training may be provided and by whom so that the best of holistic care may be made available.

REFERENCES

Baldacchino DR (2006) Nursing competencies for spiritual care. *Journal of Clinical Nursing* 15:885–96.

Burnard P (1988) Self-evaluation methods in nurse education. *Nurse Education Today* 8:4229–33.

Burnard P (1992) *Know Yourself: Self Awareness Activities for Nurses.* London: Scutari Press.

Carter EA and McGoldrick M (eds) (1980) *The Family Life Cycle. A Framework for Family Therapy.* New York: Gardner Press, Inc.

Chochinov HM (2006a) Dying, dignity, and new horizons in palliative end-of-life care. *CA Cancer J Clinicians* 56:84–103.

Chochinov HM (2006b) in Ellis HK and Narayanasamy A. (2009) An investigation into the role of spirituality in nursing. *British Journal of Nursing* 18:886–90.

Clarke J (2009) A critical view of how nursing has defined spirituality. *Journal of Clinical Nursing* 18:1666–73.

Department of Health (2002) *Guidelines of Chaplaincy and Spiritual Care in the NHS in Scotland.* Edinburgh: Scottish Executive.

Department of Health (2006) *Modernising Nursing Careers: Setting the Direction.* London: DH.

Department of Health (2007) *Our NHS, Our Future.* London: DH.

Editorial (2006) Critical reflections on the current state of spirituality-in-nursing. *Journal of Clinical Nursing* 15:801–2.

Ellis HK and Narayanasamy A (2009) An investigation into the role of spirituality in nursing. *British Journal of Nursing* 18:886–90.

Hodge DR (2001) Spiritual assessment: a review of major qualitative methods and a new framework for assessing spirituality. *Social Work* 46, Number 3.

International Council of Nurses (2000) *Code of Ethics for Nurses.* Geneva: ICN.

Jamison CA (2006) *Finding Sanctuary. Monastic Steps for Everyday Life.* Phoenix.

Koenig HG (2007) *Spirituality in Patient Care.* Philadelphia, PA: Templeton Foundation Press.

Luft J (1969) *Of Human Interaction.* Palo Alto, CA: National Press.

MacKinlay E and Hudson R (2008) A review of the literature in 2006. *International Journal of Older People Nursing* 3:139–144.

MacLaren J (2004) A kaleidoscope of understandings: spiritual nursing in a multi-faith society. *Journal of Advanced Nursing* 45:457–64.

McSherry W (2006) The principal components model: a model for advancing spirituality and spiritual care within nursing and health care practice. *Journal of Clinical Nursing* 15:905–17.

McSherry W and Ross L (eds) (2010) *Spiritual Assessment in Healthcare Practice.* Cumbria: M&K Pubs.

Narayanasamy A (1999) ASSET: a model for actioning spirituality and spiritual care education and training in nursing. *Nurse Education Today* 19: 274–85.

Narayanasamy A (2006a) The impact of empirical studies of spirituality and culture on nurse education. *Journal of Clinical Nursing* 15:840–51.

Narayanasamy A (2006b) *Spiritual Care and Transcultural Care Research*. London: Quay Books.

Neuman B (1995) *The Neuman Systems Model*, 3rd edn. Norwalk: Appleton and Lange.

Nursing and Midwifery Council (NMC) (2008) *The Code of Conduct, Standards and Ethics for Nurses and Midwives*. London: NMC.

Orem DE (1980) *Nursing: Concepts of Practice*. New York: McGraw-Hill.

Peplau HE (1988) *Interpersonal Relations in Nursing*. Basingstoke: Macmillan Education.

Puchalski C (2002) In McSherry W and Ross L (eds) *Spiritual Assessment in Healthcare Practice*. Cumbria: M&K Pubs.

Roper N, Logan WW and Tierney AJ (2000) *Roper-Logan-Tierney Model of Nursing: The Activities of Living Model*. Edinburgh: Churchill Livingstone.

Ross L (2006) Spiritual care in nursing: an overview of the research to date. *Journal of Clinical Nursing* 15:852–62.

Runcorn D (2006) *Spirituality Workbook. A Guide for Explorers, Pilgrims and Seekers*. Great Britain: SPCK.

Rungapadiachy DM (1999) *Interpersonal Communication and Psychology for Health Care Professionals*. Edinburgh: Elsevier.

Smith JK (2007) Promoting self-awareness in nurses to improve nursing practice. *Nursing Standard* 21:47–52.

Smith M (2004) *Nursing in the Community: In An Essential Guide to Practice*. Chilton S, Melling K, Drew D and Clarridge A (eds) London: Hodder Arnold Oxford University Press.

Stern J and James S (2006) Every person matters: enabling spirituality education for nurses. *Journal of Clinical Nursing* 15:897–904.

Sulmasy DP (2009) Spirituality, religion, and clinical care. *CHEST Journal of the American College of Chest Physicians* 135:1634–42.

Tanyi RA (2006) Spirituality and family nursing: spiritual assessment and interventions for families. *Journal of Advanced Nursing* 53:287–94.

Van Leeuwen R and Cusveller B (2004) Nursing competencies for spiritual care. *Journal of Advanced Nursing* 48:234–46.

Van Leeuwen R, Tiesinga LJ, Post D and Jochemsen H (2006) Spiritual care: implications for nurses. *Journal of Clinical Nursing* 15:875–84.

Vanier J (1989) Community and growth. New York Paulist Press. In Runcorn (2006) *Spirituality Workbook. A Guide for Explorers, Pilgrims and Seekers*. Great Britain: SPCK.

Weaver AJ, Koenig HG and Flannelly LT (2008) Nurses and healthcare chaplains: natural allies. *Journal of Health Care Chaplaincy* 14:91–8.

FURTHER READING

McSherry W and Ross L (eds) (2010) *Spiritual Assessment in Healthcare Practice*: Cumbria: M&K Pubs.

Rempel GR, Neufeld A and Kushner KE (2007) Interactive use of genograms and ecomaps in family caregiving research. *Journal of Family Nursing* 13:403–19.

CHAPTER

10

Collaborative working: benefits and barriers

Sally Sprung and Sue Harness

LEARNING OUTCOMES

- Explore the political drivers that inform collaborative working
- Definition of collaborative working
- Reflect on the skills required in order to collaborate effectively
- Critically reflect on interprofessional relations, including some of the barriers and constraints that can affect collaborative working

INTRODUCTION

This chapter will examine the relevance of collaborative working from the nursing perspective. Included will be a brief outline on the chronological development of this concept, with an emphasis on the importance of distinguishing the professional value of collaboration. A scenario of a complex 'end-of-life' patient will support the learning activities throughout the chapter.

Collaborative working within health services and between health services and other partners is assuming increasing importance as integrated planning and service delivery takes root in the public sector. The evidence base is growing for approaches and processes that can support good collaborative practice, and for articulating the benefits of working in partnership (Slimmer, 2003; Taylor *et al.*, 2005; Devla *et al.*, 2008; Miller *et al.*, 2008; Smith *et al.*, 2007; Suter *et al.*, 2009; Zwarenstein and Bryant, 2000). However, collaboration between different agencies or professional groups is rarely straightforward, and the consequences of engaging in collaborative networks are not always fully understood. The quality of the healthcare that is provided might be influenced by the way health professionals communicate and work together, with any difficulties resulting in concerns for patient care. There is evidence that a failure of collaboration may have tragic consequences (DH, 1994; Kennedy, 2001; Laming, 2003).

Recent governments have aspired to improve the quality of healthcare through encouraging interprofessional collaboration. There is an expectation that interprofessional collaborative working will generate health gains, and has been related to both greater responsiveness to patients (Greenwell, 1995) and efficient use of resources (Loxley, 1997). The focus to plan and implement patient-centred care that is less fragmented and facilitates the continuity of care requires a collaborative effort. Embedded in these reasons are assumed cost efficiencies and quality improvement which expect to be realized from comprehensive, coordinated and integrated care.

Achieving the objective of collaborative working is reliant on cooperation, with a focus on health professionals being responsible in meeting the rising complexity of patient care. Nurses who seek to enrich their practice do need to have a much greater understanding of how collaborative working is of benefit, not just with other professionals but with patients and their carers (Fatchett, 1996). The policy framework demands that patients and services users are involved with the planning and prioritization of service delivery.

D'Amour *et al.* (2005) claimed that health professionals throughout their education are socialized to adopt a discipline-based vision of their clientele and the services they offer. Each discipline develops strong theoretical and discipline frameworks that give access to professional jurisdictions that are often rigidly circumscribed. This constitutes the essence of the professional system. Collaborative working requires making changes to this paradigm and implementing a logic of collaboration rather than a logic of competition (D'Amour *et al.*, 2005).

POLITICAL DRIVERS

While recognizing that recent governments have stressed a need for collaborative working and joined-up thinking, it should be recognized that collaboration and team working across the professions is not a new phenomenon. However, the current prominence of working collaboratively signifies a substantial reorientation of professional working practices.

Since the late 1990s the thrust of UK government policy on health and social wellbeing has been towards developing an integrated approach to improving health and tackling health inequalities. *A Vision for the Future* (DH, 1995) set out that the aims of health professionals must be to work with each other towards common goals. The *Primary Care Act* (DH, 1997) emphasized seven areas for action, among these the inclusion of working partnerships, encouraging collaboration. The NHS Plan (DH, 2000) was a fundamental catalyst for the inclusion of collaborative working as an agenda for health and social care in the UK. It described the NHS as 'old fashioned' in its approach to care delivery and organization. In particular, it described poor team working as a huge contributor to the failure of the NHS in the past.

Rushmer (2005) discussed the reason for past failure and concluded that NHS organizations have prevented the opportunity for team work to be galvanized by constraints caused by working patterns and clinical remits of different disciplines.

Three poignant examples of poor collaborative working can be seen in the inquiries relating to Baby P (Ofsted, 2008), Victoria Climbié (DH, 2003) and the Bristol Royal Infirmary (Kennedy, 2001), which found catastrophic failures in the organizational management of two different clinical areas related to health and social care. Some core recommendations emerged from all three inquiries, including the need for health and social care professionals to have an improved network of communication and an ethos based on team work.

The UK government's rhetoric promotes the principles of choice and control for users within a seamless service (DH, 2010a). It is generally recognized that the needs of most clients are beyond the remit and expertise of any single profession and to provide a genuinely user-centred service requires collaborative working and team work. When professionals are committed to the ideal of working collaboratively, combining this with empowerment to direct energy towards achieving this goal, then this can encourage others to collaborate, overcome passive and active resistance to change, and remove organizational obstacles to progress.

The UK government is instituting major changes and investing significant resources to improve collaboration among healthcare professionals. A report by Sir David Nicholson (2010: 3) reinforces that

> by working across teams and organisational boundaries that we will achieve the quality and productivity gains we seek for our patients and service users. It is critical that in challenging economic times we work more closely with our partners – between primary and secondary care, and between health and social care – rather than retreating within our own organisational boundaries.

The importance of partnership and the interdependence between health and social care are recognized in the recent push for the NHS to invest in reablement services for vulnerable people who are adjusting to living back in their own homes after an acute episode. The UK government claims that it will be allocating additional significant resources to NHS commissioners to invest in seamless provision between health and social care (DH, 2010a). The White Paper also asserts that patients and users do not recognize a divide between health and social care and as health professionals we should not allow organizational boundaries to get in the way of high-quality care. The focus on collaborative working is set to continue, with the recent proposals contained within the Health and Social Care Bill putting the duty to encourage collaborative working in the hands of the NHS Commissioning Board and Health and Wellbeing Boards (DH, 2011).

AN UNDERSTANDING OF WHAT IS MEANT BY COLLABORATIVE WORKING

Owing to the nature of increasing complexity of health problems it is imperative that we acknowledge and develop our understanding of collaborative working in order to improve the delivery of healthcare to patients and service users. Throughout our working lives there are collective environments with sustained interactions with others. The idea that we share collective action by working towards a common purpose in a supportive trusting environment with other professionals is representative of effective collaborative working.

Collaboration is a complex and multifaceted concept (Henneman *et al.*, 1995). Makowsky *et al.* (2009: 169) defined collaborative care as a 'joint communicating and decision-making process with the goal of satisfying the patient's wellness and illness needs while respecting the unique abilities of each professional'. Oandasan *et al.* (2006) assert that working collaboratively has the potential to improve patient care, enhance patient safety and reduce workload pressures that can cause burnout among healthcare professionals. A common thread running through these concepts is that of collective efficacy; that is, a shared objective of the necessity for group members to believe that the combined group efforts are not only necessary to obtain the desired goal but also that each member is capable of and willing to do their share of the work.

However, the term is often considered synonymous with other modes of interaction such as cooperation, compromise, teamwork, alliancing, joint planning, inter-multidisciplinary, interprofessional, multi-agency and intersectoral. This lack of clarity has resulted in the term collaborative working being used in a variety of inappropriate ways. For example, it is often considered synonymous with other modes of interaction such as cooperation or compromise. Unfortunately, this ambiguity in the meaning of collaborative working may account for the lack of consistency reported by healthcare practitioners about the amount of collaboration occurring in the clinical setting (Baggs *et al.*, 1992).

A significant number of personnel and environmental factors influence whether or not collaboration occurs. The failure of healthcare practitioners being able to work collaboratively may be because a number of antecedents must happen prior to the occurrence of collaboration. Additional to this is the need for these antecedents to be in place within all parties that are involved, which may further complicate the ability to achieve collaboration. Many of these antecedents depend on the readiness of an individual to engage in this type of interpersonal activity. This readiness may result from a number of factors such as educational preparation, maturity and prior experience. In addition, it is important for individuals to have their own role and level of expertise. Confidence in one's ability as well as recognition of the boundaries of one's discipline are critical to the understanding of collaborative working. This confidence generally stems from feelings of competence in one's own area of expertise and prior recognition of worth by other members of the team. Feelings of security about one's own discipline allow the individual to see better how that discipline contributes to the whole (Mariano, 1989).

A significant attribute of collaborative working is that two or more individuals must be involved in a joint venture. This cooperative endeavour is one in which the participants willingly participate in planning and decision-making. Collaborative working requires that individuals view themselves as a team by contributing to a common goal. All participants offer their expertise, share in the responsibility for outcomes, and are acknowledged by other members in the group for their contribution to the process (Mailick and Jordan, 1977). One of the important factors of collaborative working is that the relationship between individuals involved is non-hierarchical. Power is shared and is based on knowledge and expertise as opposed to title or role. The value of working in a trusting and honest environment is recognized as facilitating good collaborative working relationships. It is important that the group recognize collective accomplishments rather than individual effort and that emphasis is placed on cooperation as a mode of dealing with issues rather than competition.

Effective group dynamics play a pivotal role in the promotion of collaborative working. Factors that promote collaboration include excellent communication skills, respect, sharing and trust. The ability to communicate effectively is an important antecedent to collaboration in which members listen to each other's perspectives yet are assertive in presenting their point of view. Effective communication allows team members to negotiate constructively with one another and is a critical antecedent in that it serves as the vehicle for articulating other important precursors to collaboration such as respect, sharing and trust. Mutual respect implies recognition for the body of knowledge, talents, skills and uniqueness of each discipline (Evans and Carlson, 1992). Trust between members of a group is an essential element for collaborative working. This requires that the group begin to know and communicate effectively with each other and over time trust and respect each other.

Leaders of organizations that encourage collaborative working promote shared visions and a commitment to shared objectives. They offer a unified direction to a group, yet foster creativity and autonomy in decision-making. Organizations benefit in that collaborative working fosters maximum productivity and effective use of personnel, as members utilize their talents and skills in a cooperative and non-competitive way. Lank (2006) advocates that by learning from experience both the organization and the employee will develop a continuous improvement culture and by evaluating the return on investment through improved patient outcomes. Retention and satisfaction of employees is enhanced when individuals feel that their contribution is valued and share in planning and decision-making (Molyneux, 2001).

COLLABORATIVE WORKING DEFINED

Interprofessional collaborative working is the process in which different professional groups work together to positively impact healthcare. Collaborative working involves a negotiated agreement between professionals that values the expertise and contributions that various healthcare professionals bring to patient care. In this way issues that arise due to different professionals working together, such as problematic power dynamics, poor communication patterns, lack of understanding of one's own and others' roles and responsibilities, and conflicts due to varied approaches to patient care (Devla *et al.*, 2008; Kvarnstrom, 2008; Miller *et al.*, 2008; Sheehan *et al.*, 2007; Suter, 2009).

Individuals who are involved in collaborative working benefit from the supportive and nurturing environment it creates. Collaboration substantiates the unique and important contribution made by an individual, hence reinforcing feelings of competence, self-worth and importance. The win–win attitude, which accompanies collaborative working, promotes a sense of success and accomplishment in meeting individuals as well as group objectives. Collaborative working promotes interprofessional cohesiveness and can be useful in further clarifying interactive roles with other professionals. Most importantly, perhaps, is the role that collaboration plays in enhancing collegiality and respect among professionals (Miccolo and Spanier, 1993).

Collaboration is a complex, sophisticated process. It requires competence, confidence and commitment on the part of all parties involved. Respect and trust both for oneself and others are key to collaborative working. As such, patience nurturance and time are required to build a relationship to the point where collaboration can occur. Although organizations can be instrumental in supporting collaboration, they cannot ensure its success. Collaborative working is in fact a process that occurs between individuals, not institutions, and only the people involved can ultimately determine whether or not collaboration occurs. Nurses play an important role in the promotion of collaborative working and are essential as nursing continues to add to its knowledge base, it will be better prepared to make its contribution to the 'whole' of patient care.

CASE STUDY

Jenny Jacobs, a nurse, is a 45-year-old lady with newly diagnosed breast cancer with widespread metastases. Her husband Chris is her main carer; he works as a self-employed builder. Jenny and Chris have two children. Luke, aged 14 years, has recently been playing truant from school and complaining of headaches. Each morning Chris has struggled to get Luke motivated and finds that he is reluctant to go to school.

Lucy, aged 8 years, has always enjoyed school and belongs to a small group of friends. However, her teacher has noticed that Lucy has recently become withdrawn and weepy in class and in the playground.

The family are owner-occupiers of a three-bedroomed semi-detached house. Situated in an urban area, the family have a small group of close neighbours with whom they are friendly. Jenny's parents live over 200 miles away, although Chris's parents live in the next town.

Jenny has completed her final chemotherapy treatment and has been told by her consultant that active treatment is no longer an option available to her.

For the past week Jenny has complained of severe headaches with some visual disturbances, which have been quite distressing. Jenny has not had much appetite recently and her clothes are becoming quite loose. She is also feeling tired due to not sleeping and is worried for her family.

As the main carer for Jenny, Chris is finding it difficult to cope, both emotionally and financially. He has also found it difficult to support both children, and has recently discovered Luke has been self-harming. Luke appears angry and refuses to talk to his Dad. Chris has not spoken to Jenny about this for fear of upsetting and worrying her further.

THE INTERFACE OF COLLABORATIVE CARE

Jenny, Chris, Luke and Lucy will all have individual health needs. The diverse wellbeing of multiple-generation family members is rarely delivered by one provider.

Therefore, in managing the healthcare of this family, it is essential to include all the relevant health, social and voluntary services that they may need, which can be identified through ongoing holistic assessment.

The World Health Organization believes that collaboration occurs when 'multiple health workers from different professional backgrounds work together with patients, families, carers and communities to deliver the highest quality of care' (WHO, 2010: 13). The level of intervention provided by health and allied services will depend on the tangible requirements of the personal healthcare needed by the Jacobs family.

ACTIVITY 10.1

Reflection point
Reflect on the case study. What care services do you think Jenny, Chris, Luke and Lucy may require?

Kenny (2002) identified the importance of nursing values in interprofessional collaboration. Weis and Schank (2000) indicate a list of such values as the 'hallmark' of professionalism – care giving, accountability, integrity, trust, freedom, safety and knowledge. In relation to the Jacobs family, these features of professionalism can be used to guide and inform the collaborative process.

Care giving is about working together for patients. The Nursing and Midwifery Council states that a nurse must 'work cooperatively within teams and respect the skills, expertise and contributions of your colleagues' (NMC, 2008).

You may have identified several *care givers* required by the family – district nurse, GP, community mental health nurse, health visitor, school nurse, Macmillan nurse, practice nurse, hospital teams and social workers. This list is not exhaustive, however; to maintain a continuity of appropriate care, it is essential for the practitioner to have an awareness of the roles and responsibilities of others required to meet the expectations of an integrated care approach. Carefully matching the patient care requirements to the service provider who can best meet these needs is fundamental to collaborative care management (DH, 2008).

As the care manager, the district nurse is likely to include the GP for advice and support and anticipatory prescriptions for Jenny. The GP will be informed of the progress of family members but the GP might not necessarily be directly involved in care. Discussions with the health visitor and school nurse will initiate any care needs required by the children, Luke and Lucy. The health visitor might know the family and could provide additional help and support. The school nurse will be able to liaise with teachers and see that the children's wellbeing in the school environment is met. The Macmillan nurse is central to providing advice and support to the interprofessional team involved in a palliative episode of care. However, like the GP, the Macmillan team may not necessarily be required to see Jenny and her family. The level of interaction will vary depending on the requirements of Jenny, Chris and their children. The community mental health nurse can support Chris, Luke (and the wider health team) to enable them to be of assistance in recognizing and understanding the difficulties experienced by them.

Accountability is a professional requirement for all personnel involved in the care of Jenny and her family. For example, the district nurse must be able to account for why he/she has involved others in the care of this family. Practitioners are personally accountable for practice and must be able to defend clinical decision-making (NMC, 2008). It is likely that multiple services will be involved (as listed above); however, the consent of each family member must be sought to enable a good working relationship and constructive interaction to occur.

McDonald and McCallin (2010) recognize that complex scenarios involving the wider healthcare context, of Jenny and her family for example, are the driving force for interprofessional collaboration. Team interactions are required here for effective and efficient patient-centred care to take place as the knowledge and skills of many services will be required.

Appreciation of roles and respect for colleagues is paramount if healthy collaboration is to work. For example, Chris has confided that he is experiencing financial difficulties. He is unable to work because he is the main carer for Jenny. The social worker may be able to assist him to claim for benefits he could be entitled to. During your discussions with Chris, he agrees for you to make a referral. At this point, it would be unwise for you to make any promise or pinpoint a date and time that the social worker would visit as you are unaware of the social worker's priorities and workload. This information can be provided once there has been some dialogue with the social worker involved.

Integrity places the Jacobs family needs first. The family must be able to trust the practitioner with their health and wellbeing. This means treating them as individuals and respecting their dignity when working with others to promote health (NMC, 2008). Jenny will rely on you to access the knowledge and skills of a variety of experts for herself and her family. However, McDonald and McCallin (2010) warn of the risk of the identification of superfluous problems, purely since a collaborative team is accessible. Ongoing holistic assessment will guide the practitioner to make appropriate referrals based on need.

While Jenny's condition is stable, it is useful to examine her wishes for a 'good death'. This requires well-developed communication skills. Impending death is a difficult topic to talk about. This topic can be initiated at an appropriate time when Jenny is ready, and preferably when the conversation can take place in private without interruption. Jenny's hopes, fears, requests and expectations must be respected and documented to inform an advanced care directive. As Jenny's condition deteriorates, it is the role of the practitioner to advocate for Jenny to ensure that her recorded wishes are met (NMC, 2008). *The End of Life Care in the NHS Operating Framework* (DH, 2010b) requires all services to work across boundaries to respond positively to patients' needs.

Trust involves having a firm belief in the reliability of a person, and in this case Jenny will develop trust in the interprofessional team as long as they demonstrate appropriate and sensitive interpersonal skills and a good communication manner. Baldwin (2007) recognizes that partnership working usually occurs within teams. In this scenario, the team is a wider group of people than the community nursing team.

Placing the patient and family at the centre of a care plan relies on the patient being involved in the collaborative process at every level.

Veracity and openness form the basis of a good working relationship with patients, within teams and the wider interprofessional team (Beauchamp and Childress, 2008). It is essential that Jenny and her family are kept fully informed and have their questions answered openly and honestly.

Freedom is the quality of not being controlled. Although it is important to provide a firm evidence base to support the care plan designed for Jenny, it is important that she has the freedom to make personal choices. Collaborating with Jenny, means working with her to meet her personal needs, not taking over, and not avoiding sensitive difficult areas of discussion. Decisions should be supported and not made on behalf of patients unless the patient lacks the capacity to make decisions. In this situation the fourth principle of the Mental Capacity Act (2005) – 'best interests' – will apply, unless an advanced directive has been drawn up. If an advanced directive exists that applies to the situation which has arisen, the advanced directive decision will prevail (Dimond, 2008).

Safety is the key feature for patient care. Risks can be obvious or hidden. They can relate to people or environments and can be the result or consequence of acts and omissions. Rigorous risk assessment is essential to maintain the wellbeing of Jenny and her family. It is also required to safeguard the visiting services who may be involved in the care of Jenny and her family. All healthcare providers are bound by policy and guidance to minimize risk and promote safety, for example if any risks are identified that may pose harm; this information must accompany the referral made to other services.

There are known risks associated with chemotherapy. The practitioner can provide advice and support for Jenny in relation to this. Additionally, vulnerable visiting staff must be aware of any issues that may pose a hazard or risk, for example to a pregnant member of staff. As Jenny's disease process progresses, it is vital that the risk assessment is evaluated and updated along with the care plan. Any changes will need to be disseminated to all those involved in visiting the Jacobs family.

Knowledge is the theoretical or practical understanding of a subject. In relation to Jenny and her family, it applies to the utilization of widely accepted evidence-based practice performed by a variety of professional and allied healthcarers. All direct clinical interventions, advice, support and education must be evidence based and from a valid and reliable source. When working with patients like Jenny, sometimes they access information online that may not be from a recognized reliable source. In this context, the practitioner must encourage the use of widely accepted reliable information sources such as NHS direct; however, they are still obliged to maintain a non-judgemental attitude if the patient chooses to use a non-evidence-based remedy that claims to be a miracle cure. They are not, however, obliged to administer any lotion, potion or any other treatment that is not prescribed by a doctor or nurse prescriber. When patients make such requests, this should be clearly documented in the care plan along with any advice given. This will safeguard the patient and guide other staff visiting the family (NMC, 2008).

SKILLS NEEDED TO COLLABORATE EFFECTIVELY

Healthcare context drives interprofessional collaboration with referrals made to others services, usually as the result of a holistic health needs assessment. Collaboration therefore is purposive. It is a process that produces the result that no single service provider could achieve autonomously.

Communication is an essential component of collaboration (Laming, 2003). Poor communication between services and personnel was cited as a fundamental flaw by Lord Laming, who reported on the Victoria Climbié inquiry. Sharing information with other services requires that we send and receive information; yet, communication is a multifarious concept. The two-way sharing of information can be face to face, but as teams and services are generally widely geographically spread health professionals liaise in a face-to-face context less frequently. They increasingly rely on information technology where the interpersonal nature of verbal cues and body language are lost. Donnelly and Neville (2008) depict four dimensions of communication, described by Cox and Hill (2010) as:

> Mechanistic – transmitted by machine, phone, fax, email, blog where interpersonal skills are not required. However, this method is reliant on clear verbal or written information being provided for accurate interpretation by the recipient.

> Psychological – emotionally charged dialogue that is written or spoken where emotive language can make clarity less factual and less objective.

> Social constructivism – where the same problem can be interpreted in different ways, depending on the area that the health professional is working. Different priorities emerge as the health professionals involved interpret the need of the patient within the commissioning framework of their specific service delivery.

> Systemic – how communication is provided by an organization, and within an organization. Often there are differences in the way in which information is cascaded and shared both within an organization and to other organizations and services.

ACTIVITY 10.2

In considering the care services required by Jenny, Chris, Luke and Lucy in the last exercise, now think about how those services will communicate with each other.

Using the four dimensions of communication discussed in the last paragraphs, examine how these dimensions are used by health professionals providing care for the Jacobs family.

Preceding sections of this chapter have discussed why healthcare professionals are required to work collaboratively, what it means to collaborate and with whom we are required to work. This section is about the skills required to collaborate effectively. Using the case study of Jenny, Chris, Luke and Lucy, scenarios will be drawn out to demonstrate the range of skills that are fundamental to effective collaboration.

COLLABORATIVE ATTITUDES

Collaboration is a word used widely in nursing and healthcare. Attitudes of those involved in team working can influence the collaborative process. Key attitudinal skills can make or break the sustenance and progression of a successful shared care episode. Clarridge and Ryder (2004) describe these professional attributes as relational skills.

Relational skills include readiness, willingness and trust, and these are thought to be the basic skills required for collaborative work (Freeth *et al.*, 2005). However, an expansion on these core skills can include other factors such as

* listening
* use of suitable language
* respect
* fairness
* sensitivity
* empathy
* courtesy
* honesty/openness.

All of these characteristics are required for the development and maintenance of professional relationships with patients, carers, healthcare professionals and organizations allied to health.

ACTIVITY 10.3

In terms of nurse–patient relational skills, what factors do you think contribute to the issues raised in the following scenario?

Jenny discovers that a lesion on her breast that she thought was a pimple has developed into a wound that is leaking odorous fluid. She tells the district nurse. The district nurse assesses the wound and tells Jenny that the wound is unlikely to heal and it will need to be re-dressed every day. During a subsequent outpatient appointment, another nurse tells Jenny that her breast is fungating and it is likely that the 'smell' could become a problem. Jenny becomes distressed and later in the day she rings the district nurse and indicates that she has had enough and wants to 'end it all'.

The district nurse visits Jenny and during their conversation reassures her that the wound can be managed to maintain her comfort and dignity. Jenny seems much happier with this information and advice.

You may have considered that the outpatient department nurse has provided too much information. However, this information may have been given in response to Jenny asking questions. Conversely, while maintaining good relational skills with patients, the nurse could have contacted the district nurse (as Jenny's care manager) to alert her to the sensitive nature of the conversation the nurse had had with Jenny.

Although it is wholly appropriate to be open and honest, there is always the need to be sensitive and empathetic. Also, the use of therapeutic language can cause alarm to patients and perhaps if the word 'fungating' had been replaced with more suitable language, the distress caused to Jenny may have been minimized. However, both nurses work in different settings. Each will have a different job description, yet both will be working within the same professional code and striving to meet the same goals in meeting patients' needs. Therefore, there must be respect for the roles and responsibilities of others and relational skills apply to professional relationships too.

CONCLUSION

This chapter has offered an insight into the nature of collaborative working and how the scenario highlights that the delivery of care to patients can often be complex. It recognizes that individual healthcare professionals involved in the scenario will use different skills but share a common goal of providing a comprehensive service tailored to meet the needs of the patient and family. The success of collaborative working will require that individuals must be able to acquire a vision and to develop common goals.

Policy initiatives and the needs of those who use services and resources will continue to steer the collaborative working agenda. In order for new policies to operate effectively they need the commitment of healthcare professionals to work collaboratively together with the ability to critically evaluate practice and work in partnership with patients and service users.

Critically evaluating your understanding of collaborative working within your practice and how this can be incorporated will help you to become an effective practitioner.

REFERENCES

Baggs JB, Ryan SA, Phelps CA, *et al.* (1992) The association between interdisciplinary collaboration and patient outcomes in medical intensive care. *Heart and Lung* 21:18–24.

Baldwin D (2007) Some historical notes on interdisciplinary and interprofessional education and practice in health care in the USA. *Journal Interprofessional Care* 21:23–27.

Beauchamp T and Childress J (2008) *Principles of Biomedical Ethics,* 6th edn. Oxford: Oxford University Press.

Clarridge A and Ryder E (2004) Working collaboratively. In Chilton S, Melling K, Drew D and Clarridge A *Nursing in the Community: An Essential Guide to Practice.* London: Hodder Arnold.

Cox CL and Hill MC (2010) *Professional Issues in Primary Care Nursing.* Chichester: Wiley-Blackwell.

D'Amour D, Ferrada-Videla L, Rodriguez SM and Beaulieu, MD (2005) The conceptual basis for interprofessional collaboration: core concepts and theoretical frameworks. *Journal of Interprofessional Care* 19:116–31.

Department of Health (DH) (1994) *The Report of the Enquiry into the Care and Treatment of Christopher Clunis.* London: HMSO.

DH (1995) *A Vision for the Future*. London: HMSO.

DH (1997) *National Health Service Primary Care Act*. London: HMSO.

DH (2000) *The NHS Plan: A Plan for Investment, a Plan for Reform*. London: HMSO.

DH (2003) *The Victoria Climbié Inquiry: Report of an Inquiry by Lord Laming*. London: HMSO.

DH (2008) *End of Life Care Strategy – Promoting High Quality Care for All Adults at the End of Life*. London: HMSO.

DH (2010a) *Equity and Excellence: Liberating the NHS*. London: HMSO.

DH (2010b) *The Operating Framework for the NHS in England*. London: HMSO.

DH (2011) *The Health and Social Bill*. London: HMSO.

Devla D, Jamieson M and Lemieux M (2008) Team effectiveness in academic primary health care teams. *Journal of Interprofessional Care* 22:598–611.

Dimond B (2008) *Legal Aspects of Nursing*, 5th edn. Harlow: Pearson Education.

Donnelly E and Neville L (2008) *Communication and Interprofessional Skills*. Exeter: Reflect Press.

Evans SA and Carlson R (1992) Nurse-physician collaboration: solving the nursing shortage crisis. *Journal of American Cardiology* 20:1669–73.

Fatchett A (1996) A chance for community nurses to shape the health agenda. *Nursing Times* 92:40–2.

Freeth D, Hammick M, Reeves S and Barr H (2005) *Effective Interprofessional Education. Development, Delivery and Evaluation*. Oxford: Blackwell Publishers.

Greenwell J (1995) Patients and professionals. In Soothill K, Mackay L and Webb C (eds) *Interprofessional Relations in Health Care*. London: Edward Arnold, pp. 313–31.

Henneman EA, Lee JL and Cohen JI (1995) Collaboration a concept analysis. *Journal of Advanced Nursing* 21:103–9.

Kennedy I (2001) *Learning from Bristol: The Report of the Public Inquiry into Children's Heart Surgery at the Bristol Royal Infirmary 1984–1995*. London: The Stationery Office.

Kenny G (2002) The importance of nursing values in interprofessional collaboration. *British Journal of Nursing* 11:65–8.

Kvarnstrom S (2008) Difficulties in collaboration: A critical incident study of interprofessional healthcare teamwork. *Journal of Interprofessional Care* 22:191–203.

Lank E (2006) Collaborative Advantage: How Organisations Win by Working Together. London: Palgrave Macmillan.

Lord Laming (2003) *The Victoria Climbié Inquiry: Report of an Enquiry by Lord Laming*. (Accessed 10 December 2010) www.victoria-climbie-inquiry.org.uk/finreport/finreport.htm.

Loxley A (1997) *Collaboration in Health and Welfare. Working with Difference*. London: Kingsley Publishers Ltd.

Mailick M and Jordan P (1977) A multimodel approach to collaborative practice in health settings. *Social Work Health Care* 2:445–54.

Makowsky MJ, Schindel TJ, Rosenthal M, *et al.* (2009) Collaboration between pharmacists, physicians and nurse practitioners: A qualitative investigation of working relationships in the inpatient setting. *Journal of Interprofessional Care* 23:169–84.

Mariano C (1989) The case for interdisciplinary collaboration. *Nursing Outlook* 37:285–8.

McDonald C and McCallin A (2010) Interprofessional collaboration in palliative nursing: what is the patient-family role? *International Journal of Palliative Nursing* 16:285–8.

Mental Capacity Act (1995) London: The Stationery Office.

Miccolo MA and Spanier AH (1993) Critical care management in the 1990s: making collaborative practice work. *Critical Care Clinics* 9:443–53.

Miller KL, Reeves S, Zwarenstein M, *et al.* (2008) Nursing emotion work and interprofessional collaboration in general internal medicine wards: a qualitative study. *Journal of Advanced Nursing* 64:332–43.

Molyneux J (2001) Interprofessional teamworking: what makes teams work well? *Journal of Interprofessional Care* 15:29–35.

Nicholson D (2010) A letter to NHS Chairs, Chief Executives and Directors of Finance. p. 3.

Nursing and Midwifery Council (NMC) (2008) *The Code: Standards of Conduct, Performance and Ethics for Nurses and Midwives.* London: NMC.

NMC (2010) Record keeping: guidance for nurses and midwives. London: NMC.

Oandasan I, Baker GR, Barker K, *et al.* (2006) Teamwork in healthcare: promoting effective teamwork in healthcare in Canada. (Accessed 24 November 2010) www.chsrf.ca.

Ofsted (2008) *Report into the Death of Baby P in the London Borough of Haringey.* London: Ofsted.

Rushmer R (2005) Blurred boundaries damage interprofessional working. *Nurse Research* 12:74–85.

Sheehan D, Robertson L and Ormond T (2007) Comparison of language used and patterns of communication in interprofessional and multi-disciplinary teams. *Journal of Interprofessional Care* 21:17–30.

Slimmer L (2003) A collaborative care management programme in a primary care setting was effective for older adults with late life depression. *Evidence-Based Nursing* 6:91.

Smith SM, Allwright S and O'Dowd T (2007) Effectiveness of shared care across the interface between primary and speciality care in chronic disease management. *Cochrane Database of Systematic Reviews* Issue 3:CD004910.

Suter E, Arndt J, Arthur N, *et al.* (2009) Role understanding and effective communication as core competencies for collaborative practice. *Journal of Interprofessional Care* 23:41–51.

Taylor KI, Oberle KM, Cruthcher RA and Norton PG (2005) Promoting health in type 2 diabetes: nurse–physician collaboration in primary care. *Biological Research for Nursing* 6:207–15.

Weiss D and Shank MJ (2000) An instrument to measure professional nursing values. *Journal of Nursing Scholarship* 32:201–4.

World Health Organization (2010) *Framework for Action on Interprofessional Education and Collaborative Practice.* (Accessed 3 January 2011) www.who.int/hrh/resources/framework_action/en/index.html.

Zwarenstein M and Bryant W (2000) Interventions to promote collaboration between nurses and doctors. *Cochrane Database of Systematic Reviews* Issue 2:CD000072.

FURTHER RESOURCES

Gold Standards Framework Toolkit – The Gold Standards Framework (GSF) is a systematic evidence-based approach to optimizing the care for patients nearing the end of life delivered by generalist providers. It is concerned with helping people to live well until the end of life and includes care in the final years of life for people with any end-stage illness in any setting. www.goldstandardsframework.nhs.uk/TheGSFToolkit (accessed 3 January 2011).

Macmillan – Macmillan and cancer backup merged in 2008. Together they provide free high-quality information for cancer patients, their families and carers. www.macmillan.org.uk/Cancerinformation/Cancerinformation.aspx (accessed 3 January 2011).

NHS Direct – an evidence-based resource for patients. www.nhsdirect.nhs.uk/ (accessed on 3 January 2011).

Approaches to acute care in the community

Linda Watson

LEARNING OUTCOMES

- Explore the spectrum of conditions that might be considered acute in community care
- Discuss and analyze the theory required to support the community nurse caring for acute conditions
- Identify and rationalize the skills required to support the community nurse caring for acute conditions
- Recognize pharmacology knowledge and interventions to manage acute conditions
- Discuss the concept and elements related to discharge planning and avoiding hospital admission

INTRODUCTION

The aim of this chapter is to examine approaches to managing acute care in the community. Traditionally 'acute care' is a term that can be used to describe how and where specialized healthcare is provided in the case of an emergency or as a result of having been referred for further investigation, surgical intervention, complex tests or other care that historically has not been done or available in the community. The use of the term acute care emerged and was used to describe care provision in instances of sudden, severe or emergency care in hospital prior to returning home to the community. Traditionally acute care was the term usually used to describe treatment provided for a short period, continuing until the individual is well enough to be supported and cared for in the community again (Health Foundation, 2010). However, considering the shifting balance of care to the community, this definition needs to be reconsidered. For the purpose of this chapter, acute care in the community refers to a short episode of care for a new condition or an exacerbation of an existing long-term condition.

Nurses are key to successful management and delivery of care in the healthcare setting. Nurses plan, negotiate and coordinate care for patients in a range of settings, including large hospitals, community hospitals, general practices, community pharmacies, schools, urgent care centres and out-of-hours care (Richards and Tawfik, 2002; Naidoo and Wills, 2009).

Some of the issues and areas of care noted as having potential to positively impact the delivery of acute care in the community have included:

- use of IT and video links/phones to link to hospital services
- provision of hospital services in the home
- provision of intravenous therapy in the home
- provision and management of anticoagulant therapy in the community
- care coordinators/facilitators to manage and signpost people to appropriate services
- additional educational support/training for community staff
- avoiding total reliance on local appointments with specialists
- avoiding reliance of adding specialist to community teams
- avoiding total reliance on sharing care with acute sector/hospitals
- not relying on GPs to deliver minor surgery in community (Norridge, 2011).

The cost of delivering all healthcare services remains a key concern of those involved in design and delivery of health services. Redesigning healthcare delivery models can, as described below', positively impact healthcare costs and enhance the services delivered. Careful exploration of the services delivered, and the professions delivering those services, has the potential to save money, streamline services and enhance patients experiences and outcomes. For example, moving care previously delivered in the acute setting and expanding the roles of those within the healthcare team to facilitate delivery of care previously the remit of the GP has the potential to reduce costs, enhance care and the patient's experience of receiving care (Pulse, 2011).

Performance of minor surgical procedures by GPs has been shown to reduce the cost of such procedures compared with the cost if the procedure had been carried out in the secondary care hospital setting. The online general practice resource *Pulse Today* (2008) notes that the total saving can be around £150 000 per year. This saving could be further enhanced by expanding and advancing the skills of the community nursing team to enable completion of some minor surgical procedures, since the hourly rate of pay for nurses is less than that of the GP.

ACTIVITY 11.1

Reflection point

As a nurse working in the community, reflect upon your practice patients who have presented as acutely unwell, but whose illness was not considered life threatening.

Identify the causes of the illness.

- Consider what clinical skills and theoretical knowledge were required to assess, diagnose and manage the condition.
- Reflect upon your own knowledge and skills, identify and list the additional skills and knowledge required over and above your existing knowledge and skills, to facilitate management of these conditions.
- Develop an action plan to identify how you can and will acquire the knowledge and skills required to manage these conditions.

ACUTE CONDITIONS IN THE COMMUNITY

'Minor injuries' is a term used to define non-life-threatening injuries. Traditionally, individuals have sought care for minor injuries at Accident and Emergency centres when treatment could be delivered just as well and more than likely quicker by a community-based service. 'Minor illness' can be defined as the less critical non-life-threatening illness or exacerbations of a long-term condition that could be managed by a well-performing community healthcare system, reducing the chances of admission to an inpatient bed (University of Sheffield, 2008). There are many conditions which can be managed well by the community-based nurse. Managing these conditions may become more challenging if they progress into a more acute condition or stage or when the patient experiences an acute exacerbation of a chronic condition. Some examples can be seen in Table 11.1. You may have experience of some other conditions that have developed acute presentations – please add these to the list. It may become appropriate for the community nurse to develop additional and/or advanced skills in order to help manage these unexpected acute episodes of care.

Table 11.1 Common chronic conditions

Respiratory conditions such as COPD and emphysema. Psychiatric disorders. Neurological conditions. Genetic conditions such as cystic fibrosis, arthritis, allergies, endocrine disease
Common minor illness/injuries that can become more severe/acute
Common cold/flu, tonsillitis, sickness and/or diarrhoea, cuts, minor trauma including head trauma, eye infections, urinary tract infections
Other
Substance abuse/misuse, kidney disease, liver disease, blood-borne viral infections, blood dyscrasias, cardiac disease

THEORY REQUIRED TO SUPPORT THE COMMUNITY NURSE CARING FOR ACUTE CONDITIONS

Thurtle *et al.* (2006) identified that primary care and community nurses wish to deliver skilful clinical care that is supported by holistic principles rather than focusing solely on an approach based on technical skills. To facilitate this, community staff must be knowledgeable and receptive to change. A flexible approach is required to meet the evolving demands of primary health while embedding a culture supporting ongoing professional development.

Holt (2008) describes role transition as arising from a single event and extending to the core elements of professional practice and development in relation to varying areas of practice. The literature supports a variety of ways to develop staff, including approved and endorsed work-based learning, recognized preceptor programmes and work-based courses (Drennan *et al.,* 2006).

Engaging in active personal development is important in identifying the learning needs and goals of individual practitioners, thereby enhancing established clinical skills and experience maximizing the usefulness of the practitioner. Evolving models of community care, such as the community matron (DH, 2005), will support development and encourage innovation in healthcare delivery and fostering development of advanced practice, management and leadership skills (Roberts and Kelly, 2007). Learning in practice is valued and viewed as integral to the development of advanced practice skills (Thurtle *et al.*, 2006).

In addition to generic areas of core skills and knowledge, areas for continuing professional development for nurses required to deliver care to patients who present with increasingly complex healthcare requirements may include history-taking skills and assessment, consultation skills, counselling, anatomy/physiology/patho-physiology, epidemiology, decision-making, independent prescribing, pharmacology, laboratory investigations/X-ray interpretation, organizational management, finance, risk assessment and audit (DH, 2005; RCN, 2010).

Research around the development of new roles that may involve providing acute care in the community is scant, but one exception is discussed by Bird *et al.* (2004) in an Australian study around the 'care facilitator' role. This role is aimed at those who are nurses or community healthcare professionals. The study reviewed elderly individuals who had attended A&E on a minimum of three occasions in a 12-month period. Those who had been appointed a care facilitator were 20% less likely to present at A&E, and 25% less likely to become an inpatient, having 20% fewer days in hospital. The researchers concluded that care facilitators who coordinated patient care across existing services, streamlining access to community health services, lowered the demand for acute care services. In the UK the community matron and case managers are similarly concerned in coordination of care, but unlike the Australian care facilitator, community matrons are required to cope with additional responsibility such as carrying a clinical case load. The Australian role differs in that it is focused solely on coordination of care and facilitating access to appropriate healthcare services.

In England, the development of the community matron role was aimed at reducing episodes of unplanned and unexpected admission to hospitals, in particular for those living with long-term conditions, and has required those wishing to undertake the role to engage in additional training, education and workplace learning (DH, 2005). There have been some inconsistencies in and differing interpretations of what the role entails, with some viewing the role as that of a case manager, whereas others understand the role to be more of a community matron or advanced practitioner type of role. The UK government intended that those undertaking the community matron role would assume responsibility for organization of healthcare needs, collaboration and negotiation of care plans with patients, negotiation and management of the services required by each patient as and when needed and clinical intervention as indicated (Gravelle *et al.*, 2006). So this new role would require the practitioner to be both an advanced clinical practitioner and an effective manager and care planner (DH, 2005). The educational development required to support those moving into the community matron role is significant. The role requires the community matron to have specialist preparation in the community role, generalist advanced practice and requires the assimilation of skills and knowledge previously held by medical practitioners. Expanding and deepening the boundaries and scope of practice required for this role (Woodend, 2006). Chapter 13 also considers the role of the community matron.

Jolly *et al.* (1998) discuss British research identifying that having a care coordinator or liaison nurse enhances the follow-up care provided to those discharged from hospital with cardiac issues. Studies note that provision of such care in the community helps focus the nursing role on assisting users to continue behaviour changes, and encourages service users to engage in shared decision-making, promoting concordance with agreed care plans and medication regimens (Jolly *et al.*, 1998). This practice differs from the traditional primary prevention practices of the community nurse, where the emphasis is on risk reduction and facilitation of change.

Development of advanced practice roles has the potential to further enhance the streamlining and delivery of acute care in the community, providing opportunities for nurses to work autonomously in assessing, diagnosing and developing management plans, and prescribing and reviewing relevant medications. It would seem relevant therefore that community nurses working at an advanced level need to be independent prescribers. This is an example of how changing the nature of 'acute' care provided by community nurses is not merely about changing the setting of the delivery of that care, but will also require the development of new knowledge, skills and competencies. There is little conclusive evidence-based research to show what these skills and competencies should be, but they should benefit the population, be sustainable and evidence based (DHSSPS, 2010; NES, 2008).

ACTIVITY 11.2

Reflection point
Reflect on the following scenario:

Mrs Smith has developed a sore throat, which began 3 days ago and is worsening. She describes signs and symptoms characteristic of the common cold: she has an elevated temperature but denies having a headache, nausea/vomiting, aversion to bright lights (photophobia) or a rash. She has managed to drink fluids and her appetite has not been affected. She denies having difficulty swallowing, but notes that swallowing is painful. She has no cough. She admits to feeling very stressed at the moment, having started a new job and feeling as though she is expected to know everything about this new job. She does not want to take sick leave as her work will accumulate, so she is worried that her symptoms are getting worse.

What knowledge and skills can you identify that would be required to assess and diagnose this patient's illness?

Some of the skills/knowledge used to assess, diagnose and manage this patient are:

• consultation (history and assessment)
• exploration of patient's motivation and expectation
• clinical examination skills
• clinical medicine
• knowledge of pathophysiology
• pharmacology – antibiotics
• National Institute of Clinical Excellence (NICE), Scottish Intercollegiate Guidelines Network (SIGN) Guidelines
• laboratory investigations
• diagnosis/differential diagnosis
• decision-making
• leadership
• management
• education/teaching skills
• education/counselling

In Activity 11.2 it is essential that the history and physical examination findings are interpreted and evaluated. For example, how would the practitioner identify whether the symptoms were caused by a viral or bacterial infection? You as the healthcare provider have to know what questions to ask, and which examinations/ skills are required to facilitate this. In this scenario, it is the history of the common cold type of symptoms and the absence of systemic illness identified from your findings of the clinical examination that suggest a diagnosis of viral sore throat. Differential diagnosis based on information gathered during your consultation and examination would assist you in confirming your diagnosis.

How will you know how to manage this condition? Are there any diagnostic tests or investigations that you might have considered using to assist you in your diagnosis? If so, which tests are they? Do you know how this condition is treated? Would you consider prescribing anything for this patient?

Identify what theory and resources you would access to assist you in your diagnostic decision-making.

Would you be confident that you gathered had sufficient information from the history and examination of your patient to make a diagnosis without the need for further tests?

How would you know that you had gathered sufficient information?

Having reflected upon the above, what are the areas you would need to develop further knowledge and skills? Consider how and why achieving this additional knowledge and skill will enhance your practice and ability to meet the healthcare needs of patients with acute conditions.

Some of the skills you may identify as being required in the community may traditionally have been areas that only doctors were allowed to carry out. There is however increasing evidence that nurses who expand their scope of practice to include skills previously considered only the domain of a doctor can provide healthcare at a level more satisfying to patients than the care they receive from their doctor. Nurses in advanced roles appear to provide healthcare that is equal to and in many areas better than that provided by doctors. Research supports that advanced practice nurses can identify 'physical abnormalities' more often, give more information than doctors, keep more accurate patient records and communicate more effectively than doctors (Horrocks *et al.*, 2002; De Geest *et al.*, 2008; Pulse, 2011).

SKILLS REQUIRED TO SUPPORT THE COMMUNITY NURSE CARING FOR ACUTE CONDITIONS

ACTIVITY 11.3

Identify the enhanced skills you will require to facilitate delivery of acute care in the community in the following areas:
* clinical
* leadership
* management
* educational.

It is important that community nurses have experience of managing care across the lifespan. Community nurses, like all nurses, will be expected to demonstrate up-to-date knowledge and practice, delivered with a non-judgemental sensitive approach when working with individuals from differing backgrounds (NMC, 2008, 2010). Community nurses require an understanding of anatomy and physiology of the human body (NMC, 2010), relevant to their specific role within the community team, and should have or be developing consultation, physical assessment and history-taking skills. Community nurses providing acute care should be competent and able to diagnose, treat, manage and when required refer some psychological problems such as anxiety, depression and addictions. For example, Patient Health Questionnaires can be useful to assist the practitioner in assessing the severity of depression or anxiety (Depression Primary Care, 2006).

In addition to development of enhanced and advanced clinical skills such as auscultation and percussion, the community nurse must become proficient at recording and documenting clinical findings. Two models often used are the problem-oriented medical record (POMR) and the subjective, objective, assessment and planning (SOAP) structure introduced by Lawrence Weed (1961). Use of these approaches can add structure to recording collected data.

The palliative/provoking, quality, radiation, severity, timing (PQRST) symptom analysis mnemonic outlines a framework by which to structure questioning (Walsh, 2005; Budassi Sheehy, 1992; Montgomery *et al.*, 2008; Ryan, 1996).

Use of PQRST

* P: Provocation/palliation
  – What initiates, starts or causes it?
  – What helps, improves or makes it better?

- – What does not help or makes it worse?
- – *What seems to set this off? Stress? Position? Certain activities? Arguments?*
- – *Does it seem to be improving, worsening, or is it remaining the same?*
- – *What helps or relieves it: changing food? Altering position? taking medicines? activity? rest?*
- – *What aggravates or causes the problem to worsen?*
- Q: Quality and quantity
  - – How does it feel, look or sound?
  - – How much is there?
  - – *Is it sharp, dull, piercing, burning, crushing, throbbing?*
  - – *Allow the patient describe the pain, sometimes they say what they think you want them to say.*
  - – *If describing an exudate: amount, smell, consistency, colour, clear cloudy?*
- R: Radiation
  - – Where is it?
  - – Does it spread?
  - – *Where does the pain spread to?*
  - – *Does it say in one place?*
  - – *Did it start somewhere else and move?*
  - – *Is it now in one or many places?*
  - – *If pain, does it travel:*
  - – *If so where to?*
  - – *Your back?*
  - – *Arms?*
  - – *Neck?*
  - – *Legs?*
- S: Severity
  - – Does it interfere with activities?
  - – Rate the severity on a scale of 1 to 10
  - – *When worst, how severe is it?*
  - – *Does it limit your activity?*
  - – *How long does it last?*
- T: Timing
  - – When does it begin?
  - – How often does this happen?
  - – Is it sudden or gradual?
  - – How long does it last?
  - – *What time did/does it begin?*
  - – *When did this first happen?*
  - – *What were you doing?*
  - – *How often does this happen? Weekly, dailyhourly?*
  - – *What time of day does it usually occur?*
  - – *Does this ever wake you up?*
  - – *Do you get any other symptoms at the same time?*

You can use this approach to assess alternative presentations and to identify knowledge deficits and learning needs.

CASE STUDY

Ryan presents to you complaining of stomach pain. You notice that he is walking slowly, is holding (guarding) his stomach and is slightly hunched over. He tentatively sits down again, protecting his stomach and abdomen with his hands and arms. He is obviously uncomfortable. On collection of the history of stomach pain (the complaint), he informs you that it began 3 days ago.

- Note 10 PQRST-based questions you would ask to facilitate a *diagnosis (e.g. When did the pain start, is it constant, where exactly is the pain and has or does it move, does anything make the pain better or worse, does eating or opening your bowels affect the pain, are you or have you had any nausea or vomiting, have your normal bowel habits changed, have you recently lost weight, have you been taking any medications, have you had any blood on your stools?)*

On further questioning, to help you further clarify, you discover that when the stomach pain started, it was in the 'middle of the stomach', but that since yesterday morning the pain is now on the right lower side of the abdomen. Ryan denies vomiting and has no change in bowel habit or diarrhoea or constipation. The pain comes and goes, and apart from the pain he feels otherwise well.

- Note the anatomical sections of the abdomen *(right upper, right lower, left upper, left lower quadrants. Alternatively you may opt to use nine anatomical segments).*
- If confirming appendicitis, what would you expect to find on examination? If you are unfamiliar with this condition – you may – as you will for any presentation you are not familiar with – have to seek help, a second opinion and access further learning resources around this subject. *(Pain in right iliac fossa, might have pyrexia. Digital rectal examination to right side will elicit pain.)*

Your examination findings lead you to suspect Ryan has appendicitis. You call the admitting healthcare professional. You discuss the case, and he/she agrees to see Ryan. You send Ryan with a letter to the A&E department, where he is admitted. The following week you see Ryan for removal of his appendectomy sutures. You receive a discharge summary letter confirming Ryan's appendectomy. Post-operatively he does very well.

- What factors can lead to some cases of appendicitis being missed?*(Signs and symptoms can be confused with viral gastroenteritis, food allergy/poisoning, IBS.)*

- Explore the possible consequences of missing the diagnosis of appendicitis. *(Possible consequences include rupture and peritonitis.)*

- List some differential diagnoses of abdominal pain *(appendicitis, cholecystitis, gastroenteritis, irritable bowel syndrome, biliary colic, duodenal ulcer, hiatus hernia, dyspepsia, gastro-oesophageal reflux, stress related symptoms, urinary tract infection, kidney stone, pancreatitis).*

Suggested answers are in italics.

ACTIVITY 11.4

Reflection point
Reflect on the case study and identify any gaps in your knowledge. Develop an action plan to meet these learning needs.

PHARMACOLOGY KNOWLEDGE AND INTERVENTIONS

Medicine management is an integral element of nursing practice in both hospital and community settings. However, it is all the more crucial to have an understanding of pharmacology to ensure safe management of medications in the community, as patients do not remain under the constant observation of a healthcare professional. Having been identified as a healthcare need in the Cumberlege Report in 1986, one of the most influential additions to the nurse's role has been the introduction of nurse prescribing (DHSS, 1986).

As a nurse responsible for monitoring, administering and possibly prescribing medication, it is essential that the community nurse is competent and can maintain safe medication practice, promoting and monitoring maintenance of adequate and safe drug levels in the body (NMC, 2007, 2008).

ACTIVITY 11.5

Reflection point
Reflect on the following and identify any personal knowledge deficits and develop an action plan to identify how you will access and achieve the knowledge and skills required to facilitate safe and competent prescribing.

- How do drugs exert their action and effect?
- What term is used to describe this process?
- Describe the processes of absorption, distribution, metabolism and excretion.
- What term is used to describe the action drugs exert on the body? Discuss/explain this process.
- What disease processes and factors affect how medications interact with the body's physiology?

If and when the community nurse is required to prescribe, it will be relevant for the community nurse to develop and maintain currency of their knowledge of recommended pharmacological regimens, development, manipulation and review of management plans and completion of a recognized prescribing course (NMC, 2006).

There are three types of non-medical prescribing:

- Independent prescribing for nurses, pharmacists and optometrists.
  As of May 2006, Nurse Independent Prescribers, previously known as Extended Formulary Nurse Prescribers, were permitted to prescribe any medicine for any condition within their area of practice and competence, including a selection of controlled medications. Pharmacists who independently prescribe are eligible to prescribe in a similar way, with the exception of controlled drugs. Optometrist Independent Prescribers can prescribe any medicine licensed for ocular conditions

which may affect the eye and/or surrounding tissue. Optometrists are not permitted to prescribe any controlled drug. Independent prescribers are autonomous practitioners, and are often advanced practitioners responsible and accountable for consultation and assessment of patients with undiagnosed and diagnosed conditions and formulating decisions regarding the clinical management required, including prescribing.

- Nurse Prescribers' Formulary for Community Practitioners
  Community Practitioners, historically referred to as district nurses and health visitors, can prescribe independently from a formulary of a limited selection of medicines, dressings and equipment commonly used in community settings.
- Supplementary prescribing
  Facilitates qualified and registered nurses, pharmacists, physiotherapists, chiropodists or podiatrists, radiographers and optometrists to prescribe any medicine including controlled drugs, according to a prepared and agreed management plan, in collaboration and consultation with the patient and doctor.

ACTIVITY 11.6

Reflection point

Reflect upon how being a nurse prescriber can enhance your practice, identifying the benefits this can have on your ability to autonomously manage your patient care.

Note the benefits this can provide to your patient and employer.

Non-medical prescribing has supported nurses in enabling them to take leading roles in the introduction and development of new and innovative services, such as minor illness clinics, long-term condition management, and has the potential to become a large component of the community nurse role, as suggested in Chapter 18. It is useful for all nurses working in evolving and developing roles to acknowledge the skills and knowledge they bring to the role. These transferable skills will remain key elements of their individual practice, but it is equally important for the nurse to continually reflect upon and identify knowledge deficits and skills required for the role.

ACTIVITY 11.7

Community nursing continues to evolve and develop, and to ensure competency the skills required of the community nurse must be constantly updated and reviewed.

Review the list of common acute exacerbations (Table 11.1) and generate a list of the types of medications that an independent prescriber would prescribe for these conditions.

If you identify any medication classes (i.e. beta-blockers, ACE inhibitors, calcium channel blockers, all used to treat hypertension) that you are unfamiliar with, formulate an action plan to identify how you access and develop further knowledge regarding these medications.

DISCHARGE PLANNING AND AVOIDING HOSPITAL ADMISSION

Well-considered and successful discharge benefits patients and their families, carers and also healthcare professionals and providers. It can minimize delays to discharge, inopportune readmission, and has the potential to maximize cost-effective use of hospital beds.

If at all possible, discharge planning should begin prior to or on admission to hospital, thereby ensuring the efficient provision and coordination of essential services. The main aim of discharge planning is to provide seamless care, assessing, formulating, coordinating and reviewing patient-focused, evidence-based and cost-effective care for patients leaving hospital (NIHII, 2008a).

With increasing pressures as a result of staff shortages and an increasingly high turnover of patients in and out of hospital, discharge planning has become particularly topical. Poor communication between hospital and community staff has historically been a source of problems (Salter, 2001). To avoid unnecessary delays and failures to communicate, developing effective working relationships between the multidisciplinary and primary healthcare teams should be encouraged.

The community nurse is ideally placed to participate in and facilitate discharge planning. Many patients require complex care, and may need careful assessment to decide whether they are ready to go home. Patients, carers and healthcare providers liaise during the planning of the discharge. Families and care providers may also require assessment of their needs

Community nurses have the potential to support a patient and their carer's physical, social and psychological needs when planning the discharge of a patient (Box 11.1). A patient's individual beliefs and culture requirements should be assessed and considered. Case and family conferences should be arranged and should include community staff (Salter, 2001).

Box 11.1 Activities community nurses lead in the discharge process

- Provision of education
- Nominated contact in the discharge planning process
- Promotion of timely, safe and effective discharges
- Review, evaluation and updating the discharge plan
- Prevention of delays to discharge and inappropriate readmissions
- Facilitation of clinical governance via audit, review or research
- Provision of written information and visual information to assist in the discharge process
- Promotion and facilitation of networking with multidisciplinary teams

---

The community nurse should attend regular meetings with hospital colleagues to facilitate patient discharge, and in uncomplicated cases the community nurse might be the main resource. In more complex cases, community nurses may become coordinators and facilitators of the discharge process. Instances of complex care might require a high level of nursing care or a care package that involves a variety of community providers and organizations (Mave, 2001; Scottish Government, 2010).

Other examples of complex discharge include when a patient's needs in the community change from before being admitted. Additional resources may need to be coordinated on discharge, and family and carer needs may intensify and require consideration and inclusion in the discharge process.

The increasing trend of unplanned admissions, especially among the older patient population, has presented as a significant source of pressure on National Health Services. The increase in 'bed days' used as a result of unplanned inpatient admissions during the last 20 years or so has been entirely for service users aged 65 years and over, with the significant majority being accounted for by patients over 80 years (ISD, 2006).

In reality, researchers have found that an ageing population contributes only a small part of the increase in unplanned admissions in older people. Changes in the health of the older population are not responsible for the increase, with evidence suggesting that older people are healthier today than they were 20 years ago (ISD Scotland, 2003; Department of Works and Pensions, 2009).

Social and cultural evolution – including improvements in standards of living and improved access to care – may provide some explanation. Issues external to the historical system of health and social care delivery go only a short way in explaining the upsurge in unplanned admissions.

In an attempt to explain and rationalize the increase, explanations may be found by examining the health and social care delivery system. The way care has been modelled and delivered recently underlies the majority of unplanned admissions. Failure to integrate and coordinate delivery and an absence of anticipatory care focusing on long-term conditions meant the structure of delivery was to wait until unplanned/unanticipated medical events occur. Unplanned admissions are invariably a short-term solution and often not the best option for the patient or for the healthcare system. Fragmentation of the healthcare system has meant that problems are often bumped from one part of the system to another, leading to overloading a part of the system, and culminating in the refusal of unplanned admissions in oversubscribed areas of healthcare delivery. One positive which can be taken from this is that a future change in population demographics involving increases in the number of elderly people does not necessarily have to result in increases in the number of emergency admissions and to overloading the acute system, a key component of the role described in the community matron role profile (DH, 2005).

The majority of the increases in unplanned admissions were for fewer than 5000 elderly individuals over 80 years of age admitted more than three times a year. Therefore, this rather small group of patients would appear to be the largest contributing factor to increased pressure on hospitals, resulting in an increased burden in other areas, such a waiting times and delay in discharging patients.

This has been attributed to this cohort of patients not having been in receipt of appropriate, personalized, coordinated and integrated community-based care. In addition to resulting in detrimental consequences for the healthcare system in its entirety, increased unplanned admissions often predispose to longer stays in hospital and delayed discharge.

Innovation and advances in the ways in which healthcare is delivered to elderly people have the potential to have significant positive impact across the system, and has been a key objective noted by healthcare policy-makers in all four UK countries (ISD, 2006).

The NHS and Social Care Long Term Conditions Model is based upon the large quantity of data collected around experiences and innovations, intended to enhance the health and quality of life of individuals living with a long term condition(s). The NHS and Social Care Long Term Conditions Model mirrors our experience of existing resources. The 'chronic care model' researched and applied by Professor Wagner and colleagues in Seattle, USA, illustrates how patients, healthcare providers and community organizations can work together to deliver improved models of care. It is founded on and relates to the 'pyramid of care' conceived by the American health provider Kaiser Permanente, which streamlines patients with long-term conditions into three discrete groups based on the extent of their condition of need. The model reflects the established models of care and services, especially in primary and community care. The aim of the model is to enhance the health and quality of life of individuals suffering from long-term conditions. This will be achieved by ensuring individual, yet methodical, continuing support for patients, founded on what works best for NHS patients (DH, 2005). This was the model of care first used to implement the community matron role (Lillyman, 2009).

Development and application of risk prediction methodology has the potential to be useful if applied in areas identified for change or improvement. Increase in unplanned/emergency admissions in the older population and increasing willingness to acknowledge that better management of long-term conditions is instrumental in improving healthcare provision, but with the growing threat of demand for healthcare outstripping capacity (NIHII, 2008b). The inability to match variations in capacity and demand for healthcare is one of the key facts which leads to waiting lists, increasing workload and implementation of the community matron role. This can result in increased waiting lists and times to access care and secure an appointment will also increase.

Comparing and assessing the value of providing ongoing follow-up in the community after hospital discharge as an alternative to outpatient visits is indicated. People discharged from hospital may be asked to attend outpatient clinics to check on their progress and continue treatment. Outpatient visits may involve a single acute episode, such as removing sutures, or be ongoing, particularly when patients have terminal or chronic conditions. This follow-up care may be appropriately provided by community nurses, community matrons and care managers, or in other instances may not be required.

More recently the virtual ward, a new concept, has been developed and introduced to help healthcare providers recognize when a patient is at high risk and to facilitate development of expertise related to management of healthcare needs within the community in a more proficient manner. The virtual community ward replicates the positive features of an acute setting within the community by implementing a multidisciplinary team model of healthcare delivery. The concept is considered 'virtual' because the ward is not a reality, and patients remain at home.

The essential members of the team are the GP, community matron and ward clerk, who participate in weekly meetings to simulate the 'ward round'; weekly multidisciplinary meetings include district nurses, community nurses, specialist nurses, physiotherapists, occupational therapists, social workers, pharmacist and any additional allied healthcare role appropriate to the case. Additional information and collective decisions regarding healthcare plans are then shared with the patient's general practice. Use of the virtual ward model is intended to enhance communication between primary care doctors, the acute care setting and the community, reducing unplanned and unnecessary admissions to the acute care setting. The intended outcomes are improvements to patients' health and increased levels of patient satisfaction regarding their healthcare services. Additional intended benefits are a reduction in duplication of healthcare services planned and provided to patients, thereby maximizing available resources and increasing the levels and availability of support for community nurses (Rankin, 2010).

CONCLUSION

In summary, community nursing continues to evolve in responses to changes to service provision and in the type and acuity of the patients cared for in the community.

To facilitate appropriate, personalized coordinated care and to increase the number of patients who can remain in the community receiving care, community nurses and employers are required to ensure that they keep up to date with theory and knowledge and are competent at providing the skills required to care for their patients.

REFERENCES

Bird S, Kurowski W and Dickman G (2004) Evaluating a model of service integration for older people with complex health needs. *The Australasian Evaluation Society.* www.aes.asn.au/.

Budassi Sheehy S (1992) *Emergency Nursing. Principles and Practice, 3rd edn.* St Louis, MO: Mosby.

De Geest S, Moons P, Callens B, *et al.* (2008) Introducing advanced practice nurses/nurse practitioners in health care systems: a framework for reflection and analysis. *Swiss Medical Weekly* 138:621. www.smw.ch/docs/pdf200x/2008/43/smw-12293.PDF.

Department of Health (DH) (2005) *Supporting People with Long Term Conditions: An NHS and Social Care Model to Support Local Innovation and Integration.* London: DH. www.dh.gov.uk/en/Publicationsandstatistics/Publications/PublicationsPolicyAndGuidance/DH_4100252.

Department of Health and Social Security (DHSSPS) (1986) *The Cumberledge Report.* Belfast: DHSSPS.

DHSSPS (2010) *A Northern Ireland Strategy for Nursing and Midwifery 2010–2015.* Belfast: DHSSPS.

Department of Works and Pensions (2009) *Older People Living Longer, Healthier Lives.* (Accessed 10 April 2011) www.dwp.gov.uk/previous-administration-news/press-releases/2009/january-2009/pens097-290109.shtml.

Depression Primary Care (2006) *Patient Health Questionnaire.* www.depression-primarycare.ouk/images.PHQ-9.pdf.

Drennan V, Goodman C, Humphrey C, *et al.* (2007) Entrepreneurial nurses and midwives in the United Kingdom: an integrative review. *Journal of Advanced Nursing* 60:5.

Gravelle H, Mark D, Sheaff R, *et al.* (2006) Impact of case management (Evercare) on frail elderly patients: controlled before and after analysis of quantitative outcome data. *British Medical Journal* 334:31.

Health Foundation (2010) *Acute Care.* London. www.health.org.uk/areas-of-work/topics/acute-care/acute-care/.

Holt I (2008) Role transition in primary care settings. *Quality in Primary Care* 16:117–26.

Horrocks S, Anderson E and Salisbury C (2002) Systematic review of whether nurse practitioners working in primary care can provide equivalent care to doctors. *British Medical Journal* 324.

ISD Scotland (2003) *Increasing Emergency Admissions among Older People in Scotland: a Whole System Account.* Whole System Project Working Paper 1. wwwisd.scot.nhs.uk/isd/files/Whole_System%20_WP1_text.pdf.

ISD Scotland (2006) *SPARRA Report.* Information Services Division, NHS National Services Scotland. www.isdscotland.org/Health-Topics/Health-and-Social-Community-Care/SPARRA/SPARRA-History/SPARRA_Report.pdf.

Jolly K, Bradley F, Sharp S, Smith H and Mant D (1998) Follow-up care in general practice of patients with myocardial infarction or angina pectoris: initial results of the SHIP trial. Southampton Heart Integrated Care Project. *Family Practice* 15:548–55.

Lillyman S, Saxon A and Treml H (2009) An evaluation of the community matron: a literature review. *Journal of Health and Social Care and Improvement.* www.wlv.ac.uk/Deafult.aspx?page=21809.

Montgomery J, Mitty E and Flores S (2008) Resident condition change: should I call 911? *Geriatric Nursing* 29(1):15–26.

Naidoo J and Wills SJ (2009) *Health Promotion: Foundations for Practice*, 3rd edn. Edinburgh: Bailliere Tindall.

National Institute for Health Innovation and Improvement (NIHII) (2008a) *Discharge Planning*. (Accessed 26 September 2011) www.institute.nhs.uk/quality_and_service_improvement_tools/quality_and_service_improvement_tools/discharge_planning.html.

NIHII (2008b) *Demand and Capacity: A Comprehensive Guide.* (Accessed 26 September 2011) www.institute.nhs.uk/quality_and_service_improvement_tools/quality_and_service_improvement_tools/demand_and_capacity_-_a_comprehensive_guide.html.

NHS Education Scotland (2008) *Capability Framework for the Advanced Practitioner*. Edinburgh: NES.

Norridge E (2001) Policy Exchange. *Implementing GP Commissioning*. www.policyexchange.org.uk/images/publications/pdfs/Implementing_GP_Commissioning_-_Apr__11.pdf.

Nursing and Midwifery Council (NMC) (2006) *Standards of Proficiency for Nurse and Midwife Prescribers*. London: NMC.

NMC (2007) *Standards for Medicine Management*. London: NMC.

NMC (2008) *NMC Code of Conduct*. London: NMC.

NMC (2010) *Standards for Pre-registration Nursing Education*. London: NMC.

Pulse (2011) Private firms turn to nurses ahead of 'expensive' GPs. (Accessed 19 September 2011) www.pulsetoday.co.uk/newsarticle-content/-/article_display_list/12704127/private-firms-turn-to-nurses-ahead-of-expensive-gps.

Pulse Today (2008)*Practical Commissioning – Why it Pays to Fund extra GP training in Minor Surgery*. London. www.pulsetoday.co.uk/story.asp?storycode=4117317.

Rankin S (2010)*Wandsworth Community Virtual Wards*. The King's Fund. (Accessed September 2011) www.wandsworth.nhs.uk.

Richards DA, Tawfik J, Meakins J, *et al.* (2002) Nurse telephone triage for same day appointments in general practice: multiple interrupted time series trial of effect on workload and costs. *British Medical Journal* 325:1214.

Roberts S and Kelly C (2007) Developing a career pathway within community nursing. *British Journal of Community Nursing* 12:225–22.

Royal College of Nursing (RCN) (2010) *Advanced Nurse Practitioner Competencies*. (Accessed 25 September 2011) www.rcn.org.uk/__data/assets/pdf_file/0003/146478/003207.pdf.

Ryan CW (1996) Evaluation of patients with chronic headache. *American Family Physician* 54(3):1051–7.

Salter M (2010) Planning for a smooth discharge. *Nursing Times* 97:32.

Scottish Government (2010) Proactive planned & co-ordinated care management in Scotland. (Accessed 11 September 2001) www.scotland.gov.uk/Publications/2010/04/13104221/1.

Thurtle V, Saunders M and Clarridge A (2006) Advancing practice by developing a primary care nursing programme. *British Journal of Community Nursing* 11:167–73.

University of Sheffield (2008) Performance indicators for emergency and urgent care.

Walsh M (2005) *Nurse Practitioners: Clinical Skills and Professional Issues,* 2nd edn. Edinburgh: Elsevier Health Sciences.

Weed LL (1969) *Medical Records, Medical Education and Patient Care. The Problem-oriented Record as a Basic Tool*. Cleveland, OH: Case Western Reserve University.

Woodend K (2006) The role of the community matrons in supporting patients with long term conditions. *Nursing Standard* 20:51–4.

FURTHER RESOURCES

Websites about long-term condition improvement tools:

www.knowledge.scot.nhs.uk/ltc

www.nodelaysscotland.scot.nhs.uk/ServiceImprovement/Tools/Pages/IT194_lean.aspx

www.institute.nhs.uk/quality_and_service_improvement_tools/quality_andservice_
   improvement_tools/lean.html

www.institute.nhs.uk/building_capability/general/lean_thinking.html

www.bqbvindicators.scot.nhs.uk/

www.dh.gov.uk/en/Healthcare/Medicinespharmacyandindustry/DH_121604

Guidelines

www.nice.org.uk

www.sign.ac.uk/

www.earcarecentre.com

www.entnursing.com

www.patient.co.uk

www.depression-primarycare.co.uk

CHAPTER 12

Emerging issues in long-term conditions

Rose Stark

LEARNING OUTCOMES

- Define long-term conditions and identify contributing factors
- Critically analyze the potential impact of long-term conditions on individuals, their families, the health and social care community broadly and nursing in particular, demonstrating awareness of current government policy
- Appraise the resources available to enable and empower professionals and service users
- Compare and contrast the various roles, skills and interventions involved in the management of long-term conditions
- Discuss the emerging role of the community nurse in addressing mental health issues in long-term conditions

INTRODUCTION

There has been a tendency to define long-term conditions (LTCs) as those without cure, but more recently there has been a different approach, for example describing LTCs as

> the irreversible presence, accumulation, or latency of disease states or impairments that involve the total human environment for supportive care and self-care, maintenance of function and prevention of further disability.
>
> *(Curtin and Lubkin, cited in Larsen and Lubkin, 2009: 5)*

The crucial role of nursing is stressed by Larsen and Lubkin (2009), who suggest that LTC care is largely within a nursing rather than a medical domain. Not least among the challenges is the fact that many people have multiple or complex conditions.

The purpose of this chapter is to explore a number of principles that are pertinent to working with people with LTCs, their carers and their families. Themes to be raised in this chapter include patient/user focus, including self-care, promoting and supporting behaviour change, medicines management, aspects of mental health, issues of vulnerability and case management.

POLICY DRIVERS AND GOVERNMENT STRATEGY

Individuals with LTCs present an increasing focus for health and social care professionals and society as a whole because of factors such as longer life expectancy and improved technological and medical advances. It is estimated that 17.5 million people are living with an LTC in this country and that many more are undiagnosed (DH, 2005b). This focus, therefore, includes not only the management and care of individuals with LTCs, but also prevention, early diagnosis and engagement, which need to be profoundly patient centred in order to achieve better health outcomes.

The underpinning philosophy is that individuals prefer to be cared for in their own homes, wishing to avoid hospital admissions, and that they will have a choice about their care from diagnosis to end of life and to remain as autonomous as possible. This is not only for the patient's benefit (and not all patients will concur), but also because of the increasing cost to society. Despite living longer, the population is not living healthier. This is even more significant for those who are less affluent. Marmot (2010) points out that there is a 13-year difference in disability-free life expectancy between the rich and poor in our society.

Government policy documents have reflected the complexity and breadth of addressing conditions for more than two decades; an example of this is *The National Service Framework for Long-term Conditions* (DH, 2005a). This document is the culmination of a series of National Service Framework (NSF) publications which were published by the previous government from 1999. Although it was developed to address neurological LTCs, its 14 Quality Requirements (QRs) are transferable to other conditions and specific groups. The QRs address prevention, early diagnosis, quality care provision, optimizing patient choice, provision of rehabilitation and appropriate end-of-life care. This reflects the idea of a pathway or continuum of care, in which community nurses have a significant contribution at nearly all levels (DH, 2005a).

The purpose of these strategy documents and policies has been to set out standards of care and managementthat provide frameworks on which can be built a network of relevant services. The National Institute for Clinical Excellence (NICE) is a key source of information and guidance. Please see Further resources at the end of this chapter for more advice. In most cases, documents relating to England have been referred to for convenience in this chapter, although materials from other countries will be included (see www.dh.gov.uk). Specific information from other parts of the UK can be accessed on the following websites: www.wales.nhs.uk; www.dhsspsni.gov.uk; www.scot.nhs.uk.

Despite some directional change, the new coalition government has included specifications for delivering and monitoring LTC care in the recent White Paper, *Liberating the NHS – Legislative Framework and Next Steps* (DH, 2010a). An NHS Outcomes Framework is set out that has five domains, the second of which is called *Enhancing Quality of Life for People with LTCs*. Other domains are also concerned with LTCs. The domains are underpinned by 150 quality standards that have been or will be developed by NICE, one of which will be the subject of an activity below.

The three domains of quality to be assessed together include effectiveness, safety and patients' experience of treatment and care.

The focus on user involvement, patient choice and self-care has resulted in a number of documents that are worth consulting as they set the scene for LTC management which is ongoing. They include *Our Health Our Care Our Say* (DH, 2006a), *Supporting People with Long-Term Conditions* (DH, 2005b) and *Supporting People with Long-term Conditions to Self Care* (DH, 2006b).

A number of other pieces of legislation and policies apply. These include the Human Rights Act (1998), the Mental Capacity Act (2005) and the Equality Act (2010). The Nursing and Midwifery Council (NMC) is a vital source of information for the Standards of Conduct, Performance and Ethics for Nurses and Midwives (2008). The NMC also provides invaluable guidance on consent, confidentiality, data protection, record keeping, safeguarding adults and medicines management.

PATIENT PERSPECTIVE AND PSYCHOLOGICAL RESPONSES TO DIAGNOSES

A diagnosis of an LTC can be devastating. When the individual has been experiencing symptoms for some time and anxiously awaiting results, there may be a period of feeling relieved. However, depending on personal perspectives and circumstances, together with the nature of the condition, the diagnosis normally means that the person's life will never be the same again. Learning to live with the exigencies of the condition can pose major challenges: disability, pain, anxiety, fear and lack of knowledge and understanding are just some. Many losses can be incurred: independence and status, financial stability, and social connections, particularly if employment is affected. Body image may be affected and personal relationships may suffer. Individual coping mechanisms will vary and a range of emotions is likely to occur.

Nichols (2003) describes various responses following diagnosis, including shock, denial, distress with symptoms and interventions, exaggerated independence alternating with collapse into dependency. Emotionally there may be feelings of stress, guilt and resentment. Nichols also discussed three levels of intervention. Level 1 includes health professionals' awareness and understanding and ability to communicate with patients. Level 2 involves monitoring, providing support, counselling, advocacy and referral. Level 3 refers to specialist therapeutic interventions.

ACTIVITY 12.1

Reflection point
The first activity invites reflection on what may be needed to guide you as a health professional, but starting with a patient's view.

Scenario
You have recently been diagnosed with type 2 diabetes. Please access the Diabetes UK website www.diabetesuk.org and reflect on how helpful this could be for you. Do you discover more about the condition and what to expect in

terms of care and support? Do you feel that it gives you some more confidence in discussing your condition with healthcare professionals? Navigate through the various parts of the site and consider the presentation and content. You may wish to look at specific aspects that interest you; for example, if you have visual impairment or perhaps you want to know more about healthy eating.

Reflection

Is the site useful for you as a health professional?

How might this resource complement the management provided by the healthcare team?

How can you make this information available to patients who do not have access to the Internet?

DEVELOPING A PATIENT-CENTRED APPROACH: SELF-CARE AND SELF-MANAGEMENT

'The term self management has been defined as: whatever we do to make the most of our lives by coping with our difficulties and making the most of what we have' (Martyn, 2002, cited in DH, 2006b: 1). Self-care refers to a range of activities by the patient that can include lifestyle change or taking greater responsibility for medicines or dressings. Some patients will get involved in Expert Patient Programmes or other structured education programmes designed to deal with specific issues.

Self-care has become a major aspect of LTC management. The Health and Social Care Model (Fig. 12.1) illustrates the levels of dependency of patients on health and social care professionals. The base of the pyramid and the second level contain more

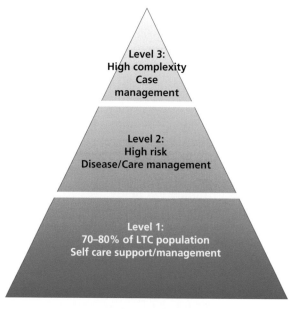

Figure 12.1 Health and Social Care Model (DH, 2005b).

than 80% of the population who are affected by LTCs. This is where opportunities for self-care predominate. However, even for the top 20% who suffer from complex conditions, there is potential for some degree of self-care. The purpose of this section of the chapter is to introduce ideas that will encourage community nurses to reflect upon and enhance their communication skills. The Health and Social Care Model will be further alluded to below in the discussion on case management

Despite its importance, there are many barriers to patients adopting self-care skills. Health professionals need to question their approach to patients. Morrison and Bennett (2006) remind us that in most situations the health professional maintains control. Advice and standard information are often imparted to patients, who are expected to act on this. People respond in various ways to a diagnosis and their attitudes are likely to vary over time. In order for LTC management to be more effective, the patient's or carer's perceptions must be the starting point. In some situations, the patient may not wish to alter their behaviour; the elderly man with severe lung disease for example who may be adamant that he will not quit smoking no matter what intervention is offered. This may indeed be his ultimate decision but the required skill for the health professional is in knowing where change is possible and what actions to take. This will be discussed in the section on helping people to change behaviour.

Levels of literacy and numeracy combined with beliefs about health and ability to process information are highly variable. Factors include age, gender, culture, religion and social class. It is a sobering thought that a significant percentage of the population of the UK has a literacy capacity that is below the level needed to discuss a condition effectively with a doctor. In the UK, one adult in six does not have the literacy skills of an 11 year old whereas one adult in two does not have even this level of functional numeracy. Adapting behaviour and increasing the level of self-care are both dependent upon effective communication. Skilled for Health provides information and resources to promote literacy (www.continyou.org.uk). It is worthwhile considering how literacy and numeracy can be improved at individual, local and national levels.

HELPING PEOPLE TO CHANGE BEHAVIOUR, INCLUDING MOTIVATIONAL INTERVIEWING

The Health Belief Model, proposed by Rosenstock (1966) and modified by Becker (1974), cited in Naidoo and Wills (2009), describes a set of functions that impacts on decision-making. The person's perceptions in terms of their susceptibility to a condition and severity of a disease will be modified by demographic and sociopsychological variables. The knowledge base and perceived threat are combined with triggers such as familial attitudes and media influence that will ultimately determine whether the person will take a specific action. The person's confidence is also a factor: what is their 'locus of control'? (Morrison and Bennett, 2006). Do they believe that the events that govern their lives are initiated from within or outside themselves? Does he or she feel they have the ability to make desired change? An appropriate level of support may make the difference.

This can be addressed further by assessing the person's 'readiness to change'. The Stages of Change model was originally formulated by Prochasta and Di Clemente (1984, cited by Naidoo and Wills, 2009). Basically there are four stages in this model. The first is pre-contemplation, where the individual is not yet ready to make the change; second is contemplation, where the person is open to altering behaviour. The remaining stages involve planning for and maintaining change. This is ultimately about patient choice. The skilled communicator senses when the person has made their 'final' decision about an aspect of behaviour change and will leave the 'door open' so that the issue can be approached again if desired.

There are times though when intervention can result in a shift from pre-contemplation. Motivational interviewing (MI) may provide a the key to this. Often, when faced with the notion of making lifestyle changes, a person will feel a degree of conflict about whether to take action. It is in this area of ambivalence that the MI practitioner seeks to make a difference. MI was developed by William Miller in the 1980s. He and his colleagues were psychologists working in the area of substance abuse. More recently, it has been found to be useful in many situations where behaviour change is desirable. The central idea is that the partnership between the patient and health professional includes exploration of this ambivalence to see if there is a way of moving forward by taking account of 'change talk' expressed by the patient. This includes such statements as 'I wish I could...' 'It would be better if ...'. Careful listening and clarification, combined with a non-judgemental, empathic and encouraging attitude, will lead the patient to discover and believe in their own motivation and abilities and make plans for taking action. Rollnick *et al.* (2008) set out the four Guiding Principles (resisting the righting reflex, understanding patient motivation, listening to and empowering the patient). Three Core Skills are crucial to achieving this (asking, listening and informing). These are all underpinned by the spint of MI, which has three components (collaboration, evocation and patient autonomy). The authors continue by discussing the desired client-centred counselling skills.

Community nurses may wish to develop such skills to enable them to have more effective relationships with patients who are grappling with the challenges of behaviour change. Reading a relevant textbook will raise awareness, so too will accessing websites (see www.motivationalinterview.org) where information is available on formal training. Some will feel it is unnecessary to undergo such training, although it may be enough to include features of the techniques into their own practice. Consider whether setting up local workshops is feasible, possibly with multidisciplinary involvement.

CASE MANAGEMENT AS PART OF THE HEALTH AND SOCIAL CARE MODEL

The principle of this particular model of case management is that there is a 'person who acts as both provider and procurer of care and takes responsibility for ensuring that all health and social care needs are met, so that the patient's condition stays as stable as possible and well being is increased'.

(DH, 2005b)

Within the UK, principles of management are common, although different approaches have been adopted in terms of service structure and delivery. The English and Scottish models will be referred to below.

ACTIVITY 12.2

This activity is designed to highlight the needs of the patient with multiple or complex conditions and increase awareness of the resources available to provide support in the community.

Scenario

Mr A is a new patient in the practice. He is a 70-year-old man with chronic obstructive pulmonary disease (COPD) and has been referred to the practice nurse because he is having some difficulty in using his inhaled medication. He has had several hospital admissions and also suffers from Parkinson's disease, has high blood pressure and rheumatoid arthritis. What skills are required to undertake a full assessment? What resources will be required to provide ongoing care, including input from other nurses, health professionals and agencies? How will he be referred and who will coordinate his care? Which policy documents underpin and support relevant standards of care?

In recent decades, as greater longevity has combined with increasing levels of illness and disability, health and social care strategists in several countries have sought to address the complex needs of those individuals with serious or multiple medical conditions. Companies such as Evercare and Kaiser Permanente in the United States, for example, have developed integrated systems to deliver intensive services for people with LTCs. For more background on this, please see Snodden (2010). Despite differences between the configuration of healthcare provision – especially in terms of funding – between the UK and other countries, it was felt that much could be gained by adopting similar approaches. National Service Frameworks and other standards documents were frameworks within the UK system on which to develop locally relevant systems of care.

Mr A is an example of a patient at the top of the Health and Social Care pyramid; he has highly complex needs. His assessment and ongoing care will require a high level of expertise and support from various professionals and agencies. In order to improve health outcomes and quality of life for the patient, and also aiming to reduce the level of unnecessary hospital admissions, a number of advanced nursing roles were developed in England following the publication of the document *Supporting People with Long-term Conditions* (DH, 2005b). One of these roles is the community matron (CM). The Scottish model for managing complex conditions will be described at the end of this section.

The CM (or equivalent practitioner) will be competent both in terms of advanced clinical (or social work) practice and case management. The skills required include advanced assessment skills, competence in LTC management. The CM will be an independent prescriber. The CM is an autonomous practitioner with scope for high-level decision-making to support Mr A. CMs normally will have been senior nurses from specialist hospital settings and from community nursing.

In terms of direct management and care, the CM's skills and depth of knowledge will ensure that Mr A's condition is closely monitored. For example, the CM will have a major role in medicines management. Mr A will potentially be taking several medicines for each of his conditions, including pain relief. In accordance with the regulations set down in *Standards for Medicines Management* (NMC, 2007/2010), the CM can make prescribing decisions according to individual competence. An example of this is management of COPD where the CM can work closely with the patient, supporting concordance and effective use of medication. These patients often suffer from exacerbations of their condition which require hospital admission. However, the CM can encourage self-care not only by teaching and providing information but also by prescribing a 'rescue pack' for the patient to use when he feels his condition is deteriorating. The pack consists of antibiotics and steroids, thus a hospital admission is avoided.

Mr A will require input from several other professionals. The CM is also likely to be his case manager. The CM is not always a case manager. Depending upon the patient's needs, a mental health professional, allied health professional or social worker may fulfil this role. This means that the CM will coordinate Mr A's care. This includes referral to other health departments and wider agencies. The skills required for this include developing effective networking and fostering collaborative relationships with others, at times breaking down traditional barriers. For example, referrals from the CM will be accepted by hospital consultants.

The virtual ward is another example of case management for heavily dependent patients. This is also discussed in Chapter 11. Tools for predicting which patients are likely to be re-hospitalized have emerged in recent years (see www.kingsfund.org.uk for further information). Some community trusts have developed virtual ward environments for those who have a high risk of readmission. The community nurse is at the centre of this and still has a major role in monitoring and coordinating care. The 'ward' mirrors an actual hospital setting but the patient remains in their own home, with ward rounds including involvement of the relevant professionals who network 'electronically' making decisions and plans for ongoing care.

The Scottish government reported on a review of community nursing in 2007 which introduced an integrated service model based on 'seven elements of nursing in the community'. The elements focus on care and support including self-care, multidisciplinary and agency collaboration, prevention and service coordination. This was part of a review of the health system as a whole that included LTC care and provision for those with complex conditions. This is documented in *Delivering for Health* (Scottish Executive, 2005), where measures similar to those in other parts of the UK are recommended, but the role of care coordinator is unspecified. The role of general practice is highlighted, although it is stated that a local decision should be taken as to who is best placed to deliver this element. It could be a GP, nurse, allied health professional or social worker. For readers in Scotland, it would be useful to explore how this role has developed within nursing and other disciplines.

EXPLORING MENTAL HEALTH ISSUES IN LONG-TERM CONDITIONS CARE

The community nurse who does not have formal learning in mental health may find this a challenging area of care. Yet it can no longer be ignored in LTC management. Depression is two to three times more common in patients with LTCs, affecting approximately 20% of them (NICE, 2009). Severe mental health conditions will continue to be managed by mental health teams, but recently much work has been carried out which shows that with a skilled, collaborative approach, mild to moderate levels of depression can be managed by non-mental health professionals.

For community nurses this may be daunting but it is important to consider that an assessment which does not include mental health is arguably not holistic, and a separation of the physical and mental aspects of the individual renders them less than a person and the assessment incomplete. The National Collaborating Centre for Mental Health (NCCMH) suggests that 'treating depression in people with long term physical health problems has the potential to increase their quality of life and life expectancy' (NICE, 2009: 6). Gask *et al.* (2009) cite the work of a number of writers who continue to research and survey the skills of general practitioners and nurses in the community who are seeking opportunities for improved working within and between teams and are calling for greater training to enhance this.

To enable this, the nurse needs to develop appropriate skills to be able to determine whether assessment, advice and support are enough to ensure adequate care or whether the patient needs referral elsewhere, usually via the GP. NCCMH (NICE, 2009) has produced clear guidance on how a non-mental health professional can conduct a depression assessment. The practitioner is advised to ask the following questions:

- During the last month, have you often been bothered by feeling down, depressed or hopeless?
- During the last month, have you often been bothered by having little interest or pleasure in doing things?

The practitioner is also advised to ask whether the person has contemplated suicide. If the patient answers 'yes' this will warrant immediate referral to mental health services.

ACTIVITY 12.3

Access the NICE document referred to above on www.nice.org.uk/CG91. Read the document, particularly the early sections from pages 1–24. Discuss the guidelines with your team leader and clarify what your team's position is on this – you may wish to include it as an agenda item in a team meeting.

What do the team feel is their role in terms of depression in LTC care?

Is there collaboration with the wider healthcare team, especially the GP?

Is there affective working between the primary healthcare team, mental health professionals and other statutory and non-statutory agencies?

What relevant self-care or expert patient programmes are available for your local population?

How can you and your colleagues gain competence and confidence in this area of practice?

The purpose of this section of the chapter is to stimulate reflection on what skills and underpinning knowledge will be needed to ensure that patients receive optimum mental healthcare. There are two ways in which community nurses can address management of mental health. The first is by striving to develop effective working relationships with mental health colleagues and being aware of when it is appropriate to refer to the service. The second is to explore how their own skills can be developed.

CARING FOR PEOPLE WITH DEMENTIA

Dementia presents an increasing problem for our society. Currently, there are 700 000 people with dementia in the UK (DH, 2009). Projected figures for the condition suggest that the cost to society will rise considerably. Today's figures are estimated to cost £17 billion. In 2038, there are likely to be 1.4 million sufferers at a cost of over £50 billion.

Dementia is prevalent in all ethnic groups and both genders, and although it is most common in the over 65 age group, there are at least 15 000 sufferers in younger age groups. One of the reasons why the numbers are increasing in this group is that those living with certain congenital conditions, for example Down's syndrome, are living longer and they are at higher risk of developing dementia. There are different types of the disease, of which is Alzheimer's disease is common; a more detailed account of dementias and general advice can be found at www.alzheimers.org.uk.

The condition presents significant challenges not only for individuals but also for care providers for several reasons. Issues of vulnerability and mental capacity can be difficult to assess and can be highly sensitive. For example, the person with dementia may wish to make decisions about financial matters or end-of-life care in advance of losing the ability to do so. However, their wishes may not be realistic if matters subsequently take an unpredicted course. Risk assessment is often required on a daily basis. One carer, mindful of her spouse's quality of life, prefers the term risk–benefit assessment as she 'allows' him out alone rather than confining him to the house as he loves the outdoors.

It can be particularly distressing for family members and carers who feel they have lost the person. One of the many dilemmas described by carers is that the person may 'time travel' to a time when they were young, their parents were alive, children were yet to be born and the carer was perceived to be young and desirable – so who is the 'grey-haired old woman' who has invaded the household? Or the reflection in the mirror presents as an intruder, especially when they start waving their arms around in a threatening manner. The person with dementia may ask when his or her mother is coming home. The brutal truth may be inadvisable, as the person is likely to mourn over and over again. Discussing aspects of the person's mother with the patient until he or she is satisfied can be a better approach. Carers have described the experience of living with a person with diminishing life skills and cognition as being extremely painful emotionally, and can be even physically risky at times. A carer addressed the problem of the patient passing urine onto the toilet floor. Through close observation, she discovered that the visual deficiency that can develop was preventing her husband from differentiating between the white toilet mat and the white floor. When she removed the mat, the problem eased. Removing mirrors from the home also reduced the issue of mistaken identity.

What is being highlighted here is the crucial importance of listening to and supporting the patient and carer. *The National Dementia Strategy* (DH, 2009) sets out a 5-year plan for dealing with dementia. This is made up of three key steps and 17 objectives, which include early diagnosis, as this leads to better treatment options, ensuring better knowledge about the condition and the setting up of improved accessible services, better support and ongoing research.

THE IMPACT OF A LONG-TERM CONDITION ON A YOUNGER FAMILY

ACTIVITY 12.4

The purpose of this exercise is for the new community nurse to explore, reflect upon and address potential risks for the family.

Scenario

A 45-year-old woman (Mrs B) has been referred to you for assessment. She has been diagnosed with multiple sclerosis, having had distressing neurological symptoms for some weeks. She is having problems going out as she tends to lose her balance and she is very concerned about difficulties she has with continence. Prior to her diagnosis, she had been the main wage earner in the household, and was employed as an administrator in a local government department. She has a husband and two children aged 13 years and 9 years.

Consider your assessment of this woman and what risks there may be in terms of her physical and psychosocial wellbeing. What are the risks for her husband and children? How can these risks be addressed by community nursing, the wider health and social care agencies and non-statutory sector? It may help to create a mind map or spider diagram of the various teams who need to be involved.

In the distressing and complex situation in Activity 12.4, there are numerous aspects to consider. The physical aspects alone present profound implications for life change. They include disability, risk of falls, loss of sensation, pain fatigue, and difficulties in getting to the toilet. Is the physical environment suitable? Later, there may be problems with tissue viability.

Psychological aspects are at least as challenging. Will Mrs B be able to continue working? If not, there may be an economic risk to the family. What about the home environment? What about her status within the family, the local community and the workplace? Will her relationship with her husband be threatened? Will a sexual relationship still be possible? What are her concerns for her health in future – how will she deal with the unpredictable nature of her condition? What are Mr B's needs? Is he prepared for potential caring responsibilities?

There are a number of risks in this situation. The responses of any of the individuals affected can vary. There may be some very positive outcomes, high levels of support and care within the family for instance. But by contrast, there may be relationship or family breakdown, substance misuse or domestic violence. Children's schooling may be disrupted. Morrison and Bennett (2006) discuss caring in some detail, describing 'helpful and unhelpful caring'. The former can result in better outcomes including increased levels of satisfaction for the carer and higher levels of self-care for the patient. The latter can lead to physical health problems but also severe emotional and psychological problems, for example feeling resentful and trapped or disappointed that life expectations have been thwarted.

The community nurse needs to be fully aware of the various agencies that can offer support in this situation, but sensitive ongoing monitoring of the situation is required. What is the appropriate action if domestic violence is suspected?

See Further resources for websites providing useful information.

DEVELOPING COMPETENCE IN LONG-TERM CONDITIONS MANAGEMENT

This chapter has been designed to reflect current thinking in terms of how healthcare services will be provided by nurses and their multidisciplinary and interagency colleagues, both now and in future. The vision is to promote patient and carer focus and involvement together with wider team collaboration to enhance shared learning, desired health outcomes and improved quality of life patients and those close to them. In *Modernising Nursing Careers: Setting the Direction* (DH, 2006c), the Chief Nursing Officer stressed the need for a change in thinking about how nursing care is to be delivered in future throughout the UK, partly in recognition of the impact of LTCs.

There are several community nursing disciplines involved and many roles continue to be developed. Some roles are designed to actively prevent LTCs. Consider, for example, the work of the school nurse with childhood obesity or the general practice nurse with management of asthma. Other roles focus more specifically with care and treatment, for example district nurses, specialist nurses and community matrons. Other roles which are vital include mental health nurses and community children's nurses. It may be useful to discover which roles, teams and wider networks have been set up in your local area.

Learning resources include formal education programmes provided by higher education institutes, skills training delivered by various bodies both within the NHS and privately. Details of competencies required in specific areas of care can be accessed from the Skills for Health website, which informs job descriptions and Knowledge and Skills Framework outlines for those working in the NHS (www.skillsforhealth.org.uk). The Royal College of Nursing library is a rich source of information (www.rcn.org).

It is also important to assess current abilities and to reflect on learning from colleagues and patients. Local organizations will have developed strategies and formularies based on national guidelines; these usually include tissue viability, palliative care, continence, nutritional assessment tools and more. Linked to these, further useful direction is provided in the recently updated *Essence of Care* documents (DH, 2010b).

It may be useful to revisit theoretical models of nursing. The Model of Living and the Model of Nursing provide a comprehensive guide to assessing individuals at all stages in terms of their daily activities and quality of life in the context of maintaining a safe environment (Holland *et al.*, 2008). Finally, do consider the research, supervisory, leadership and influencing skills that are required in this area of healthcare.

CONCLUSION

The ideas and discussion that have been presented in this chapter are the tip of the iceberg in terms of LTCs. The aim has been to introduce the new community nurse to various contemporary and urgent issues which are evolving, not only for nursing but for health and social care and society as a whole. If the challenges posed by LTCs are to be successfully tackled, their management requires a radical overhaul in thinking. It is imperative that the new generation of nurses in all sectors consider their role in terms of prevention, advocacy, support and care for individuals, families and groups who are affected by LTCs. It is vital that these professionals acquire, maintain and update their skills in integrating the best of traditional ways of working with proficiency in developing more appropriate techniques for the future healthcare environment. This includes enhancing opportunities for collaborative and partnership working with health and social care colleagues and constantly reflecting on what patient focus really means when addressing the needs of those who are experiencing the effects of LTCs. It is imperative that professionals who work with those affected by LTCs have a deep appreciation of self-care so that patients and carers can be fully supported to gain improved quality of life, despite the condition and its challenges.

REFERENCES

Department of Health (DH) (2005a) *The National Service Framework for Long Term Conditions.* London: The Stationery Office.

DH (2005b) *Supporting People with Long-Term Conditions: liberating the talents of nurses who care for people with long-term conditions.* London: DH.

DH (2006a) *Our Health Our Care Our Say.* London: DH.

DH (2006b) *Supporting People with Long-Term Conditions to Self Care.* London: DH.

DH (2006c) *Modernising Nursing Careers: Setting the Direction.* London: DH.

DH (2009) *The National Dementia Strategy.* London: The Stationery Office.

DH (2010a) *Liberating the NHS – Legislative Framework and Next Steps.* London: The Stationery Office.

DH (2010b) *Essence of Care.* www.dh.gov.uk/cno.

Gask L, Lester H, Kendrick T and Peveler R (2009) (eds) *Primary Care Mental Health.* London: Royal College of Psychiatrists Publications.

Holland K, Jenkins J, Solomon J and Whittam S (2008) *Applying the Roper Logan Tierney Model in Practice,* 2nd edn. London: Churchill Livingstone/Elsevier.

Larsen PD and Lubkin I (2009) *Chronic Illness: Impact and Intervention*, 7th edn. London: Jones and Bartlett Publishers.

Marmot M (2010) *Fair Society Healthier Lives: The Marmot Review.* www.marmotreview.org (Accessed January 2011).

Morrison V and Bennet P (2006) *An Introduction to Health Psychology.* Harlow: Pearson/ Prentice Hall.

Naidoo J and Wills J (2009) *Foundations for Health Promotion,* 3rd edn. London: Bailliere Tindall/Elsevier.

National Institute for Health and Clinical Excellence (NICE) (2009) National Collaborating Centre for Mental Health. *Depression in Adults with a Chronic Physical Health Problem.* Clinical Guideline 91. London: NICE.

Nichols K (2003) *Psychological Care for Ill and Injured People – A Clinical Guide.* Maidenhead: Open University Press.

Nursing and Midwifery Council (NMC) (2007/2010) *Standards for Medicines Management.* London: NMC.

Rollnick S, Miller WR and Butler C (2008) *Motivational Interviewing in Health Care: Helping Patients to Change Behaviour.* New York: The Guilford Press.

Scottish Executive (2005) *Delivering for Health – Section Two. Making Improvement Happen.* (Accessed 14/9/11) www.scotland.gov.uk/Publications/2005/11/02102635/26372.

Scottish Government (2007) *Visible, Accessible and Integrated Care Report of the Review of Nursing in the Community in Scotland.* (Accessed 17 November 2011) www.scotland .gov.uk/Publications/2007/07/16091605/4.

Snodden J (2010) *Case Management of Long Term Conditions: Principles and Practices for Nurses.* Oxford: Wiley Blackwell.

FURTHER READING

Carrier J (2009) *Managing Long Term Conditions and Chronic Illness in Primary Care.* Abingdon: Routledge.

Margereson C and Trenoweth S (2010) (eds) *Developing Holistic Care for Long Term Conditions.* Oxford: Routledge.

McVeigh H (ed.) (2009) *Fundamental Aspects of Long Term Conditions*. London: Quay Books.

Presho M (2008) *Managing Long Term Conditions: A Social Model for Community Practice*. Chichester: Wiley Blackwell.

FURTHER RESOURCES

There is an infinite number of relevant materials available via textbooks and websites. Community nurses are advised to keep up to date with developments in LTCs by accessing the DH website regularly. In addition to the websites mentioned below, it is worth noting that almost all conditions will have at least one dedicated website. Some will have several, with a number more relevant for health professionals, for example the British Thoracic Society www.brit-thoracic.org.uk

(www.nmc-uk.org/nurses-and-midwives)

(see www.expertpatients.co.uk)

(www.learndirect.co.uk)

Most consumer-led sites are involved in advocacy and campaigning. Good examples are www.mind.org.uk and www.ageuk.org

Patient and carer focused sites include:

www.carersuk.org

NHS Choices at www.nhs.uk

www.patient.co.uk

www.mssociety.org.uk;

Clinical information can be accessed at the following sites:

www.cks.nhs.uk

www.library.nhs.uk

www.thecochranelibrary.com

www.nice.nhs.uk

Providing quality in end-of-life care

Gina King

INTRODUCTION

The term 'end-of-life care' (EoLC) has become a new phenomenon and it encompasses all aspects of care at the end of an individual's life. Rather than describing care as palliative, supportive or terminal, EoLC is now the preferred term when identifying a person who is in the final stages of life, which may last years, months, weeks or days. The importance of this term is that it helps professionals acknowledge and more actively plan ahead for the care that may be needed to optimize quality of life and focus on living rather than dying. The six steps of the end-of-life (EoL) pathway outlined in the EoLC Strategy (DH, 2008) have been used to structure this chapter and each one will be discussed in turn.

Each year in England around half a million people die, of which two-thirds are aged over 75 years. Most deaths (58%) occur in NHS hospitals, with around 18% occurring at home, 17% in care homes, 4% in hospices and 3% elsewhere. The evidence suggests 56% would prefer to die at home (DH, 2008), demonstrating a vast difference in preferences and actual place of death. There are several contributing factors that can influence this outcome. The older the population, the more likely it is that they have complex needs and require integrated care packages (Ellershaw and Murphy, 2005). It addition, the need for hospital admissions increases due to disease progression and carer crises, all of which reduce the patient's and family's confidence and ability to cope with dying at home (Munday *et al.,* 2007). The number of deaths is set to increase by 17% between 2012 and 2020 in England and Wales (Ellershaw and Murphy, 2005), which will have a significant impact on community service provision and nurses will need to be equipped with the appropriate knowledge and skills so they can offer high-quality care (DH, 2009a).

The aim of high-quality EoLC is to support all individuals with advanced, progressive and incurable illnesses regardless of diagnosis, stage or setting, to live as well as possible until they die, therefore to be able to live with a quality of life and have mechanisms in place to enable discussions and make informed decisions about their preferences and choices so they die where and how they choose (DH, 2008). The National Council for Palliative Care (NCPC) stresses the importance of identifying the supportive and palliative needs of both patients and family throughout the last phase of life and into bereavement, which includes the management of pain and other symptoms and provision of psychological, social, spiritual and practical support (NCHSPCS, 2002).

Over the past century the demographics of dying in relation to age profile, cause and place of death has changed fundamentally, as previously a greater number of deaths either occurred in childhood or as young adults. As a result, the public's social contact with dying has been reduced and an experience of someone dying that is close to them does not tend to occur until later in their own lives (Hanks *et al.*, 2010). The stigma associated with dying in society today means that we do not tend to discuss death and dying openly, causing difficulties in communication when end of life approaches either for the individual concerned or someone close to them (Seymour *et al.*, 2010).

Each individual has their own perspective in terms of what constitutes a 'good death', and the majority agree that it is about

- being treated as an individual, with dignity and respect
- being without pain and other symptoms
- being in familiar surroundings
- being in the company of close family and/or friends (DH, 2008).

These elements of high-quality EoLC are important to achieve for the individual concerned and especially for the family if we respect the words of Dame Cecily Saunders, the founder of the Hospice movement, when she stated 'How people die remains in the memory of those who live on' (Saunders, 1989).

ACTIVITY 13.1

Reflection point
Reflect on a patient that you have cared for who has died. Consider what you felt about their quality of life and the care received.

END-OF-LIFE CARE STRATEGY

The end-of-life care strategy was produced in July 2008 by the Department of Health and was the first ever paper to identify that there was a need for equitable and standardized care for all individuals regardless of their diagnosis, setting or stage (Gray, 2011). Historically, those with a cancer diagnosis had easier access to care, resources and services (NAO, 2008). Other reports and White Papers, such as the NICE guidance for improving palliative and supportive care (NICE, 2004), *Our Health, Our Care, Our Say* (DH, 2006), *Transforming Community Services* (DH, 2009b) *Dementia Strategy* (DH, 2009c) and *EoLC and Neurological Strategy* (2010), have reinforced the call for all health, social and voluntary care professionals and organizations to examine their service provision in order to provide good-quality EoLC.

The EoLC Strategy (DH, 2008) provides processes and themes for organizations and individual professionals involved in the provision of EoLC to use in developing practice and improving the delivery of care over a 10-year plan (Gray, 2011). Its overall aim is to provide high-quality care for all at the end of life, not just within hospices and specialist palliative care services but in other care settings as well (Gray, 2011). The paper is based on the following 12 principles:

1 Raising the profile on death and dying
2 Strategically commissioning services to provide the best quality care
3 Identifying people approaching the end of life
4 Care planning
5 Coordination of care
6 Rapid access to care
7 Delivery of high quality services in all locations
8 The last days of life and care after death
9 Involving and supporting for carers
10 Education and training and continuing professional development
11 Measurement and research
12 Funding to support these principles

(DH, 2008)

In community nursing practice, the six steps of the EoL Pathway outline in the EoLC strategy is a useful tool to help apply theory to practice (Fig. 13.1).

Step 1: Discussions as EoLC approaches: identification of people approaching the end of life and initiating discussions about preferences for EoLC

The key aspect of the EoL pathway is to identify those patients who are approaching the end of their life. Historically, this has presented a challenge not only in relation to prognostic tools that can be complex to use, but also in acknowledging the time when care becomes palliative as opposed to curative. However, unless all members of the multidisciplinary team (MDT) work together to identify patients regardless of their diagnosis, discussions around preferences and options will not take place, families and friends will not be appropriately supported and patients will not achieve a good death (Hubbard, 2011). The Gold Standards Framework advocated by the *End of Life Care Strategy* (DH, 2008) has produced a 'Prognostic Indicator Guidance' which outlines the Karnofsky Performance Status Score, the three main disease trajectories (cancer, neurological conditions and dementia/frailty) and, mostly importantly, recommended the adoption of the 'surprise question', Would

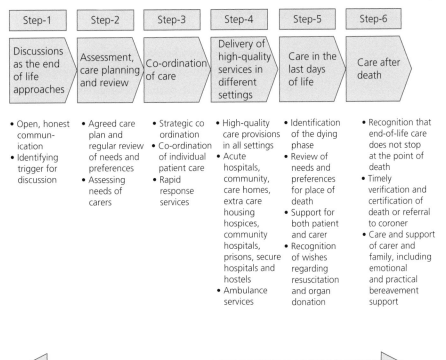

Figure 13.1 The six steps of the EoL Pathway outlined in the EoLC Strategy (DOH, 2008). With kind permission from the National End of Life Care Programme.

you be surprised if this patient were to die in the next 6–12 months? (GSF, 2008). This question has been regarded as one of the most effective instruments in identifying EoLC because of its simplicity and application to any diagnosis or just old age (Boyd and Murray, 2010).

Good communication skills are essential not only to initiate conversations and discussions with patients and their families as EoLC approaches but also to provide support, help and advice to them along their journey and to help them feel valued (Munday *et al.*, 2007). This can be a challenging prospect for many health professionals as it may provoke professional discomfort based on many influencing factors, such as the professional's accountability and responsibility; their knowledge, skills, attitude and expertise; their workload pressures; and the fear of getting or creating upset for patient/family (Watson *et al.*, 2009; Barclay and Maher, 2010). Four aspects of awareness (closed, suspicion, mutual pretence and open) were identified by Glaser and Strauss in 1965 (Cope, 1998) which may influence discussions between professionals and patients. Closed awareness is where professionals are aware of the patient's prognosis but refrain from disclosing the information and use methods to avoid initiating or engaging in a conversation (Seale *et al.*, 1997). The patient therefore may become 'suspiciously aware' and try to use tactics such as cues to find the truth. If the professional does not recognize it, this can lead on to 'mutual pretence', where both parties are aware but do not openly discuss and acknowledge the dying trajectory (Cope, 1998). Lastly, 'open awareness' is when both parties are able to engage in conversation in relation to what the patient knows and understands (Seale *et al.*, 1997).

It is everyone's responsibility to encourage discussions and the patient's identified needs and wishes need to be communicated and coordinated within the MDT as part of the care planning process. If the discussion has not taken place then the MDT need to decide who will open the dialogue with the patient (Hanks *et al.*, 2010).

Communication is fundamental to good EoLC (Watson *et al.*, 2009) and Table 13.1 can help facilitate difficult conversations.

Table 13.1 How to promote good communication (Heyse-Moore, 2009; Watson *et al.*, 2009; NEoLCP, 2010a; Fallowfield, 2010; Barclay and Maher, 2010)

Factors to Consider	Guidelines	Example
The environment	Privacy, no interruptions	Quiet room, arranged time
Body language	Understanding how your posture may reflect barriers in communication Observing the patient's body language	Barriers: arms and legs crossed, tapping of a foot, clenching of hands
Non-verbal communication	Personal space, posture, gestures	Relaxed facial expressions, eye contact
Verbal communication	Use of simple language and open-focused questions	How have you been feeling since your last visit to the doctor?
Listening	Use of silence and use of body language to acknowledge that you have 'heard'. Also what is being said. What is the meaning behind the words and the non-verbal communication to identify triggers and cues for further exploration	Gentle nodding of head You sound very angry about what has been happening to you
Demonstrating empathy	Acknowledge feelings	I understand how difficult this must be for you
Reflection	Assess level of understanding and document/share with MDT for further discussion – seamless care	So from what you were saying I understand that …
Barriers	The patient may have internal and external factors that are affecting the communication process	Disease progression, tiredness, lack of understanding, language, environment, feelings of loss

Sensitivity and respect should be displayed around the discussion as some individuals may not feel ready to have the dialogue at that particular point in time (Barclay and Maher, 2010). There is no particular point on the EoL pathway that is the optimum time to initiate a discussion around EoLC; however, the 'earlier the better' is advocated to allow the patient the opportunity to make an informed choice and support the process of Advance Care Planning (ACP) (Barclay and Maher, 2010).

ACP is a process of discussion between an individual and their care provider irrespective of discipline. If desired by the patient, family and friends are included. With the individual's agreement, this discussion should be documented, regularly reviewed and communicated to key people involved in their care (Henry and Seymour, 2007). The difference between ACP and general care planning is that the purpose of ACP is to clarify a patient's wishes and decisions (e.g. preferred place of death) and for these to be incorporated into a general care plan so the MDT can provide appropriate care and support on their EoL pathway (NEOLCP, 2010d).

The two key terms used in ACP are an advance statement and an advance decision (Table 13.2). A statement can be either verbal or written and identifies the individual's wishes, preferences, beliefs and values. It is not legally binding but must be taken into account when the person loses capacity to advocate their wishes and preferences in their best interests. An Advance Decision states that specific medical treatment is to be refused in the circumstances that are stated and is written by the individual with support from professionals, relatives or carers. It becomes effective once the individual has lost capacity by giving consent or refusing treatment even if it puts their life at risk. However, it cannot be prepared if the individual has lost capacity and therefore must meet all the requirements of the Mental Capacity Act and will be legally binding for social and healthcare professionals (NEOLCP, 2008).

Table 13.2 Taken from Advance Decisions to Refuse Treatment (ADRT) – A guide for health and social care professionals (NEOLCP 2008) with permission from the National End of Life care Programme

Patient Considerations	Family/carers and Professional
It is a voluntary process and may be initiated by the patient	Family members, carers, partners may be involved if requested by the patient
Must be aged 18 and over and have capacity to discuss the options available and be able to agree to them	Professionals supporting the patient must follow the appropriate guidance 'Advance decisions to refuse treatment – A guide for health and social care staff'
The individual's responsibility is to keep the ADRT up to date and to keep professionals involved in their care informed and up to date	To establish whether an advance decision is valid and applicable, healthcare professionals must try to find out if the person: - has done anything that clearly goes against their advance decision - has withdrawn their decision - has subsequently conferred the power to make that decision on an attorney - would have changed their decision if they had known more about the current circumstances

ACTIVITY 13.2

Consider who you feel is the most appropriate member of the MDT to initiate discussions for a patient approaching EoLC and why.

Step 2: Assessment care planning and review: care planning: assessing needs and preferences, agreeing a care plan to reflect these and reviewing these regularly

A holistic common assessment (psychological, spiritual, physical and social) of the patient and family needs is essential to ensure that all the individual's wishes are taken into account and helps to identify any unmet areas of care (King's Fund, 2007). The MDT can then coordinate and communicate the best possible care dependent on the level and availability of the services (Hanks *et al.*, 2010). This is a joint assessment with the individual that involves their consent. It should be based on the principles of person-centred care and is a continuous process, as information cannot always be gathered at one visit (NEOLCP, 2010b).

The most important aspect of the holistic assessment is verifying the individual's and their family's levels of understanding of their diagnosis, treatment options and prognosis (NCAT, 2007). This knowledge then enables discussions in relation to their preferences and choices at the end of life, development of a proactive plan of care and anticipation of crises to prevent readmission to hospital (NEOLCP, 2010d). There are five domains of the assessment, which are background information and assessment preferences, physical needs, social and occupational needs, physical wellbeing, and spiritual wellbeing and life goals (NEOLCP, 2010c). This forms an essential part of the Gold Standards Framework (GSF).

The Gold Standards Framework

The Gold Standards Framework is a system-focused approach formalizing best practice for individuals in their last year of life (Gray, 2011). It provides tools and resources to identify, assess and plan care in a more coordinated and communicated way so that all professionals feel empowered to give the best possible care (Thomas, 2003; GSF, 2009). It originated initially in GP practices in 2001 and is now being adopted in care homes and acute hospitals across the UK (Munday and Dale, 2007). The key aspect of the GSF is that it enables the MDT, at regular meetings, to proactively plan ahead, anticipate possible crises, assess carers' needs and manage bereavement concerns of the family/relatives. It involves the holistic assessment of the individual and their family, advance care planning and care of the dying (Thomas, 2003; GSF, 2009). The GSF in the community setting has been paramount in changing how professionals plan care and involve other members of the MDT (for example specialist palliative care, allied health professionals, social care, receptionist) who are involved in the patient's pathway (Munday and Dale, 2007).

The GSF comprises One aim, Three Steps, Five Goals and Seven Cs (Table 13.3).

Table 13.3 Taken from Community Nurses' GSF Factsheet 1. (National Gold Standards Framework Centre May 2009). With kind permission from Professor Keri Thomas.

Five goals	Seven Cs
1. Consistent high-quality care	Communication
2. Alignment with patients' preferences	Coordination
3. Pre-planning and anticipation of needs	Control of symptoms
4. Improved staff confidence and team work	Continuity of care
5. More home-based, less hospital-based care	Continued learning
	Care support
	Care of the dying

One aim

To deliver a 'gold' standard of care for all patients nearing the end of life.

Three Steps *(Fig. 13.2)*

To **identify** the last year of life (6–12 months) and list those identified patients on a GSF Register for the MDT to proactively plan care. Their disease trajectory is predicted by using the Needs Based Coding (Fig. 13.3) to estimate their stage to plan their care needs.

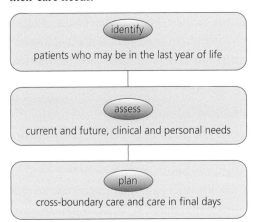

Figure 13.2 The three steps of the Gold Standards Framework. With kind permission from Professor Keri Thomas.

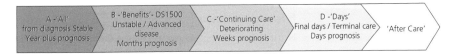

Figure 13.3 Needs-based coding–using the 'surprise question' to predict main areas of need and support required. With kind permission from Professor Keri Thomas.

To assess through a holistic common assessment including their benefits – patients may be entitled to claim for non-means-tested benefits, e.g. DS1500 to support Disability Living allowance/Attendance allowance. Assess the patient's possible needs such as anticipatory care and prescribing including ACP. Most of all, early assessment of carers' needs is advocated (formal assessment) along with provision of written information.

To plan general care generated from the holistic common and carers assessment, the ACP discussions and any recorded wishes/choices. It is about thinking proactively and anticipating possible crises, by ordering medication and equipment and coordinating and communicating with the MDT especially out of hours (OOH) services. Identification and allocation of a key worker can support the patient and family in the EoL Pathway and guide the MDT discussions (GSF, 2009).

ACTIVITY 13.3	Consider how you would implement and/or evaluate the GSF into your GP practice and what resources you would need to achieve this.

Step 3: Coordination of care

Coordinating an individual's care is one of the key aspects at the end of life. If their wishes and preferences are not respected, the individual and their family may feel devalued and experience unnecessary anxiety. The GSF is one tool that can ensure that the MDT is communicating and coordinating care (Munday and Dale, 2007). The importance of every health and social care professional being involved in an integrated care plan that is regularly reviewed is essential to ensure the patient's needs are supported (NEOLCP, 2010c). Communication links with the out-of hours services such as medical 'hubs' and evening and night community nursing services are paramount as there is more likelihood of a crisis happening at that time. The patient and family feel more vulnerable and isolated at home when carers' or professionals' visits and contact is less frequent (Munday *et al.*, 2007). By using the tools within the GSF such as the OOH communication tool or special notes on electronic systems, community nurses can inform these services that the patient is now end of life and outline any possible predicament. In some areas of the UK, the MDT use an End of Life Locality register, which is a template comprising a checklist. This lists all the key information surrounding decisions and actions in the last 6–12 months of life in a tick box format (Social research Institute, 2011).

As a community nurse it is necessary to involve and include the MDT resourcefully such as specialist palliative care dependent on how much the patient and family require or want their involvement (Boyd and Murray, 2010). The key component is that every person is an individual with changing needs and feelings. It is important to remember that although patients may decline support or refuse equipment at certain points along the pathway, their needs still exist and it is the nurse's role to encourage and support the individual regardless and enable them to maintain independence, choice and control (Barclay and Maher, 2010). As outlined in the communication section, just listening and encouraging the patient to express their feelings and anxieties can initiate discussions about dying and alleviate their feelings of isolation and loneliness. However, it is important to respect the person's privacy as it is their home, their environment and their space. Family members and carers, friends and neighbours play an essential part in a person's pathway and need to be included in joint discussions and decisions (NEOLCP, 2010d).

ACTIVITY 13.4	Reflect on how you can assess whether all the services are communicating and coordinating care.

Support for carers, both during a person's illness and after their death

Many family members become unpaid carers and there are around half a million people who provide care for a terminally ill relative or friend in the UK (Payne, 2010). The role is an intricate one as although they are still the individual's relative they are dealing with an unpredictable journey, providing intimate care that they would never have envisaged and experiencing the emotional strain that they will eventually be bereaved. Also, they are often 'thrown' into this role without any previous knowledge or experience (Payne, 2010). The ongoing pressure of the caring role is one of the key reasons why patients are admitted to hospital during their pathway and at the end of life (Jack and O'Brien, 2010). Therefore, many carers need respite, support, guidance and information to help them cope with their daily lives (NAO, 2008). Although for some it may be a temporary role, it can still affect the carer's work and impact on the rest of their life with regard to their future role in life (for further information refer to Chapter 9). It is important that the community nurse assesses, coordinates and supports the care in a proactive way to ensure that the carer is involved and able to cope with the ever changing circumstances at the end of life (Jack and O'Brien, 2010; Milne *et al.*, 2007).

ACTIVITY 13.5	Joan is 78 years old and has been married to Harold for 60 years. She has had dementia for 3 years, with a history of arthritis in her hands. Harold is her main carer and has been finding it increasingly difficult to cope recently as Joan is unable to communicate her needs and has begun wandering at night. The GP has referred Joan to an Alzheimer Adviser/Admiral Nurse for further support and information for Harold. How can you as a community nurse assess Joan and Harold's needs in coordination with the Alzheimer Adviser/Admiral Nurse to identify the cause of Joan's change in condition? What other support is available to Harold to ensure he feels he is able to manage?

Step 4: Delivery of high-quality services

Patients and families may need to use a combination and range of services from across different organizations and settings, and it is imperative that they should receive high-quality and equitable care regardless of its origin (NEOLCP, 2010d). The role of the community nurse is to make certain that all information is documented and shared with all the professionals involved in the patient's care. The key aims of this chapter are to ensure that the community nurse is aware of EoLC tools and the EoL Pathway in order to provide a high standard of care. It is, however, an individual practitioner's responsibility to be aware of their own and the team's training needs, to meet these learning needs and to develop their practice (DH, 2009d).

ACTIVITY 13.6

Reflection point
Reflect on a patient you have recently cared for and for whom you felt the care could have been better managed. What personal and professional development needs can you identify that would help you feel more effective in the future?

Step 5: Care in the last days of life

The dying process

Supporting the family through the dying process is a sensitive and emotional experience. Being aware of the general issues that an individual may experience will enable the community nurse to prepare the family to deal with the changes (EoLCP, 2010b). For further guidance refer to *Care of the Dying: A Pathway to Excellence* (Ellershaw and Wilkinson, 2003).

The Liverpool Care Pathway

The Liverpool Care Pathway (LCP) was introduced in the late 1990s to standardize and improve care in the last hours and days of life (Dee and Endacott, 2011). The model originated from the Hospital Specialist Palliative Care Team at the Royal Liverpool and Broadgreen University Hospital NHS Trust and staff from the Marie Curie Hospice in Liverpool who identified that the majority of patients died in hospital (60%). As a result, they wanted to transfer best practice from a hospice setting to a hospital setting (Taylor, 2009). The key features are illustrated in Table 13.4. They developed a tool that encompassed an assessment and care plan for patients who were identified as dying (last hours/days of life). The decision to start using the LCP will usually be made by the GP, district nurse and other members of the MDT. The patient and/or the family should also be included. It provides guidance for staff on how to achieve ongoing high-quality palliative care by providing goals in the form of a checklist and symptom control algorithms (Ellershaw and Wilkinson, 2003). It also helps staff to record clearly and simply the care that has been given and the observed condition of the patient, which is critical as the care may become more complex with more involvement from the MDT required (Jack and O'Brien, 2010).

Table 13.4 Key Features of the Liverpool Care Pathway

Key Features	Example
Anticipatory prescribing of medication	Analgesia, anti-emetics, anti-secretic, sedative
Discontinuation of inappropriate measures	Blood tests, identification of resuscitation status
Communication and coordination	Informing the MDT, especially OOHs
Checking the patient's and family's understanding	Planned care, prognosis, dying phase
Comfort measures	Providing supportive and palliative care
Symptom control	Care planning: ongoing assessment
Psychological and spiritual care	Initial and ongoing assessment
Care of the family	Before and after death

The LCP is designed to monitor the patient's condition every 4 hours and if a goal has not been met, the healthcare professional has to provide a rationale for the disparity known as a 'Variance' (V). If the goal has been met then it is documented as 'Achieved' (A) (Ellershaw and Wilkinson, 2003). It is important that the patient's status is reviewed regularly as they may need to be taken off the LCP. In 3% of cases signs of improvement have been demonstrated. They can always be placed back on the LCP if their condition starts to deteriorate again (Taylor, 2010).

The LCP has been criticized in some literature for supporting euthanasia, for not effectively meeting spiritual and religious needs and for not adequately preparing or training staff to use the tool (Taylor, 2010). However, supporting evidence has found that it has helped to improve the care of dying patients and provide positive outcomes for the MDT in changing attitudes and methods of working (Paterson *et al.*, 2009).

ACTIVITY 13.7

Consider how you would implement or evaluate the LCP into your work place for a patient you have identified as 'dying'.

Step 6: Care after death – bereavement

What to do when someone dies

When a patient dies, even though it is expected, it can be a difficult, emotional and stressful time for the bereaved relatives and for the community nurse. Each individual's family situation is different and sometimes complex due to previous psychosocial issues within the family's matrix (Watson *et al.*, 2009). Table 13.5 provides an aide-memoire for this time based on information provided in 'What to do after a death in England and Wales' (DWP 2009) . The most vital component is to reassure, support and offer comfort to those present and allow privacy if desired and, if no one is present, to notify the family as quickly as possible. The LCP is a

Table 13.5 'What to do after a death in England or Wales' (2009) Department for Work and Pensions

Process	Example
Provide information to the family on what to do next	'What to do after a death in England and Wales' and a localized bereavement leaflet
Inform services of the death	GP practice, Out of Hours Service
Verify the death	The death can be verified (if certified competent) or refer to the doctor who will verify and certify the death
Informing the coroner	Unexpected death or patient not seen by the GP for 14 days. (GP and police to be informed first)
Request for a post-mortem	An unexpected death that the coroner decides needs further investigation
Contacting the funeral director	Once the death certificate is issued
Registering the death	Within 5 days and then a burial or cremation certificate will be issued by the registrar

useful tool to support this process as it guides the community nurse through the care after death and ensures that families are supported in an equitable and standardized way (Ellershaw and Wilkinson, 2003).

The bereavement process

There are some well-known theories that explore and explain grief which may help community nurses understand the process and support the bereaved person. However, as each bereavement is individual and unique it is often difficult to theorize. It is sometimes difficult to make sense of the emotions involved that may pose challenges for health and social care professionals (Alpack, 2010). This section will not explore the grief process in detail but will provide further guidance.

The grieving process does not always begin when the person dies; for many it begins when the prognosis is given or when it becomes apparent the person dying. This is why it is important to identify the EoLC phase earlier in the pathway to allow time for the patient and family to go through the process of grieving and have opportunities to discuss their feelings and to identify any 'unfinished business' (Heyse-Moore, 2009). Grief is a normal response to bereavement or a significant loss in a person's life and their experience varies dependent on the relationship or the impact of the loss (Watson *et al.*, 2010). Individuals need to process their loss at their own pace. Although each journey is unique, Kubler-Ross (1969) was recognized for her work on identifying the five stages (denial, anger, bargaining, depression, acceptance) that people might enter. However, since then this work has been criticized by other researchers who state that there is no particular sequence that the bereaved may experience, and that some people may experience several emotions at one time (Freidman and James, 2008). However, not all emotions in bereavement are negative, as some individuals have a positive response when they feel they have done as much as they possibly could in the dying phase (Davies *et al.*, 1998; Koop and Strang, 2003). Over a period of time, individuals should be able to recover from the loss and return to the daily functions of life and establish a new way of living without their loved one. The role of the community nurse is to identify those who are less likely to cope and at risk of complicated grief and signpost the bereaved to appropriate care such as their own GP or bereavement services. For further reading please refer to Chapter 15.6 in Hanks *et al.* (2010).

ACTIVITY 13.8

Reflect on a family that have been bereaved. What emotions were displayed and how did you feel they coped with them? What strategies did you use to manage the situation?

CONCLUSION

This chapter has outlined the importance of the provision of good quality EoLC in the community setting by using the six steps from the EoL Pathway as a framework for best practice. It has highlighted the need for earlier discussions in the pathway, even for the public to start thinking about having conversations before identification of EoLC occurs. It has also identified the essential need for ongoing communication and ACP throughout the pathway around the patient's identified wishes and preferences. Ongoing assessment, care planning and review of the patient and family, with involvement of the MDT across different services, can ensure coordinated care. Finally, EoLC tools that have been discussed can guide, reinforce and document care but cannot dictate the delivery as only the community nurse can determine the level of care they provide.

REFERENCES

Alpack J (2010) Sorrow profiles: death grief and crisis in the family. London: Karnac Books.

Barclay S and Maher J (2010) Having difficult conversations about end of life care. *British Medical Journal* 341: c4862.

Boyd K and Murray SA (2010) Recognising and managing key transitions in end of life care. *British Medical Journal* 341: c4863.

Cope G (1998) A review of current theories of death and dying. *Journal of Advanced Nursing* 28:382–90.

Davies B, Deveau E, De Veber B, *et al.* (1998) Experiences of mothers in five countries whose child died of cancer. *Cancer Nursing* 21:301.

Dee JF and Endacott R (2011) Doing the right thing at the right time. *Journal of Nursing Management* 19(2): 186–192.

Department for Work and Pensions (2009) *What to do after a death in England or Wales.* London: Department for Work and Pensions.

Department of Health (DH) (2006) *Our Health, Our Care, Our Say: A New Direction for Community Services.* London: The Stationery Office.

DH (2008) *End of Life Care Strategy: Promoting High Quality Care for all Adults at the End of Life.* London: The Stationery Office.

DH (2009a) *Common Core Competences and Principles for Health and Social Care Workers Working with Adults at the End of Life. National End of Life Care Programme, Skills for Health, Skills for Care.* London. The Stationery Office.

DH (2009b) *Transforming Community Services.* London: The Stationery Office.

DH (2009c) *Dementia Strategy.* London: The Stationery Office.

DH (2009d) *End of Life Care Strategy Quality Markers and Measures for the End of Life.* London: The Stationery Office.

EoLC and Neurological Strategy (2010).

Ellershaw J and Murphy D (2005) The Liverpool Care Pathway (LCP) influencing the UK national agenda on care of the dying. *International Journal of Palliative Nursing* 11:132–4.

Ellershaw J and Wilkinson S (eds) (2003) *Care of the Dying: A Pathway to Excellence.* Oxford: Oxford University Press.

Fallowfield L (2010) Communication and palliative medicine. In *Oxford Textbook of Palliative Medicine*, 4th edn. Oxford: Oxford University Press.

Freidman R and James JW (2008) The myth of the stages of death, dying and grief. *Skeptic* 14:37–42.

Gold Standards Framework (GSF) (2009) *Community Nurses GSF.* Factsheet 1. London: National Gold Standards Framework Centre.

GSF (2008) *Prognostic Indicator Guidance*. London: National Gold Standards Framework.

Gomes B and Higginson I (2006) Factors influencing death at home in terminally ill patients with cancer: systematic review. *British Medical Journal* 332: 515–21.

Gray B (2011) *England's Approach to Improving End-of-Life Care: A Strategy for Honoring Patients' Choices. Issues in International Health Policy*. London: The Commonwealth Fund.

Hanks G, Cherny N, Christakis NA, *et al.* (2010) *Oxford Textbook of Palliative Medicine*, 4th edn. Oxford: Oxford University Press.

Henry C and Seymour J (2007) *Advance Care Planning: A Guide for Health and Social Care Staff*. London: The Stationery Office.

Heyse-Moore L (2009) *Speaking of Dying*. London: Jessica Kingsley Publishers.

Hubbard G (2011) The surprise question in end of life care. *British Journal of Community Nursing:* 16:109.

Jack B and O'Brien M (2010) Dying at home: community nurses' views of the impact of informal carers on cancer patient's place of death. *European Journal of Cancer Care* 19: 636–42.

King's Fund (2007) *Holistic Common Assessment of Supportive and Palliative Care Needs for Adults with Cancer*. London: Department of Health.

Kissane I and Zaider H (2010) In Hanks G, Cherny N, Christakis NA, *et al.* (eds) *Oxford Textbook of Palliative Medicine*, 4th edn. Oxford: Oxford University Press.

Koop PM and Strang VR (2003) The bereavement experience following home-based family care giving for persons with advanced cancer. *Clinical Nursing Research* 12:127.

Milne A, Hatzidimitriadou E, Chryssanthopoulou C and Owen T (2007) *Caring in Later Life: Reviewing the Role of Older Carers* (Executive summary). London: Help the Aged.

Munday D and Dale J (2007) Palliative care in the community (Editorial). *British Medical Journal* 334:809.

Munday D, Dale J and Murray S (2007) Choice and place of death, individual preferences uncertainty and the availability of care. *Journal of Social Medicine* 100:211–15.

National Audit Office (NAO) (2008) Patient and carer experiences regarding End of Life care in England. Leeds: OVE ARUP and Porters Ltd.

National Cancer Action Team (2010) *Holistic Common Assessment of Supportive and Palliative Care Needs for Adults Requiring End of Life Care*. London: National Cancer Action Team.

National Council for Hospice and Specialist Palliative Care Services (NCHSPCS) (2002) *Definitions of Supportive and Palliative Care*. London: NCHSPCS.

National Institute of Clinical Excellence (2004) *Guidance on Cancer Services: Improving Supportive and Palliative Care for Adults with Cancer*. London: NICE.

NHS National End of Life Care Programme and the National Council for Palliative Care (2008) *Advance Decisions to refuse treatment: A Guide for Health and Social Care Professionals*. Leicester: NHS National End of Life care Programme.

NHS National End of Life Care Programme (NEOLCP) (2010a) *Support Sheet 2: Principles of Good Communication*. Leicester: National End of Life Care Programme.

NEOLCP (2010b) *Support Sheet 8: The Dying Process*. Leicester: National End of Life Care Programme.

NEOLCP (2010c) *Differences Between General Care Planning and Decisions Made in Advance*. Leicester: National End of Life Care Programme.

NEOLCP (2010d) *Route to Success in Care Homes*. Leicester: National End of Life Care Programme.

Paterson BC, Duncan R, Conway R, *et al.* (2009) Introduction of the Liverpool Care Pathway for end of life care to emergency medicine. *Emergency Medicine Journal* 26:777–9.

Payne S (2010) Following bereavement, poor health is more likely in carers who perceived that their support from health services was insufficient or whose family member did not die in the carer's preferred place of death. *Evidence Based Nursing* 13:94–5.

Saunders C (1989) Pain and impending death. In Wall PD and Melzak R (eds) *Textbook of Pain*, 2nd edn. Oxford: Churchill Livingstone, 624–31.

Seale C, Addington-Hall J and McCarthy M (1997) Awareness of dying: prevalence, causes and consequences. *Social Science Medicine* 45:477–84.

Seymour J, French J and Richardson E (2010) Dying matters: Let's talk about it. *British Medical Journal* 341:c4860.

Social Research Institute (2011) *End of Life Locality Registers Evaluation Interim Report*. London: Ipsos MORI.

Taylor H (2009) Liverpool Care Pathway. Bevan Britan: This article was previously published in the February 2010 edition of *Health Care Risk Report*.

Thomas K (2003) *Caring for the Dying at Home: Companions on the Journey*. Abingdon: Radcliffe Medical Press.

Watson M, Lucas C, Hoy A and Wells, J (2009) *Oxford Handbook of Palliative Care*, 2nd edn. Oxford: Oxford University Press.

FURTHER RESOURCES

www.mcpcil.org.uk/liverpool-care-pathway/

www.goldstandardsframework.nhs.uk/

www.endoflifecareforadults.nhs.uk/tools/core-tools/preferredprioritiesforcare

www.terminalillness.co.uk/understanding-grieving-process.html

www.dyingmatters.org

www.nhs.uk/carersdirect

www.ageuk.org.uk/HomeCare

www.helpthehospices.org.uk

www.macmillan.org.uk

www.endoflifecareforadults.nhs.uk/tools/core-tools/rtsresourcepage

www.publicguardian.gov.uk/mca/code-of-practice.htm

14

Organization and management of care

Jill Gould

LEARNING OUTCOMES

- Explore work organization and care delivery in the primary care setting
- Critically reflect on prioritization, delegation and skill mix
- Discuss principles and methods of service review
- Analyze the role of community nurses in influencing service provision

INTRODUCTION

Nursing in the community setting is varied, complicated and challenging (Drennan *et al.*, 2005; Barrett *et al.*, 2007). Community nurses work in a dynamic and constantly changing care environment with potentially limitless demands. On this 'ward without walls' it can be difficult to apply restrictions to the number or complexity of patients and there is little control over increased workload or new referrals (Haycock-Stuart *et al.*, 2008). Practitioners need to be responsive to fluctuating workload demands and unpredicted wide-scale crises such as flu epidemics. In addition to managing the risks associated with a continually shifting caseload, community nurses are responsible for safeguarding vulnerable groups, seeking health needs and actively identifying potential clients/patients, employing a proactive, pre-emptive approach to service provision (DH, 2008a, 2010a; Kane, 2008; NMC, 2009). This chapter focuses on the care organization of district nurses, health visitors and school nurses, as these community practitioners largely address the wide-ranging needs of the most vulnerable of the population, requiring well-honed assessment, prioritization and leadership skills.

Some practitioners in primary care such as practice nurses or community matrons are likely to have a more clearly defined patient population or can 'close' when their lists or 'virtual ward' is full. This is not normally an option for those providing universal services, or caring for the more vulnerable or housebound population, making prioritization and work organization a critical element of their role. Professional accountability encompasses clinical decision-making, delegation and the need to raise concerns if care delivery could be viewed as 'unsafe or harmful' (NMC, 2008a; NMC, 2010a; DH, 2010b). With the constantly changing work environment, community nurses are routinely responsible for individual care decisions but must also seek, identify, appraise, communicate and respond to the needs of their wider populations. The management of care, prioritization and directing resources towards areas of greatest need are a professional obligation as well as being vital to the cost-effectiveness and high quality of care provision in primary care.

As illustrated in Table 14.1 there is a great range of community nurses with new services, roles and job titles emerging in response to localized identified need and the progression towards patient-led services (DH, 2010a, 2011a,b). While the diversity of services in primary care is vital, district nurses, health visitors and school nurses have extensive responsibility for the population's health through the lifespan and are expected to have higher levels of judgement in clinical practice, leadership, management, care organization and service development (NMC, 2001, 2004; DH 2008b, 2010c). District nurses provide one of the few 24-hour services in primary care and manage the acute, chronic, complex and palliative care needs for a diverse

Table 14.1 Example nursing services in primary care

Population	'Core' services	Supplementary or 'specialist' services	
Child and Family	Midwifery Health visiting School nursing	Family Nurse Partnerships; Sure Start Centres	
		Youth Offending Services	
		Children not in mainstream education (i.e. PRUs)	
		Family Planning/Sexual Health Services	
		'Specialist' nurses:	Safeguarding leads
			Continence/bowel care
			Children's community nurses
			Learning disabilities
Adult	District nurses Practice nurses	Community matrons/case managers	
		Occupational health nurses	
		Nurse consultants/advanced practitioners—out-of-hours, primary care centres or minor injuries clinics	
		'Intermediate care'/Step-down units	
		'Specialist' nurses:	Chronic disease: e.g. Diabetes, CHF/ CHD, COPD/Respiratory, Neurological
			Continence
			Tissue viability etc.
Mental Health	Community Mental Health	Alcohol and Drug Dependency Services, Outreach Teams, CAHMS etc.	
ALL	Public Health department(s), NHS Direct; Smoking cessation services; Community Hospitals/Minor Injuries, Community Outpatients, Maternity Units, etc.		

CAHMS, Child and Adolescent Mental Health Services; CHF/CHD, Congestive Heart Failure/ Coronary Heart Disease; COPD, chronic obstructive pulmonary disease; PRU, Pupil Referral Units and often vulnerable, housebound population. Health visitors and school nurses are responsible for 'universal services' throughout the lifespan, also providing care coordination and intervention for higher risk individuals and families (DH, 2011c). This chapter explores the practical application of care organization, particularly for district nursing services, and considers the wider context of practitioners' need to minimize risk, be responsive to changes, influence service provision and act as leaders of quality-care provision in the community.

WORK ORGANIZATION AND CARE DELIVERY IN PRIMARY CARE

The practicalities of work organization and prioritization differ between discrete disciplines in primary care. These distinct roles have been affected to a varying extent by the emergence of 'Transforming Community Services' funding streams, quality outcomes and the commissioning agenda (DH, 2009a,b, 2011b,d). Changes to primary healthcare funding have resulted in a growing need to quantify, categorize and record clinical activity and to meet defined health outcomes (DH, 2011b).Research by Haycock-Stuart *et al.* (2008) suggests that district nurses routinely prioritize direct patient care over administrative duties, although this expanding need to measure activity and increased data input has an impact on the amount of time spent on patient care. Similarly, there is pressure on health visitors and school nurses to generate more thorough and precise documentation, particularly in relation to safeguarding, also influencing the amount of time spent on direct contact. This was illustrated poignantly in the Laming report (2009: 23) with one teenager stating: 'It seems like they have to do all this form filling... it makes them forget about us.'

While the growing need for robust documentation and computer-generated records is common to most community nurses as is the need to prioritize interventions, the disciplines have discrete foci for their routine work organization. As illustrated in Table 14.2, for district nurses the emphasis on clinical need such

Table 14.2 Transforming community services reference guides (DH TCS Programme 2009b)

The Six Transforming Community Services Reference Guides		
Transforming health, wellbeing and reducing inequalities	HV/SN/DN (all practitioners)	
Transforming services for children, young people and their families	HV/SN	
Transforming services for acute care closer to home	DN	and specialist nurses
Transforming rehabilitation services	DN	
Transforming services for people with long-term conditions	DN/CM/PN	
Transforming end-of-life care	DN/MAC	

CM, Community Matrons or case managers; DN, district nurse; HV, health visitor; MAC, Macmillan nurse; SN, school nurse; PN, practice nurses.

as acute and chronic ill-health and end-of-life care can be seen as more aligned with these types of transforming community services 'streams' (DH, 2009a; 2011b,d). Conversely, health visitors and school nurses are encouraged to take a more pre-emptive public health, population-wide approach, relating to children's services, family health and public health funding streams (NMC, 2004; DH 2010b, 2011c,d).

Despite the less pronounced clinical role, public health nurses (health visitors and school nurses) are also required to respond to acute situations such as safeguarding. There is little in the literature to detail how clinical work is prioritized and delegated in these aspects of primary care, although numerous attempts have been made to measure and quantify workload (Kerr, 2004; Hurst, 2005, 2006; Baldwin, 2006; Kane, 2008; Reid *et al.*, 2008).

ACTIVITY 14.1

Reflection point

Jo is a staff nurse who is the acting team leader of a busy district nursing team. It is 9 am and she has received a sick call from Dee, who was going to do two of the daily insulin injections on her way in to the office. There is a message that one patient has a blocked urethral catheter and another message that a palliative care patient has deteriorated overnight and needs an urgent visit. There are another 30 visits of varying complexity to be delegated between Jo, two staff nurses and a nursing auxiliary.

- What would be the priorities?
- What would influence the decision-making?

Care organization, prioritization and delegation for a district nursing caseload of patients involves the scrutiny of diverse factors with varying degrees of importance (Luker and Kenrick, 1992). Theoretical models are widely applied to nursing, but Kennedy (2002: 710) found that they are not as applicable to the complex and varied nature of community nurses' knowledge. Community nurses need to be able to swiftly grasp and weigh the significance of the many variables that add to the complexity of decision-making in primary care (Kennedy, 2004). As a general starting point, prioritization is based on determining the most significant or urgent of the identified clinical needs.

However, even within the simple illustration in Activity 14.1, other factors such as 'knowing the patient' (Speed and Luker, 2004; Kennedy, 2004) could influence decision-making. For example, if the patient referred for a 'blocked' urethral catheter was known to bypass urine regularly without the catheter actually being blocked, they would not be considered as urgent unless they had expressed a symptom atypical for them. Other factors influencing care priorities and delegation include available skill mix, clinical expertise/experience, various crises, geographical location and sometimes factors such as traffic or weather conditions (Haycock-Stuart *et al.*, 2008). In addition to prioritization, the district nurse needs to consider if the referral is appropriate (Audit Commission, 1999). Some of the many influences on prioritization and delegation are outlined in Table 14.3.

Table 14.3 Prioritization/delegation – example influencing factors

Variables	DN	HV	SN	Other
Clinical need	'Urgent' (requiring rapid intervention but not deemed to be a 'medical emergency') or higher priority: i.e. Pain, discomfort, trauma, distress, potential harm if untreated End-of-life care Prevention of hospital admission Non-urgent (but still requiring a visit within 24-hours) Many examples – some wound care, medication/injection, etc. Routine: Anything that can be safely deferred	'Urgent' or higher priority: Safeguarding Emotional/Post-natal health issues) Emerging PH crises Non-urgent (but planned for a specific time) Clinics/Screening etc. Surveillance– prevention of acute issues Routine: Anything that can be safely deferred	"Urgent' or higher priority: Safeguarding Emotional or sexual health issues Emerging PH crises Non-urgent (but planned for a specific time) Drop-in clinics/ Teaching sessions/ Screening etc. Surveillance– prevention of acute issues Routine: Anything that can be safely deferred	Specialists/ Community Matrons Prevention of hospital admission Routine/support visits Practice nurses Non-routine/ urgent situations Patient clinics Community Mental Health Team Urgent or routine
	OTHER: Higher priority: refusal of referral to other services or hospital admission identified as being necessary for wellbeing/safety			
Skill mix and service configuration	Working arrangements: Referral criteria; team or individual practitioners; corporate caseload/geographical working or GP attached Delegation based on: Staff competence/skills, experience, knowledge, NMC standards; employment contracts/ policies, staff availability Liaison with other services/referral processes			
Geographic location	Visits organized to optimize efficiency within the confines of skill mix – may be GP attached or working geographically			
Traffic/weather, etc.	May need to request assistance for travel; reorganize planned care/visits			
Public health 'crises'/ disasters	I.e. flu epidemic/immunization programmes/natural disasters:organizations have contingency plans which should include policies and protocols to guide the prioritisation of care services, some use dependency scoring tools for this			

Work organization can be seen to start with the services' referral criteria, which is becoming particularly complicated in the context of the emerging commissioning agenda where organizations are in a process of change or merger. Bridging a vast range of conditions from acute to chronic, district nurses can be seen as 'the only professionals with no limit to their workload' (QNI, 2009a: 22). The varied and 'invisible' nature of the work is not helped by a lack of clearly defined referral criteria (Audit Commission, 1999; Low and Hesketh, 2002; RCN, 2003; QNI, 2006, 2009a; Jarvis *et al.*, 2006). The development of referral criteria is recommended to reduce the number of inappropriate referrals, to clarify and add legitimacy to the district nursing role and to help ensure the best use their skills and judgement (RCN, 2003; Jarvis *et al.*, 2006). The establishment and implementation of referral processes can thus be seen as a fundamental step in organizing and managing nursing care in the community setting, particularly for district nurses, who have little control over their workload (Haycock-Stuart *et al.*, 2008).

Primary care organizations (PCOs) should have documented referral criteria as a basis by which district nurses can monitor and direct the number and types of patients on their active caseload. Referrals can be received from a range of sources including General Practice (GP), acute care, residential homes, day centres, social services, family, carers and the patients/clients themselves. However, there are variations in the use of referral criteria for a number of reasons, including

- detail/specifics – inconsistency between care organizations/employers
- implementation – a lack of awareness/patchy support for their use
- the commissioning agenda – there is a growing need for services to be more 'marketable' and thus potentially more flexible/less rigid.

Some referral criteria comprise only a general outline of the types of care provided by district nursing services, whereas others are very clearly delineated. The RCN (2003: 26) recommends that referral are categorized in a way that aids prioritization:

- *urgent* – contact necessary within four hours
- *non-urgent* – contact within 24 hours and visiting date agreed
- *routine* – contact within 48 hours and visiting date agreed.

The Audit Commission Report (1999) found great variations between different geographical areas/teams of the number and types of patients on district nurse caseloads. Although there has been no recent equivalent large-scale study, indications are that these variations have continued or worsened (QNI, 2009b). Given the changes in primary care, with services being commissioned for portfolios of services rather than for professional groups (NHS Alliance and QNI, 2009b) and the diversification of roles with the advent of 'case managers', 'community matrons' and 'intervention teams', it can be asserted that disparity in district nurse caseload sizes has increased. Further to considering the appropriateness of new referrals, district nurses evaluate each of the scheduled visits on the basis of their clinical need, identifying those of higher priority. As suggested in Table 14.3, from that starting point a range of influences on prioritization and delegation are examined before decision-making occurs.

Health visitor and school nurse services also provide a range of services and show wide variations in this provision. However, health visitors have worked hard to establish clear service aims (DH, 2009c) and are recognized broadly as leaders in public health and within the Darzi stream of 'children's services' (DH, 2009a). There is reported a significant decline in the number of specialist district nurses and public health nurses (DH, 2009d; Unite, 2009; Cook *et al.*, 2009; QNI, 2009a, 2010). Recent policy in England has aimed to redress this for health visitors by denoting a target number of health visitors to be educated and employed over the next few years (DH, 2011c,d). This may be partly in response to concerns over their increased workload, with one survey finding that nearly 70% of health visitors report they no longer have the capacity to support the most vulnerable children (Unite/CPHVA Omnibus Survey, 2008). The remit to provide universal services for the health visitor (Fig. 14.1) populations and additionally target those with greater needs may be more clearly delineated than the equivalent for district nursing services, but remains highly challenging.

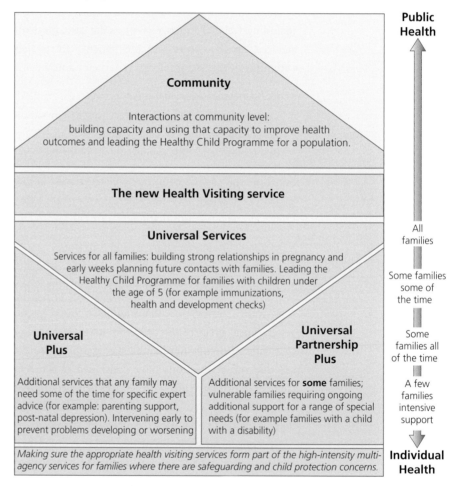

Figure 14.1 The 'Service Vision' for Health Visiting Services in England (based on the *Health Visiting Implementation Plan*, DH, 2011c).

This model suggests health visitors work in partnership with other services to provide universal care for all, as well as supporting the most vulnerable families, particularly those where there are safeguarding concerns (DH, 2011c). While there is potential for flexibility in how outcomes are achieved and services are delivered, the exigency of safeguarding can be a barrier to practice innovation (Wakefield *et al.*, 2010). Some public health or population-based health issues have an insubstantial evidence base potentially leading to variations. As with specialist district nursing practice, it is difficult to establish an evidence base to make explicit the need to 'employ health visitors rather than other workers to deliver their traditional role' (DH, 2009c: 3).

Care organization has myriad influences, some of which arise from the key contrasts between acute and primary care (Box 14.1).

Box 14.1 Supporting expert nurses to work in community settings (Drennan et *al.,* 2005)

A study commissioned by the Department of Health found that nurses new to the community 'become novice practitioners again' irrespective of their previous level of expertise (Drennan et *al.,* 2005). The four main reasons identified for this finding were:

1. The patient is in control of all decisions affecting their health and wellbeing, including their home environment.
2. The patients and their carers undertake most of their own health maintenance, treatment and care activities.
3. The multiple systems and infrastructures that support the delivery of health and social care vary between local areas.
4. The nurse has to make clinical and professional decisions, sometimes rapidly in less than ideal circumstances, at a physical distance from professional colleagues.

---

1   The centrality of the patient perspective – the care organization must take into account the clients' interpretation of their needs. Community nurses must acknowledge that 'patients at home are much more in control of their decisions' (NHS Employers, 2006: 2) and take into account their personal preferences. For instance, if a patient is relatively active and requires daily wound packing, they may prefer to be visited at a specified time. However, this consideration has to be balanced with other influences on care organization such as urgent unplanned visits, staff absence or higher priority needs.

2   Patients and carers undertake most of the care activities – unlike the acute care setting, much of the work in primary care involves ongoing identification and analysis of need and care provision or coordination of services. Integral to this is ensuring support is available to those providing the bulk of the care. It has been calculated that the economic value of the contribution made by informal carers is 'more than the annual cost of all aspects of the NHS' (Carers UK, 2007: 2). It is recognized that carers have distinct needs with the introduction of recent strategies, including support for greater personalization and improved quality of care (HM Government, 2010).

3   The multiple systems and infrastructures – care organization is highly dependent on the accessibility of services and resources. With the array of systems and structures within primary care, community nurses need to have excellent communications skills and sustain an extensive working knowledge of these resources.

4 Clinical and professional decision-making in isolation – the need to make care decisions in isolation can be daunting for practitioners new to nursing or to the community setting. The ranging skills of the nursing team demand that more experienced practitioners delegating tasks need to be assured of the skill level of each team member and must aim to minimize the risk of less experienced or skilled staff performing visits which may be outside their scope of practice.

Care organization in primary care is dependent on an variety of factors that is constantly fluctuating. The requisite skills of community nurses are wide-ranging and are seen to include 'proactively targeting services where most needed, addressing the wider causes of ill-health, managing risks associated with patients and carers making their own decisions and understanding and influencing practice-based commissioning' (NHS Employers, 2006: 2). Practitioners are responsible for maintaining a continued currency of knowledge and skills, not only in relation to assessment and prioritization, but also in the local knowledge of available services and structures, the needs of carers and an awareness of risk factors requiring a strong skill mix within teams. The next section looks more closely at this topic of skill mix, roles, responsibilities and delegation.

SKILL MIX, ROLES AND RESPONSIBILITIES

A series of policy documents has proposed that care is moved away from the acute setting and closer to the patients' homes (DH, 2008a, 2009a, 2010a, 2011d). Despite the resulting pressures on the primary care workforce, findings indicate the 'supply of skilled nurses is falling' (QNI, 2010: 2). This has developed through a combination of dilution of the workforce with practitioners who are lesser trained and the ageing workforce, with 72% of district nurses over 40 years and many nearing retirement age (QNI, 2010). The impact of this steady decline of trained nurses and specialist trained district nurses (team leaders) has not been examined or evaluated, but there are distinct implications for skill mix, roles, responsibility and accountability. The leadership role is recognized as 'pivotal' with the DH (2011a: 8) stating that, 'the strength of that leadership has an unambiguous link to the quality of care and the reputation of the profession'. While it is not unreasonable for the DH (2011a) to emphasize professional accountability for all community staff, these much larger teams coupled with ambiguous lines of leadership can present formidable challenges for less experienced community nursing staff.

Most employment contracts and the NMC standards (NMC, 2001, 2004, 2007) indicate that specialist practitioners (district nurses) remain accountable for their own practice and for the safe and conscientious delegation of work. However, with teams rapidly expanding and moving from GP attachment to larger corporate caseloads, it is challenging for these team leaders to sustain a working knowledge of the patient caseload or the competence level of individual practitioners. In some areas, caseloads of active patients (requiring regular visits) have grown to over 1400 patients with teams in excess of 20 staff members (Table 14.4). The scale of these teams and potential complexity of the caseload implies district nurses/team leaders

Table 14.4 Example variations in case load sizes in seven adjacent primary care organizations (Gould, 2010)

What is the usual/average caseload* size for district nurses in your area?					
Range	300–1500	300–1200	400+	400–500	135–500
Number of respondents	2	1	2	1	1

* Caseload is defined as the number of active patients under the care of district nurse services.

may have difficulty in maintaining the NMC standards for specialist practice (NMC, 2001) or working within the professional Code (NMC, 2008a).

A team leader district nurse takes responsibility for their defined caseload population and is accountable for the prioritization and delegation of work (NMC, 2001, 2008a). This presupposes a sufficient awareness of individual practitioners' knowledge and skills and relies on team members to articulate if they consider a task to be beyond their scope of practice (NMC, 2008a). The QNI (2010: 3) suggest that, 'the NMC and other stakeholders should explore how best to recognise community qualifications… so that employers can identify people with the right skills to lead teams' and suggest commissioning arrangements should also be reflective of these required skills.

ACTIVITY 14.2

Reflection point

Jo is a staff nurse in a rural district nursing team. It is becoming an increasingly busy caseload, especially the daily insulin injections. She is 'in charge' most days as the team leader is now based at a different geographical location. The Band 2 nursing auxiliary (Cee) has expressed an interest in learning to administer insulin injections, but Jo is unsure of Trust policy. She also has some concerns over Cee's general knowledge and understanding of diabetes.

* How might she approach these challenges?
* What are the implications in relation to professional accountability?

The DH commissioned report by Drennan *et al.* (2005) found that the requisite knowledge and skills for primary care were primarily 'covert' and needed to be made explicit in order to create clear guidelines for employers to prepare acute care nurses for community practice. An outline of the preparation needed for this transition would be of benefit to any practitioner embarking on a career in community care and the QNI (2010) and NMC (2010b) suggest that this should begin with pre-registration nursing programmes. A number of tools to assist in knowledge, skills and competence development are available, including the Skills for Health (SFH) resources website. These are cross-referenced to the Knowledge and Skills Framework (KSF) used to measure and record competence. Recent evidence suggests that KSFs could be used more effectively as there is currently variation and a non-standardized approach (Bentley and Dandy-Hughes, 2010a).

The SFH resources (Table 14.5) are flexible and potentially useful for community nurses with tools for self-assessment, skills/competence mix analysis, role design/

Table 14.5 Example Skills for Health (SFH) tools

Type of Tool	Examples
Career framework	Level 2 – Phlebotomist – 19 competencies
	Level 5 – School Nurse – 37 competencies
	Level 6 – District Nurse – 25 competencies
	Level 6 – Health Visitor – 30 competencies
	Level 7 – Specialist diabetes nurse (primary care) – 49 competencies
Competency framework	Public health – 76 individual competencies
	LTC case management – 20 individual competencies
	Continence care – 13 individual competencies
Competency	Monitor the health and wellbeing of children and young people (health visitor career framework)
	Undertake a trial without catheter (Continence Care Framework)
Other SFH tools	Self-assessment tool; Team Assessment Tool; KSF mapping tool; Workforce Reconfiguration Tool; Nursing Workforce planning tool

redesign, workforce planning, competence-based service design, staff appraisal, recruitment and selection, staff induction, training, development and continuing professional development (SFH, 2010). With greater accountability and a foreseeable need for more stringent methods of professional regulation (NMC, 2007, 2008b; TSO, 2007; Bentley and Dandy-Hughes, 2010b), it is beneficial for practitioners to find clear and effective ways to assess, verify and record their competence levels and continuing professional development.

In addition to ensuring teams working competently and effectively in primary care, there is also a need for efficiency. A suite of tools offered by the NHS Institute for Innovation and Improvement offers support for improving efficiency through 'the Productive Community Series'. Modules are available that team leaders can employ to help measure the needs of the service and resulting resource or staff education and training requirements (NHS Institute, 2011). In keeping with NMC (2001, 2004) specialist standards and the broader health policy agenda, community practitioners need to look beyond the immediate prioritization of daily work and ensure the right balance of skills and knowledge to meet the needs of their population. The next section looks at methods of service evaluation to help this process of matching skills to service need.

Principles and methods of service review

Care organization and caseload management vary according to geographical area, employer and professional discipline but can be seen broadly as focusing on the identification of need and efficient use of resources to meet this need. While community nurses may have little authority over budget management, time and other factors can be influenced to make potentially significant improvements to client care.

Health visiting has traditionally been arranged around a 'caseload' of patients, but there is very little research literature relating to this topic (Cowley and Bidmead, 2009; DH 2009c). When evaluating one health visiting workload tool, Pollock *et al.* (2002) concluded that it produced such inaccurate data it would be unsafe to use unless significant improvements were made. Problems with interpretation centred on the need for a more rigorous process for weighting elements of 'health visiting need' and scoring more accurately the wide variation in need among families (Pollock *et al.*, 2002).

This illustrates the inherent difficulties of workload assessment and dependency scoring in primary care, also substantiated by a recent systematic review of caseload management tools and models that found there was 'a poor evidence base' (Kolehmainen *et al.*, 2010: 47). This extensive review, initially finding over 2000 papers (narrowed down to 42), reported that despite 'considerable literature on caseload management' it was not possible to draw conclusions aside from a need to critically appraise methods and tools. Despite these inherent challenges, service review is recognised as an important element of care organization (Ervin, 2008; Kane, 2008).

ACTIVITY 14.3

Reflection point
Reflect on the scenario below and consider:
• How might organizational structures affect service review findings?

Scenario
Organization A has a 'traditional' pattern of employing their district nursing services in that the teams are relatively small (3–8 members) and they are attached to a single GP practice. While the GP practices range in size, the caseloads of each of the district nursing teams are proportionate, with an average of 60 patients per whole time equivalent (WTE). The team leader doesn't visit every patient on the caseload but as a coordinator and provider of care is familiar with most patients and acts as a mentor/educational resource for the team, particularly for those who are less experienced. There is a community matron who is also GP attached who has a caseload of high-intensity patients with long-term conditions (LTCs).

Organization B has moved away from the 'traditional' model, and the much larger district nursing teams work with 'corporate caseloads'. They communicate with a number of GP surgeries over the geographical patch. The staff nurses need to be more self-directed as the caseload size is so large that the team leader wouldn't necessarily be able to identify individual clients. The team leader acts as a manager in directing and delegating care, identifying educational needs and sometimes undertaking patient visits. The community matrons also work geographically and have a separate caseload of high-intensity patients with LTCs.

Organization C has moved away from the job title of 'district nursing'. The practitioners who had been district nurses in the past are now 'case managers' whose client group are housebound patients with chronic diseases. They mainly work geographically although some are GP attached. Staff nurses constitute the 'intervention teams' and are geographically based. These teams are quite large, focus on 'episodic care' and are managed by an intervention team leader who covers what would have previously been three or four district nursing teams.

How could service review be used to influence/improve service delivery and care organization?

Caseload management skills are recognized as important for primary care practitioners and it is argued that continuing education and staff development programmes need to include these competencies 'to improve the efficiency and quality of nursing care' (Ervin, 2008: 127). Caseload management and the 'process of measuring and comparing caseload information can be used to improve the quality of care' (Kane, 2008). While the process of caseload/workload assessment (profiling) can be viewed as onerous, in one evaluative study (Gould, 2010) district nurse practice teachers described service review positively in terms of its usefulness and its contribution to service organization and development (Box 14.2).

Box 14.2 Practice teacher service review survey (Gould, 2010)

In relation to service review, what is your interpretation of its purpose and scope?

- To look at the practice population and services as a whole; assess transferrable skills and how services can be developed to meet the current demands
- To provide an insight into the caseload/workload; people management; to identify unmet need; to introduce changes to practice
- To be able to get a picture of other agencies involved or required to meet the needs of individual caseloads
- The development of business skills; to enable the use of evidence and articulate need for change; 'selling the service' – how we can improve it
- To look objectively at issues from 'ground level'; to highlight issues to management

Service review can be seen as a combination of caseload profiling (the types and needs of the client group) and workload assessment that aims to measure and quantify the work or dependency of the client group. It has been long been recognized that there is a need to quantify the work of community nursing teams in order to effectively meet service requirements and to manage the needs of populations efficiently (Audit Commission, 1999). It could be argued that the quantification of community nursing work is even more essential now as services will be commissioned for their evident worth and thus 'productivity' and outcomes need to be measurable (DH, 2011b).

Basic 'caseload profiling tools' normally involve providing a 'snapshot' of the types and numbers of clients, families or patients on the caseload and may include:

- number of patients on the caseload
- referral rates (including one-off referrals)/referral source
- discharge rates
- types of patients ('case mix')
- patient profile (ages/sex) (Audit Commission, 1999; Kane, 2008).

While there is some overlap of terminology, workload tools are more concerned with quantifying the work associated with a caseload population or measuring the dependency levels of the clients. The difficulties in measuring workload have been well documented with a variety of tools and methods tried over a period of time that aim to go beyond counting contacts to provide better quality information (Bentley and Tite, 2000; Hurst, 2006; Jones and Russell, 2007; Kane, 2008; Lewis and Pontin, 2008; Kolehmainen *et al.*, 2010).

Workload tools can be 'prospective' or 'retrospective'. Prospective tools such as the 'Warrington' provide a numerical estimate of the amount of time certain procedures take (Baldwin, 2006). Retrospective tools aim to record the numbers of visits and time spent by practitioners on care-related and administrative tasks. All methods are reliant on the accuracy of the practitioner in recording activity and the complexity associated with measuring the workload of community nurses is acknowledged, with a paucity of accurate measurement systems available (Brady *et al.*, 2007, 2008).

Reid *et al.* (2008) used systematic review methodology to identify four methods of workforce planning, including professional judgement, population-based health needs, caseload analysis and dependency acuity. The conclusion was that each of the techniques on their own was flawed in some way (Hurst, 2006; Reid *et al.*, 2008), with mixed methods advocated as most useful for the purpose of developing services aimed at effectively meeting client need. These methods were then employed to successfully inform a major service redesign (Kane, 2008). The improved efficiency of the restructure was evident in the outcome of reduced administration and inappropriate referrals, along with very consistent caseload sizes.

The Community Client Need Classification System (CCNCS) appears to be the most adaptable for measuring the workload of the range of primary care disciplines as it was developed in an area where public health nurse roles encompass all age groups, with no differentiation between health visitors, district nurses or school nurses (Brady *et al.*, 2007). It demonstrated a direct correlation between measured client need in the older population and the amount of community nursing time required (Brady *et al.*, 2007: 47) and has been found to be consistently reliable (Brady *et al.*, 2008). However, the dependency classification may be perceived as too general and its transferability to other health service environments has not yet been evaluated (Brady *et al.*, 2007, 2008). Computer-based systems, such as Systmone (TPP, 2011), are becoming more widespread for recording community nursing activity. IT systems are designed to provide a 'seamless' record of community nursing interventions, care plans, caseload data and with partnerships, other information such as prescriptions (TPP, 2011).

The role of primary care nurses in influencing service provision

As alluded to in the Introduction, it can be perceived that the continuum from 'everyday' prioritization of care to the broader remit of service organization is interrelated. Just as it is necessary for community nurses to be aware of the changing needs of their populations so as to influence the way services are organized, structural systems are an influence on the everyday practice of work organization. Nurses are accountable for their own practice and as careers progress to higher levels such as specialist or advanced practice, this accountability extends beyond the confines of their individual competence towards their team, the populations they serve and in the need to influence services and resources (NMC, 2001, 2004, 2008a, 2009, 2010a).

ACTIVITY 14.4

Reflection point

Kay is a health visitor based in a socioeconomically deprived area. It is becoming an increasingly busy caseload, particularly in relation to safeguarding. She is the only qualified health visitor attached to this GP practice, working with one staff nurse health visitor and a nursery nurse. Because of the increase in the number of child protection cases, Kay has been unable to attend well-baby clinics or drop-in services for some time. Recently several mums have contacted Kay to say they are not happy with the advice they have been given at the baby clinic.

* How would you approach these challenges?
* How might service redesign help address these problems?

Community caseloads comprise the most vulnerable members of society and practitioners must always consider potential safeguarding issues (DH, 2010a; NMC, 2010a), the centrality of the patient/client and the need for empowerment and advocacy. As a primary care practitioner, this accountability necessarily extends beyond the remit of individuals to the wider structures influencing service provision. With the exception of health visiting (DH, 2011c), the need for specialist community practitioners has paradoxically not been aligned with the budget to support practitioner development, with a significant drop in the number of trained specialist community nurses (QNI, 2009a).

Highly efficient ways of working are greatly needed, as is evidence of 'productivity', both of which are achievable through service review. Access to and consistent use of reliable ICT systems that document client contact and other pertinent statistics also help provide the required evidence to demonstrate the quantity and breadth of work undertaken in the community setting. Another area where data collection and analysis may help improve services is in relation to evaluating the way services are structured, e.g. whether services are GP attached or geographical. Although some benefits have been described by health visitors changing from GP attachment to corporate caseloads (Table 14.6), there has also been a reported need for further evaluation as initial research demonstrated no improvement in staff stress levels, the quality of client service or increase in public health nursing activity (Hoskins *et al.*, 2007).

Table 14.6 GP attachment compared with geographical working/corporate caseload

GP Attachment	Geographical Working/Corporate Caseload
Care provision and documentation to all GP registered patients	Care provision for the whole population – no need for patients to be GP registered
A range of services integrated within one convenient and familiar setting	'A range of service models are challenging the central role of the GP and the practice' (Brocklehurst *et al.*, 2003)
Close communication links with the GP; direct access to notes	Communication/documentation variable – not usually direct access to 'notes'
Potential for 'integrated' team working to meet a full range of needs of the practice population	Potentially greater autonomy/ability to balance GP requests with other work; Negotiation of services
Ability to 'know the patient' with a more confined caseload; better continuity of care; less risk of communication issues; clearer lines of accountability	Potential for: lack of continuity; serious concerns and safeguarding issues being missed; and lines of accountability becoming confused (DH, 2009c)

CONCLUSION

The safe, cost-effective and efficient management of care in the community setting is one of the many challenges nurses face on a regular basis. The practitioner's accountability for care delivery extends beyond daily patient prioritization and work organization to influencing the structures and systems within which care is delivered. Integral to the decision-making are the evaluation of services and the skill mix of the team to ensure the needs of the population are identified and addressed.

REFERENCES

Audit Commission (1999) *First Assessment. A Review of District Nursing Services in England and Wales.* London: Audit Commission.

Baldwin M (2006) The Warrington workload tool: determining its use in one trust. *British Journal of Community Nursing* 11:391–5.

Barrett A, Latham D and Levermore G (2007) Defining the unique role of the specialist district nurse practitioner. *British Journal of Community Nursing* 12:442–8.

Bentley J and Dandy-Hughes H (2010) Implementing KSF competency testing in primary care Part 1: developing an appraisal tool. *British Journal of Community Nursing* 15:485–91.

Bentley J and Dandy-Hughes H (2010a) Implementing KSF competency testing in primary care Part 2: evaluation of the pilot of an appraisal tool. *British Journal of Community Nursing* 15:553–60.

Bentley J and Tite C (2000) Developing an activity measuring system in district nursing. *British Journal of Community Nursing* 9(18):2016–20.

Brady A-M, Byrne G, Horan P, *et al.* (2007) Measuring the workload of community nurses in Ireland: a review of the workload measurement systems. *Journal of Nursing Management* 15:481–9.

Brady A-M, Byrne G, Horan P, *et al.* (2008) Reliability and validity of the CCNCS: a dependency workload measurement system. *Journal of Clinical Nursing* 17:1351–60.

Brocklehurst N, Heaney J and Pollard C (2003) GP attachment versus geographical working: what's best? *Community Practitioner* 76:81–2.

Carers UK (2007) Valuing carers – calculating the value of unpaid care. http://tinyurl.com/valuing-carers.

Cook R, Sweeney K, Perkins L, Goulden A and Walsh N (2009) The future of district nursing: the Queen's Nursing Institute Debate. *British Journal of Community Nursing* 14:540–4.

Cowley S and Bidmead C (2009) Controversial questions (part three): is there randomised controlled trial evidence for health visiting? *Community Practitioner* 82:24–8.

DH (2008a) *NHS Next Stage Review: Our Vision for Primary and Community Care.* (Accessed: 25 September 2011) www.dh.gov.uk.

DH (2008b) *Framing the Nursing and Midwifery Contribution: Driving up the Quality of Care.* Chief Nursing Officer's Directorate. (Accessed 25 September 2011) www.dh.gov.uk/cno.

DH (2009a) *Transforming Community Services: Enabling New Patterns of Provision.* (Accessed 25 September 2011) www.dh.gov.uk/publications.

DH (2009b) *Transforming Community Services Programme. Transformational Reference Guides* (6 in total). (Accessed 25 September 2011) www.dh.gov.uk/publications.

DH (2009c) Unite the union, Community Practitioners' and Health Visitors' Association (CPHVA) *Action on Health Visiting Getting it Right for Children and Families 'Ambition, Action, Achievement'.* (Accessed 25 September 2011) www.dh.gov.uk/publications.

DH (2009d) Unite the Union, Community Practitioners' and Health Visitors' Association (CPHVA) *Action on Health Visiting Getting it Right for Children and Families: Defining research to maximise the contribution of the health visitor.* (Accessed 2 May 2010) www.dh.gov.uk/publications Last.

DH (2010a) *Equity and Excellence: Liberating the NHS.* (Accessed 2 January 2011) www.dh.gov.uk.

DH (2010b) *Clinical Governance and Adult Safeguarding – An Integrated Process.* National 'No secrets' NHS Advisory Group Essex NHS Operational Leads Group. (Accessed 2 January) www.dh.gov.uk/.

DH (2010c) *Advanced Level Nursing: A Position Statement.* Chief Nursing Officer's Directorate. (Accessed 2 January) www.dh.gov.uk/cno.

DH (2011a) The Government's response to the recommendations in Frontline Care: the report of the Prime Minister's Commission on the Future of Nursing and Midwifery in England. Chief Nursing Officer's Directorate. (Accessed 31 August 2011) www.dh.gov.uk.

DH (2011b) Transforming Community Services: Demonstrating and Measuring Achievement: Community Indicators for Quality Improvement. (Accessed 31 August 2011) www.dh.gov.uk.

DH (2011c) *Health Visitor Implementation Plan 2011–15.* (Accessed 2 March 2011) www.dh.gov.uk.

DH (2011d) Business Plan 2011–2015 (July 2011). (Accessed 31 August 2011) www.dh.gov.uk.

Drennan V, Goodman C and Leyshon S (2005) Supporting the expert nurse to work in community settings – Supporting Experienced Hospital Nurses to Move into Community Matron Roles Primary Care Nursing Research Unit. (Accessed 28 December 2010) www.dh.gov.uk/publications.

Ervin N (2008) Caseload management skills for improved efficiency. *Journal of Continuing Education in Nursing* 39:127–32.

Gould J (2010) Autonomous District Nursing Service Review Report – An Evaluation (Unpublished Report).

Haycock-Stuart E, Jarvis A and Daniel K (2008) A ward without walls? District nurses' perceptions of their workload management priorities and job satisfaction. *Journal of Clinical Nursing* 17:3012–20.

HM Government (Cross Government Publication) (2010) Recognised, valued and supported: Next steps for the Carers Strategy Crown. (Accessed 28 December 2010) www.dh.gov.uk/publications.

Hoskins R, Gow A and McDowell J (2007) Corporate solutions to caseload management – an evaluation. *Community Practitioner* 80:20–4.

Hurst K (2005) Relationships between patient dependency, nursing workload and quality. *International Journal of Nursing Studies* 42:75–84.

Hurst K (2006) Primary and community care workforce planning and development. *Journal of Advanced Nursing* 55:757–69.

Jarvis A, Mackie S and Arundel D (2006) Referral criteria: making the district nursing service visible. *British Journal of Community Nursing* 11: 17–22.

Jones A and Russell S (2007) Equitable distribution of district nursing staff and ideal team size. *Journal of Community Nursing* 21:4–9.

Kane K (2008) How caseload analysis led to the modernization of the DN service. *British Journal of Community Nursing* 13:11.

Kennedy C (2002) The work of district nurses: first assessment visits. *Journal of Advanced Nursing* 40:710–20.

Kennedy C (2004) A typology of knowledge for district nursing assessment practice. *Journal of Advanced Nursing* 45:401–9.

Kerr H (2004) *Adaptation of the Warrington Workload Tool.* Conwy and Denbighshire NHS Trust, North Wales.

Kolehmainen N, Francis J, Duncan E and Fraser C (2010) Community professionals' management of client care: a mixed-methods systematic review. *Journal of Health Services Research and Policy* 15:47–55.

Lewis M and Pontin D (2008) Caseload management in community children's nursing. *Paediatric Nursing* 20:18–22.

Lord Laming (2009) *The Protection of Children in England: a Progress Report.* London: The Stationery Office.

Low H and Hesketh J (2002) *District Nursing: the Invisible Workforce.* London: QNI.

Luker K and Kenrick M (1992) An exploratory study of the sources of influence on the clinical decisions of community nurses. *Journal of Advanced Nursing* 17:457–66.

NHS Alliance and Queens Nursing Institute (2009) Briefing No. 11. *Understanding Commissioning and Providing*. London: QNI.

NHS Employers (2006) Briefing: From hospital to home – supporting nurses to move from hospital to the community. Issue 26: November 2006, © NHS Employers London.

NHS Institute for Innovation and Improvement (2011) *The Productive Community Series – Releasing Time to Care*. London: NHS Institute for Innovation and Improvement 2006–2011.

Nursing and Midwifery Council (NMC) (2001) *Standards for Specialist Education and Practice*. London: NMC (Accessed 22 November 2010) www.nmc-uk.org.

NMC (2007) *Employers and PREP Advice Sheet*. (Accessed 22 November 2011) www.nmc-uk.org.

NMC (2008a) *The Code: Standards of Conduct, Performance and Ethics for Nurses and Midwives*. (Accessed 22 November 2011) www.nmc-uk.org.

NMC (2008b) *The PREP Handbook*. (Accessed 22 November 2011) www.nmc-uk.org.

NMC (2009) *Guidance for the Care of Older People*. (Accessed 2 December 2011) www.nmc-uk.org.

NMC (2010a) *Raising and Escalating Concerns: Guidance for Nurses and Midwives*.(Accessed 7 March 2011) Mwww.nmc-uk.org.

NMC (2010b) *Standards for Pre-registration Nursing Education*. (Accessed 7 October 2011) www.nmc-uk.org.

Pollock J, Horrocks S, Emond A, Harvey I and Shepherd M (2002) Health and social factors for health visitor caseload weighting: reliability, accuracy and current and potential use. *Health and Social Care in the Community* 10:82–90.

Queen's Nursing Institute (QNI) (2006) *Vision and Values – A Call for Action on Community Nursing*. London: QNI.

QNI (2009a) *2020 Vision Focusing on the Future of District Nursing*. London: QNI.

QNI (2009b) *Practice Based Commissioning – Briefing*. London: QNI.

QNI (2010) *Position Statement – Nursing People in their Own Homes – Key Issues for the Future of Care*. London: QNI.

Reid B, Kane K and Curran C (2008) District nursing workforce planning: a review of the methods. *British Journal of Community Nursing* 13(11).

Royal College of Nursing (2003) *Developing Referral Criteria for District Nursing Services Guidance for Nurses*. London: RCN.

Skills for Health (SFH) (2010) *Improve Quality and Productivity through Workforce Transformation. How Skills for Health can help you: a summary of tools, products and services*. (Accessed 3 January 2011) www.skillsforhealth.org.uk.

Speed S and Luker KA (2004) Changes in patterns of knowing the patient: the case of British district nurses. *International Journal of Nursing Studies* 41:921–31.

The Phoenix Partnership (TPP) (2011) *SystmOne*. (Accessed 31 August 2011) www.tpp-uk.com/systmone

The Stationery Office (TSO) (2007) *Trust, Assurance and Safety – The Regulation of Health Professionals in the 21st Century*. London: The Stationery Office.

Unite/Community Practitioners' and Health Visitors' Association (CPHVA) (2008) The Omnibus Survey, 2008. www.unite-cphva.org/.

Unite the Union (2009) *The Crisis in Health Visiting (Facts and Figures).* London: Unite the Union.

Wakefield S, Stansfield K and Day P (2010) Taking a solution-focused approach to public health. *British Journal of School Nursing* 5:7. (Accessed 20 November 2010) www.Internurse.com.

Clinical leadership and quality care

Caroline AW Dickson

LEARNING OUTCOMES

- Critically discuss the role of clinical leadership in the delivery quality care
- Explain the concept of practice development and consider its contribution to the wider clinical governance agenda
- Critically analyze ways of getting evidence into practice
- Critically explore ways to enable sustainable change
- Examine quality improvement processes

INTRODUCTION

The only certainty within the health service today is that change is inevitable. Change is constantly occurring in response to new policy, changing demographics and to meet the demands of patients and carers within the community. Central to current policy across the UK is 'shifting the balance of care' (DH, 2006; Scottish Government, 2007) from acute to community services. This shift, however, needs support and action from all partners within health and social care (Audit Scotland, 2007). Community nurses have a key role in delivering this new policy agenda. Strong leadership is required to shape and develop practice to ensure that service delivery is based on best evidence, delivered in a manner acceptable to service users within a culture that values the participation and involvement of all stakeholders. The means of achieving this must fit within the framework of clinical governance where responsibility for providing quality healthcare lies with every member of an organization and the organization itself. This requires effective leadership to facilitate change and development in the pursuit of quality care. This chapter will explore leadership and quality at the level of clinical practice within community nursing. The practice development model, *A Vision for Practice Development* (NHSQIS, 2006), has been used to structure the chapter as it supports clinical leaders to evidence their current service and in developing their service in response to patient/client need.

To set the scene, the concepts of clinical governance and practice development are identified. Using the framework, leadership, evidence-based practice, person-centredness, quality improvement processes, innovative and creative approaches to sustaining change, and learning and development will be explored within the context of delivering quality patient/client care in the community (Fig. 15.1).

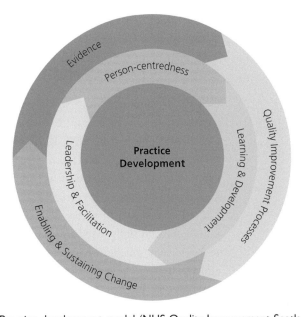

Figure15.1 Practice development model (NHS Quality Improvement Scotland, 2006) with kind permission.

Clinical governance

During the mid-1990s there was recognition of variance in the quality of care provided for patients/clients throughout the UK. Until the mid-1990s, NHS Trusts, as was, were accountable for their financial expenditure, through corporate governance, but not for the quality of care provided within their organizations. In 1997 in *The New NHS Modern and Dependable* (DH, 1998) in England, Wales and Northern Ireland and *Designed to Care* (Scottish Office,1997) in Scotland introduced clinical governance which placed responsibility and accountability for quality care on the shoulders of the chief executives. In order to carry this obligation, shared responsibility was encouraged through working in open systems and formal standards, procedures, regular monitoring and reporting were introduced (Wilkinson *et al.*, 2004). The most well-known definition of clinical governance is that of Scally and Donaldson:

> A framework through which NHS organizations are accountable for continually improving the quality of their services and safeguarding high standards of care by creating an environment in which excellence in clinical care will flourish.
>
> *(Scally and Donaldson, 1998)*

They proposed this would be the main vehicle for continuously improving the quality of patient care and developing the capacity of the NHS in England. Since then, the addition of staff governance has led to the concept of healthcare governance. This includes all three aspects: corporate, clinical and staff governance. Practice development plays a key role in meeting the clinical governance agenda. Through practice development, practitioners are also able to demonstrate accountability. This approach however is 'bottom-up', whereas clinical governance is 'top-down'.

PRACTICE DEVELOPMENT

Practice development was initially introduced as a means of developing evidence from practice to substantiate nursing as a profession in the early 1990s (Redfern and Stevens, 1996; Pearson, 1997) through the establishment of nursing and practice development units. Since then, theoretical understanding and the evidence to support practice development as a means of taking practice forward has grown considerably. In the early years, the purpose of practice development was advocated as good-quality patient-focused care achieved through the improvement of technical knowledge and skills (McCormack et al., 2004), and through the dissemination of research into practice (Kitson, 2009). Although this approach was direct and effective in working to short-term goals, it was associated with top-down change and was often an ineffective sustainable approach. According to McCormack (2004; NHS QIS, 2009) it lacked 'vision'. The work of Manley (1999), Garbett et al. (2001) and McCormack et al., 2004), McCormack and Garbett (2003), Dewing (2008) and others takes a broader, or emancipatory, view of practice development. Emancipatory practice development has been defined by Garbett and McCormack (2002: 88) as

> a continuous process of improvement towards increased effectiveness inpatient-centred care. This is brought about by helping healthcare teams to develop their knowledge and skills and to transform the culture and context of care. It is enabled and supported by facilitators committed to systematic rigorous continuous processes of emancipatory change that reflect the perspectives of service users.

It is a systematic approach that aims to help practitioners and healthcare teams to look critically at their practice and identify how it can be improved (McCormack et al., 2009). They argue, however, that development not only occurs within the confines of a project framework, but is also a means of scrutinizing the workplace culture to find new and improved ways of working. Cultures of practice where learning is encouraged and embraced are receptive to change. They will enable practitioners to consider issues for development arising from their own practice in addition to directives from policy-makers. Sustainability of change will only occur if the culture and context of care is addressed (McCormack, 2004). Fundamental to this practice development approach is person-centredness, participation and involvement of all stakeholders. Person-centredness within this context concerns all people – patients, clients, families and staff.

Elements to consider

Challenging practice is achieved through individual and team personal and professional learning and development (Manley and McCormack, 2003; Dewing, 2008). It is facilitated through critical questioning (McCormack, 2009). Through critical questioning enlightenment, empowerment and emancipation occur (Dewing, 2008: 134). The notion of emancipation or liberation from old ways of thinking and balanced participation iscrucial in recognizing areas of practice that require attention. Practice development encourages, empowers and engages individuals, teams and organizations through dynamic leadership and management in the quest to improve patient care and/or services.

The NHS Quality Improvement Scotland (2009) framework usefully illustrates the core components of practice development. Practice development is defined as a synthesis of evidence, quality improvement processes and innovative and creative approaches to sustaining change. NHSQIS advocate person-centred approaches, strong leadership and relevant programmes of learning and development as necessary to support the development and improvement of clinical practice.

LEADERSHIP

Leadership theories are concerned with who the leader is, what the leader does and in what context. Old paradigm leadership models, according to Northouse (2001), see leadership as a process that involves influencing others, occurs within a group context and involves goal attainment. Limitations of these models lie in the emphasis on one aspect of leadership, often at the detriment of the others. Conversely, new paradigm models are seen as a process of social influence that deals with the realities of constant change, and considerable emphasis is placed on the power and importance of followers (Bass and Steidlmeir, 1999). One such model is transformational leadership. Wong and Cummings (2007) systematically reviewed studies examining the relationship between transformational leadership nursing and patient outcomes. The findings provide evidence supporting a positive relationship between transformational nursing leadership practices and improved patient outcomes. This theoretical perspective is most associated with practice development and currently underpins the majority of development programmes used within the NHS. According to Barr and Dowding (2008: 60)

> transformational leaders motivate others to perform by encouraging them to see a vision which changes their perception of reality. They are committed individuals with long term vision, a need to empower others and are interested in the consequences.

Contemporary leadership

Contemporary leadership theorists claim old paradigm models are in fact management rather than leadership. In addition, they claim the evidence underpinning the new paradigm models is questionable (e.g. Alimo-Metcalfe and Alban-Metcalfe, 2005). These models are based largely on US studies of 'distant' leaders, top-level managers and chief executives, rather than those close to the realities of practice directly with their followers. An alternative model of transformational leadership was proposed by Alimo-Metcalfe and Alban-Metcalfe (2006; 2008) that examined the leadership interaction with followers. In this model of 'close' or 'nearby' leadership, there is a theme or ordinariness, rather than heroism. Follower engagement is placed at the heart of leadership and leaders are committed to building a shared vision through participation and inclusion of all stakeholders. Leaders increase followers' self-efficacy and self-worth by communicating confidence and expectation to a mission of a better future. Alimo-Metcalfe and Alban-Metcalfe (2008) claim leaders that achieve high engagement are able to achieve high levels of motivation, job satisfaction and commitment among their staff.

Models of clinical leadership are also focused on follower engagement. Through the study of nurses in one NHS Trust, Stanley (2006; 2008) developed a model of congruent leadership. He concluded clinical leaders were found at all nursing levels and tended not to be at the most senior level. Leaders are motivational, inspirational, organized, effective communicators and relationship builders. Their leadership approach is based upon a foundation of care that is fundamental to their values and beliefs of nursing care. Stanley identified the attributes of clinical leaders as clinical competence, clinical knowledge, approachability, motivation, empowerment, decision-making, effective communication, being a role model and visibility. Whereas transformational leadership is most associated with practice development, contemporary theories may offer an additional perspective useful in the development of practice.

Action-centred leadership

Another model worth the briefest of mentions is Adair's action-centred leadership. With a background in the military, Adair sees the role of leader as one of addressing the needs of the task, the team and the individual. The individual addresses these needs through different functions: planning, initiating, controlling, supporting, informing, evaluating. Although responsible for addressing the three areas of need, the leader would not be expected to perform all the functions, rather distribute them appropriately throughout the team (Adair, 2005). The language is somewhat different from that of other contemporary theorists, but Adair's work may be useful in the current context of healthcare. The challenge for community nurses within the healthcare environment is the nature of teams they lead. Interagency teams, according to Martin *et al.* (2010: 296), often work with ambiguous objectives and are composed of people from different areas of work who have different concerns and interests (Table 15.1).

Leadership skills and attributes

Continuous improvement and development of services requires sound leadership across the organization, at the strategic level and at the clinical interface. This has been recognized in a number of healthcare policy drivers in recent years (DH, 2006; Scottish Government, 2006, 2007, 2008) and in the emergence of the NHS Leadership Centre (www.institute.nhs.uk/) and a number of leadership frameworks (National Leadership Council, 2011; Scottish Government, 2005). There is a particular drive for community nurses to increase their leadership and management capacity. The challenging context of the community, where nurses practise autonomously at all levels, means team leaders must demonstrate advanced

Table 15.1 An overview of some key theories. Please see additional leadership literature for a more in-depth study of leadership theory. *Adapted from Northouse (2010).*

Old Paradigm	New Paradigm	Contemporary Leadership
Trait leadership Leaders are born, not made, and possess such traits as self-confidence, empathy, ambition, self-control, curiosity (Dawes and Handscomb, 2005)	**Transformational leadership** Individuals who stimulate and inspire followers to both achieve extraordinary outcomes and in the process develop their own leadership capacity. Transformational leaders help followers grow and develop into leaders by responding to individual followers' needs by empowering them and by aligning the objectives of the individual followers, the leader, the group, and the larger organization (Bass and Riggio, 2006: 3)	**Close/nearby leadership** A 'nearby' transformational or engaging leader is someone who encourages and enables the development and wellbeing of others, in the ability to unite different groups of stakeholders in articulating a shared vision, and in delegation of a kind that empowers and develops potential, coupled with the encouragement of questioning and of thinking which is critical as well as strategic (Amilo-Metcalfe and Alban-Metcalfe, 2008: 16)
Behavioural leadership From the studies of Lewin, Lippit and White (1939) Authoritarian, democratic and laissez-faire leadership styles were identified	**Transactional leadership** The emphasis is on mutual agreement of goals Transactional leaders clarify the role of subordinates, show consideration to them, initiate structure, reward and punish and attempt to meet social needs. Motivate by appealing to self-interest via pay or motivation (Bass, 1985)	**Congruent leadership** Leadership is a match (congruence) between the activities, actions and deeds of the leader and the leader's values, vision and beliefs (Stanley, 2006b: 132)
Situational leadership Leaders employ different leadership styles for different situations (Bourmans and Londerweerd, 1993) Leaders vary the level of guidance, direction and support depending on the follower's level of development, i.e. enthusiastic beginner, disillusioned learner, capable but cautious contributor and self-reliant achiever. Maturity of followers (Hersey and Blanchard, 1985; 1993)	**Charismatic leadership** Charismatic leaders are often found in the highest level of society and organizations. They transform followers' needs, values, preferences, and aspirations and motivation is driven by a need to serve the collective (Michaelis et al., 2009)	**Action-centred leadership** The group or functional approach where the role of leader is to address the needs of the task, the team and the individual. He/she achieves this through different functions: planning, initiating, controlling, supporting, informing, evaluating. Whilst responsible for addressing the three areas of need, the leader would not be expected to perform all the functions, rather distribute them appropriately throughout the team (Adair, 2005)

decision-making in the management of their team to ensure care is safe and effective. The management of risk is paramount in a service that sees more skill mix in the delivery of care in patients' homes.

According to Cook (2001), the nurse leader creates new ways of working, while the clinical leader is directly involved with implementing improved care. A leader utilizes understanding, knowledge and skills, communication and empathy as well as good role modelling to bring out the best in team members. He/she balances potentially conflicting needs, individuals, task and group maintenance to take a team forward (McSherry and Warr, 2008: 74). The contemporary leadership advocated in healthcare policies is based on facilitation (NHS Scotland, 2008) and is ideal for addressing the current changing context in healthcare. Facilitation, advocated in practice development, is the process of valuing a nurturing critical questioning environment that allows a team to learn and develop together (McCormack, 2004; Huber, 2010). Heron identifies modes of facilitation as planning: interventions (setting goals for the group); giving meaning (helping the group to make sense of experience); confronting (raising the group's awareness of the gap between saying and doing and tackling resistances); structuring (choosing which methods of learning are best suited to the event); and valuing (creating a climate which gives people recognition (Heron, 1999). The characteristics of facilitation in practice development and the attributes of effective leaders and practice developers are outlined in Table 15.2.

Table 15.2 Characteristics of facilitation in practice development

Simmons 5 Facilitation Characteristics (Simmons, 2004)	Attributes of Effective Clinical Nurse Leaders (Cook and Leathard, 2004)	Attributesof Practice Developers (McCormack and Garbett, 2002)
Critical thinking	Creativity	Values and beliefs: commitment to improving patient care, enabling not telling
Shared decision-making	Highlighting	Facilitative skills
Making things easier	Influencing	Energy and tenacity
Leadership of change	Respecting	Flexibility, sensitivity and reflexivity
Equity	Supporting	Knowledge
		Creativity
		Political awareness (being in the middle)
		Credibility

ACTIVITY 15.1

Think of someone you consider to be a good leader. What is it you admire about them? In relation to this, what are your strengths and what are your areas for development? Who and where will you get help in order to develop these skills?

EVIDENCE-BASED PRACTICE

Decisions made in practice and advice given by nurses must be evidence based (NMC, 2008). Crucial to leadership and developing practice is the implementation and utilization of evidence. Evidence is drawn from practice and research and drives the need for practice development. It is also generated as an outcome of practice development and must be evaluated to show performance and achievement of targets and outcomes. This can be achieved through developing robust systems of evaluation including quality audits (McSherry and Warr, 2008). Leaders in community practice striving to develop cultures where individuals and teams are open to challenge are actively seeking the best ways of doing things and are keen to demonstrate clinical effectiveness. However, ensuring practice is evidence based is challenging, not exclusively due to lack of available evidence in some areas but because the process of implementing that evidence is complex and challenging.

In 1998, Kitson *et al.* developed a conceptual framework to underpin successful implementation of evidence into practice. They identified three key factors they consider vital for successful research implementation: evidence, facilitation and context. The more robust the evidence, effective the facilitation and receptive the culture to change, the more likely implementation is to be successful. In 2002, the Promoting Action on Research Implementation in Health Services (PARIHS) framework was developed from this work by Rycroft-Malone (2002, 2004). Evidence in the new framework included clinical and patient experience, although systematically and rigorously collected. Multiple sources would contribute to 'high' evidence. Facilitation has been highlighted in the section above, but evidence and context will now be further discussed.

Evidence

Within the changing context of healthcare delivery, community nurses need knowledge and the skills to retrieve data, critique the quality of evidence, consider how to use the evidence most effectively to improve patient care and ways of dissemination of best practice. The issue with gold standard evidence is patients are individuals with individual needs, and decisions about care must be based on these needs. Many areas of nursing practice do not lend themselves to randomized controlled trials. Figure 15.2 identifies the types of knowledge required to support clinical effectiveness. Figure15.3 identifies some of the available types of evidence to inform practice.

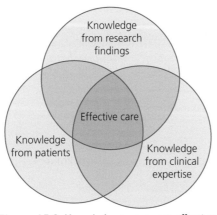

Figure 15.2 Knowledge to support effective care.

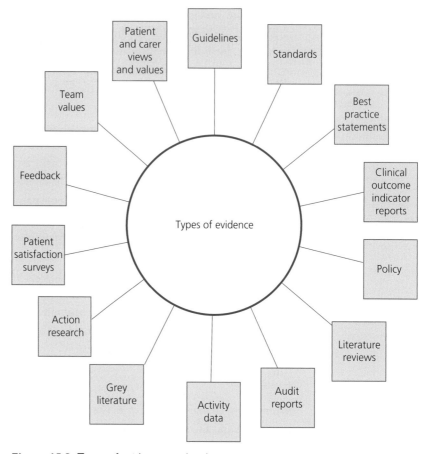

Figure 15.3 Types of evidence: spider diagram.

Context

Context is the environment or setting of practice. Important contextual factors identified in the framework are culture, leadership and evaluation. For successful implementation of evidence, the dimensions of each of these factors should be addressed. These dimensions are outlined in Table 15.3.

Table 15.3 Contextual factors. *Adapted from Rycroft-Malone (2004)*

Culture	Leadership	Evaluation
Able to define culture(s) in terms of prevailing values/ beliefs	Transformational leadership	Feedback on individual, team and system performance
Values individual staff and clients	Role clarity	Use of multiple sources of information on performance
Promotes learning organization	Effective team work	Use of multiple methods of evaluations • clinical • performance • economic

Culture	Leadership	Evaluation
Consistency of individual role/experience to value	Effective organizational structures	
Relationship with others	Democratic inclusive decision-making	
Team work	Enabling/empowering approach to learning. teaching/managing	
Power and authority		
Rewards/recognition		

ACTIVITY 15.2

How would you describe the culture of your workplace?

How well do staff work together? Who has the authority?

What leadership styles and behaviours are evident?

PERSON-CENTREDNESS

Patient and person-centredness feature greatly in current healthcare policy (Scottish Government, 2010; DH, 2006, 2008)and practitioners are charged with modelling their services whilekeeping the patient experience central. Freeth (2006) describes person-centredness as a value or philosophy of healthcare (a guiding principle) that informs policy development. The resulting policy implementations require models of care where the concept is central. The NMC Code of conduct echoes the notion of person-centredness, charging nurses and midwives to 'make the care of people your first concern, treating them as individuals and respecting their dignity'.

Nurses and midwives must treat people as individuals and their directive is:

- You must treat people as individuals and respect their dignity
- You must not discriminate in any way against those in your care
- You must treat people kindly and considerately
- You must act as an advocate for those in your care, helping them to access relevant health and social care, information and support.

(NMC, 2008: 3)

A person-centred approach is modelled on partnership and mutuality, respect and insight into others' values and beliefs and is advocated by the Practice Development Framework (NHS QIS, 2006), but this extends further than patients and clients. To lead a team effectively, treating people as individuals within that team is equally important, and therefore the concept has evolved into relationship-centredness (Andrews *et al.*, 2009). The challenge for community nurses is the interagency nature of teams involved in care and service delivery, where practitioners will have differing values and beliefs. By adopting this approach, teams will be enabled to move forward together towards a common goal.

ENABLING AND SUSTAINING CHANGE

Enabling and sustaining change is a key purpose of leadership and practice development and as identified in the sections above, facilitation and context are fundamental. Being clear about the purpose of the change, ensuring a systematic approach, having adequate resources and involving key stakeholders are also crucial in enabling and sustaining successful change. Involvement of stakeholders must be from the outset, at the identification of the issue of concern, to the dissemination of the outcome.

> It is impossible to undertake a journey, for in many respects that is what change is, without first addressing the purpose of the trip, the route you wish to travel and with whom … It is about evaluating, planning and implementing operational, tactical and strategic journeys.
>
> *(Paton and McCalman, 2008: 3)*

Change models

According to Clark (2009) it is the challenge of the team leader to negotiate the appropriate approach and timing of driving a particular planned change forward according to the team's readiness for change. In order to support this, there are a number of different change models available to facilitators in preparation for the journey of change. The models of planned change help to structure the process of change and assist with transition but are criticized as being too linear and simplistic. Probably the best known model of change was developed in 1951 by Kurt Lewin. He said that in order to prepare a team for change, the status quo must be destabilized to increase the sense of discontent with current practice. To assist with this process he recommends carrying out a force-field analysis where the driving and restraining forces of the intended change are identified by the team. This 'unfreezing' process, he argues, will increase the perceived need for change and involve stakeholders.He then identifies the 'moving' stage where the change is implemented and established. The 're-freezing' stage where the change is imbedded into the organization.

Kotter identified eight steps to successful change in his emergent model of change (Price, 2009: 54). The steps he identified are establishing a sense of increased urgency, creating a guiding coalition, developing a vision and strategy, communicating the change vision, empowering broad-based action and generating short-term 'wins'. Finally he identifies consolidating gains and producing more change. Predictive models of transformative change which are more cyclical, as opposed to linear, are more useful in developing practice. The DICE mode, currently being used within the health service, was developed by Sirkin *et al.* (2005). They state that duration (of the project), integrity (of the team), commitment (by both management and employees) and effort (demands made of employees) determine the outcome of any transformation initiative. If the project is long term, there should be short milestones and regular evaluation. The integrity of the team relates to the ability of the team to deliver the project successfully; commitment, to the support from senior management as well as 'buy-in' from those affected by the change. Sirkin and his colleagues consider that employees cannot be expected to make more than 10% increased effort above their current workload.

Reaction to change

People react to change in a number of different ways. For some people change is exciting and the very thought of it will motivate them to participate. For others, more explanation and persuasion are required before they are willing to take the plunge. Others are more reticent; they require detailed evidence and time before they can offer commitment. Other members of the team will find change threatening, at times distressing and may even try to avoid taking part. The National Institute for Clinical Excellence has produced guidance, *How to Change Practice*. The barriers to change in healthcare are identified as awareness and knowledge of the required change, motivation of individuals and teams, skills required to make change happen, acceptance and beliefs of the quality of current practice and the proposed change and practicalities in terms of resources and organizational structures. The guidance also suggests ways in which the barriers can be identified and how they can be overcome (Table 15.4).

Through the process of change, practice development recognizes a need to think of new ways of working, by challenging ritualistic practice. Different tools to encourage teams to think 'out of the box' are available to facilitators of change. Facilitation tools are available on many change management and quality improvement websites.

Table 15.4 How to change practice (NICE, 2007)

How Barriers can be Identified	How Barriers can be Overcome
Observe clinical practice in action	Educational materials
Brainstorm	Opinion leaders
Run a focus group	Clinical audit and feedback
Use a questionnaire	Reminder systems
Talk to key individuals	Educational outreach visits
	Educational meetings
	Patient-mediated strategies

ACTIVITY 15.3

Browse websites for facilitation tools and try out some in practice.

QUALITY IMPROVEMENT

Every practitioner is responsiblefor ensuring clinical effectiveness, managing risk and continuous quality improvement, although the additional leadership responsibility is in demonstrating this in practice. Lord Darzi's report *High Quality Care for All: NHS Next Stage Review* (DH, 2008) outlines quality improvement as a core element of any approach to leadership. Healthcare governance and the drive to modernize the NHS has created a culture where clinical quality indicators, performance indicators and other targets have become part of the culture of healthcare. The *NHS Performance Assessment Framework* (DH, 2000) categorizes quality indicators into six areas: health improvement; fair access; effective delivery of appropriate healthcare; efficiency; patient/carer experience of the NHS; and health outcomes of NHS care. In Scotland, HEAT (Health Improvement Efficiency Access Treatment) targets were set out in the Scottish Government's policy document *Better Health Better Care*. Achievement in practice is assessed against seven high-level targets and 15 shared national outcomes. The Quality Outcomes Framework was introduced in 2004 as part of the General Medical Services (GMS) contract (www.nice.org.uk/aboutnice/qof/qof.jsp) in England, Wales and Scotland and is a framework of performance measures that benchmark activities within general practice. Although the NHS boards and general practice are measured against these targets, teams are expected to contribute to their achievement and to use the targets to guide service delivery.

The Institute of Medicine's six dimensions of quality care (Table 15.5) have been adapted in a number of policy documents.

Table 15.5 Six dimensions of quality care

Safe	Avoiding injuries to patients from the care that is intended to help them
Effective	Providing services based on scientific knowledge to all who could benefit and refraining from providing services to those not likely to benefit (avoiding underuse and overuse). Doing the right thing for the right person at the right time
Family-centred	Providing care that is respectful of and responsive to individual patient preferences, needs and values, and ensuring that patient values guide all clinical decisions
Timely	Reducing waits and sometimes unfavourable delays for both those who receive and those who give care
Efficient	Avoiding waste, in particular waste of equipment, supplies, ideas and energy
Equity	Providing care that does not vary in quality because of personal characteristics such as gender, ethnicity, geographic location and socio-economic status

Quality improvement tools

Useful tools to guide quality improvement are widely available. The usefulness arises from the constant reviewing of practice and standard setting. Audit is a crucial component of improvements to the quality of patient care (Patel, 2010) and must be an ongoing dynamic process constantly reviewing standards to ensure they are being met (Bryar and Griffiths, 2003; McSherry and Pearce, 2011). Steps in the audit cycle are outlined in Box 15.1.

Box 15.1

Evaluate clinical practice against standards
Identify areas requiring change
Standards for practice set informed by evidence
Evaluate practice and identify variations
Implement change (development of action plan)

Adapted from Bryar and Griffiths, 2003

The 'Plan–Do–Study–Act' or PDSA cycle focuses on persistent improvement throughout the process of change and encourages teams to constantly review their practice and use the evaluation to shape the ongoing development (Nelson *et al.*, 2007). Evaluation will demonstrate effectiveness and will be fundamental evidence for the broader roll-out of any change.

Plan – Plan the change to be implemented

Do – Implement the change

Study – Evaluate the data from before and after the change

Act – Act upon information gained from change and plan further changes necessary

(NHS Institute for Innovation and Improvement, 2005)

LEAN methodology is an improvement approach advocated by the Institute of Innovation and Improvement to improve flow and eliminate waste. It is the basis of Productive Communities and Wards. Table 15.6 illustrates LEAN methodology. The goals of LEAN are: doing work on time; identifying problems before it's too late; learning by doing; being right first time, every time; matching resources to meet demand; eliminating waste; improving flow; empowering staff.

Table 15.6 LEAN methodology. *Institute for Innovation and Improvement (www.institute. nhs.uk/).*

This is achieved by	The benefits LEAN I principles can deliver are identified as:
value stream mapping	improved quality and efficiency
pull signal	higher standards of patient care
visual workplace (5s: sort, straighten/simplify, shine, standardize, sustain)	better safety and lower mortality rates
match resources to demand	shorter length of stay for patients
work standardization	reduced waste, e.g. duplication of work and re-work
staff involvement	lower costs
rapid improvement events	fewer delays
multifunctional staff	increased staff morale

| ACTIVITY 15.4 | Consider an issue in practice where you have identified evidence development is needed. Using one of the quality improvement tools, develop an outline plan indicating how it could be addressed. |

LEARNING AND DEVELOPMENT

The NHS, like all health care systems, is the sum total of the people who work in it and the day-to-day interactions they have with patients and colleagues … The way to achieve transformation is through the mobilization of our staff to drive change.

(Sir David Nicholson, NHS Chief Executives Annual Report, 2007)

Life-long learning, driven through governmental policy (DH, 2004; Scottish Government, 2006), is now rooted within practice. Organizations have the responsibility within the clinical governance framework to ensure there are systems in place to support this. As leaders, there is a responsibility to ensure the team meets all statutory and professional requirements. Amy (2008) carried out survey research to identify the contribution of leaders to learning at individual and organizational levels. She identified the required behaviours as fac ilitation, problem-solving and decision-making, communication, relating and developing. However, attending courses, study days and conferences, although useful, the resulting development of practice is not guaranteed. The facilitation of critical reflection, crucial in the development of practice, occurs through high support and high challenge in such relationships as clinical supervision (Driscoll, 2007), critical companionship (Titchenin, 2004) and action learning (McGill and Brockbank, 2003). These relationships enable practitioners to reflect on their practice and consider new ways of thinking and working. Reflection, based on Kolb's experiential learning model (1984), enables practitioners to critically evaluate their practice by combining informal (personal) theories with formal (professional and theoretical). Through this process practice continually improves keeping the person at the heart of that development. Other relationships that support personal and professional development are preceptorship, mentorship and coaching. Preceptorship programmes are now more commonplace for newly qualified staff and offer support in the consolidation of their educational preparation programme. Examples of this are NHS Flying Start (www. flyingstartengland.nhs.uk/ in England and www.flyingstart.scot.nhs.uk/ in Scotland) and the Northern Ireland Practice and Education Council for Nursing and Midwifery (https://www.nipecdf.org/). Mentorship and coaching relationships however are less commonplace and appear to be confined to senior managers and leaders.

Leadership development

Attributes of effective nurse leaders have been highlighted in the literature as stewardship, respect, caring, advocacy, honesty, confidentiality and initiating a values programme (Jooste, 2006) and as creativity, highlighting, influencing, respecting and supporting (Cook and Leathard, 2004). Development programmes offered to potential leaders within the NHS are now commonplace. The *Leadership*

Qualities Framework (NHS Institute for Innovation and Improvement, 2006) and the Scottish leadership development framework: *Delivery Through Leadership* (SE, 2005) offer support and guidance to practitioners in the development of their leadership skills and attributes. Identification of learning needs highlighted by personal development planning and review will enable practitioners to plan their learning and development activity.

> Developing the leaders of today and tomorrow will be crucial in delivering the ambitious goals that have been set for the health service.
>
> *(SE, 2005: 2)*

ACTIVITY 15.5

Access one of the leadership frameworks above. Identify the qualities you would like to develop. Compile your own personal development plan indicating how you will develop, who will help you and the resources you need.

CONCLUSION

The practice development model, *A Vision for Practice Development* (NHSQIS, 2006), provides a useful framework to consider leadership and quality in community nursing practice. Practice development is everybody's concern and therefore an understanding of the purpose and processes involved is essential for all practitioners. The essential elements of leadership, evidence-based practice, person-centredness, quality improvement processes, innovative and creative approaches to sustaining changeand learning and development have been discussed within the context of the clinical governance agenda. After reading the chapter and undertaking the activities, it is hoped the reader will develop an understanding of not only the context of their practice but themselves as leaders of community nursing practice.

REFERENCES

Adair J (2005)*How to Grow Leaders*. London: Kogan Page.

Alimo-Metcalfe B and Alban-Metcalfe J (2005) Leadership: Time for a new direction? *Leadership* 1(1):5–71.

Alimo-Metcalfe B and Alban-Metcalfe J (2008) *Engaging Leadership: Creating Organisations that Maximise the Potential of Their People*. London: CIPD.

Amy AH (2008) Leaders as facilitators of individual and organizational learning. *Leadership and Organizational Development Journal* 29:212–34.

Andrews N, Driffield D and Poole V (2009) All Together Now: a collaborative and relationship-centred approach to improving assessment and care management with older people in Swansea. *Quality in Ageing* 10:12–23.

Audit Scotland (2007) *Managing Long Term Conditions*. Edinburgh: Audit Scotland.

Barr J and Dowding L (2008) *Leadership in Healthcare*. London: Sage Publications.

Bass BM and Steidlmeir P (1999) Ethics, character and authentic transformational leadership behaviour. *Leadership Quarterly* 10:181–217.

Bryar RM and Griffiths JM (2003) *Practice Development in Community Nursing: Principles and Process*. London: Arnold.

Clark CC (2009) *Creative Nursing Leadership and Management.* United States of America: Jones and Bartlett Publishers.

Cook MJ (2001) The attributes of effective clinical nurse leaders. *Nursing Standard* 15:33–6.

Cook MJ and Leathard HL (2004) Learning for Clinical Leadership. *Dimensions of Critical Care Nursing* 24:32–4.

Department of Health (DH) (1998) *The New NHS: Modern and Dependable.* London: The Stationery Office.

DH (2000) *Human Resources Performance Framework.* www.dh.gov.uk/en/ Publicationsandstatistics/Lettersandcirculars/Healthservicecirculars/DH_4004640.

DH (2004) *The NHS Knowledge and Skills Framework (NHS KSF) and the Development Review Process.* Available at www.dh.gov.uk/en/Publicationsandstatistics/Publications/ PublicationsPolicyAndGuidance/DH_4090843.

DH (2006) *Our Health, Our Care, Our Say: A new direction for community services.* London: The Stationery Office.

DH (2008) *High Quality Care for All: NHS Next Stage Review.* London: The Stationery Office.

Dewing J (2008). Implications for nursing managers from a systematic review of practice development. *Journal of Nursing Management* November:134–40.

Driscoll J (2007) *Practical Clinical Supervision: A Reflective Approach for Health Care Professionals.* London: Balliere Tindall.

Freeth R (2006)Person-centred or patient-centred? *Healthcare Counselling and Psychotherapy Journal* 6: 36–9.

Garbett R and McCormack B (2002) A concept analysis of practice development. *NT Research* 7 :87–99.

Garbett R, Manley K and McCormack B (2001) *Practice Development: Concept, Culture and Evaluation.* Geneva: International Council of Nurses.

Harvey G, Loftus-Hills A, Rycroft-Malone J, *et al.* (2004) Getting evidence into practice: the role and function of facilitation. *Journal of Advanced Nursing* 37:577–88.

Heron J (1999) *The Facilitator's Handbook.* London: Kogan Page.

Huber D (2006) *Leadership and Nursing Care Management,* 3rd edn. Philadelphia, PA: Saunders Elsevier.

Huber D (2010) *Leadership and Nursing Care Management,* 4th edn. Philadelphia, PA: Saunders Elsevier.

Institute of Medicine (2001) *Crossing the Quality Chasm.* http://iom.edu/About-IOM.aspx.

Jooste K (2006) Leadership: a new perspective. *Journal of Nursing Management* 12:217–23.

Kitson A (2009) The need for systems change: reflections on knowledge translation and organizational change. *Journal of Advanced Nursing* 65:217–28.

Kitson A, Harvey G and McCormack B (1998) Enabling the implementation of evidence-based practice: a conceptual framework. *Quality in Healthcare* 7:149–58.

Kolb DA (1984) *Experiential Learning: Experience as the Source of Learning and Development.* London: Prentice-Hall.

Lewin K (1951) *Field Theory in Social Science.* New York: Harper.

Manley K (1999) Developing a culture for empowerment. *Nursing in Critical Care* 4(2):99–100.

Manley K and McCormack B (2003) Practice development: purpose, methodology, facilitation and evaluation. *Nursing in Critical Care* 8:22–9.

Martin V, Charlesworth J and Henderson E (eds) (2010) *Managing in Health and Social Care,* 2nd edn. London: Routledge.

Michaelis B, Stegmaier R and Sonntag K (2009) Affective commitment to change and innovation implementation behavior: the role of charismatic leadership and employees' trust in top management. *Journal of Change Management* 9:399–417.

McCormack B, Manley K and Garbett R (eds) (2004) *Practice Development in Nursing.* Oxford: Blackwell Publishing.

McCormack B, Dewing J, Breslin L, *et al.* (2009) Practice development: realising active learning for sustainable change. *Contemporary Nurse* 32:92–104.

McCormack B and Garbett R (2003) The characteristics, qualities and skills of practice developers. *Journal of Clinical Nursing* 12: 317–25.

McGill I and Brockbank: (2003) *Action Learning Handbook: Powerful Techniques for Education, Training and Professional Development.* London: Routledge Falmer.

McCormack B, Kitson A, Harvey G, *et al.* (2002) Getting evidence into practice: the meaning of 'context'. *Journal of Advanced Nursing* 38:94–104.

McSherry R and Pearce P (2011) *Clinical Governance: A Guide to Implementation for Healthcare Professionals,* 3rd edn. Chichester: Wiley Blackwell.

McSherry R and Warr J (eds) (2010) *Implementing Excellence in Your Health Care Organisation.* Glasgow: Open University Press.

McSherry R and Warr J (2008) *An Introduction to Excellence in Practice Development in Health Social Care.* Glasgow: Open University Press.

National Institute for Clinical Excellence (2004) *Quality and Outcomes Framework.* www.nice.org.uk/aboutnice/qof/qof.jsp.

National Institute for Clinical Excellence (2007) *How to Change Practice.* www.nice.org.uk/media/D33/8D/Howtochangepractice1.pdf.

Nelson E, Batalden P and Godfrey M (2007) *Quality by Design: A Clinical Microsystems Approach.* San Francisco, CA: Jossey-Bass.

National Leadership Council (2011) *The Leadership Framework.* (Accessed 14 September 2011) www.nhsleadership.org.uk/workstreams-clinical-theleadershipframework.asp.

NHS Institute for Innovation and Improvement (2005) *NHS Leadership Qualities Framework.* www.nhsleadershipqualities.nhs.uk

NHS Quality Improvement Scotland and NHS Education for Scotland (2006) *Integration, Collaboration and Empowerment – Practice Development for a New Context.* Edinburgh: NHS Quality Improvement Scotland. www.knowledge.scot.nhs.uk/media/CLT/ResourceUploads/12355/ClinicalGovernance_PDUFramework_APR09.pdf

Northouse P (2010) *Leadership: Theory and Practice,* 5th edn. London: Sage.

NHS Scotland (2008) *Leading Better Care, Report of the Senior Charge Nurse Review and Clinical Quality Indicators Project.* Edinburgh: The Scottish Government.

Nursing and Midwifery Council (NMC) (2008) *The Code: Standards of Conduct, Performance and Ethics for Nurses and Midwives.* London: Nursing and Midwifery Council.

Patel S (2010) Achieving quality assurance through clinical audit. *Nursing Management* 17:28–34.

Paton R and McCalum J (2008) *Change Management: A Guide to Effective Implementation,* 3rd edn. London: Sage Publications.

Pearson A (1997) An evaluation of the King's Fund Centre Nursing Development Unit Network 1989–91. *Journal of Clinical Nursing* 6:25–33.

Price B. (ed.) (2009) *The Principles and Practice of Change.* London: Palgrave Macmillan.

Redfern S and Stevens W (1996) Nursing development units: their structure and orientation. *Journal of Clinical Nursing* 7:218–26.

Rolfe G and Fishwater D (2001) *Critical Reflection for Nursing and the Helping Professions: A Users Guide.* Basingstoke: Palgrave.

Roussel L, Swansburg R and Swansburg R (2006) *Management and Leadership for Nurse Administrators,* 4th edn. Boston: Jones and Bartlett Publishers.

Rycroft-Malone J (2002) Getting evidence into practice: ingredients for change. *Nursing Standard* 16(37):38–43.

Rycroft-Malone J (2004) The PARIHS framework – a framework for guiding the implementation of evidence-based practice. *Journal of Nursing Care Quality* 19:297–304.

Scally G and Donaldson LJ (1998) Clinical governance and the drive for quality improvement in the new NHS in England. *British Medical Journal* 2 17:61–5.

Scottish Government (2005) *Delivery Through Leadership: NHS Scotland Leadership Development Framework.* www.scotland.gov.uk/Publications/2005/06/28112744/27452.

Scottish Government (2006) *DeliveringCare, EnablingHealth: Harnessing the Nursing, Midwifery and Allied Health Professions' Contribution to Implementing Delivering for Health in Scotland.* www.scotland.gov.uk/Publications/2006/10/23103937/0.

Scottish Government (2007) *Better Health Better Care: Action Plan.* www.scotland.gov.uk/Publications/2007/12/11103453/0.

Scottish Government (2008) *Leading Better Care: Report of the Senior Charge Nurse Review and Clinical Quality Indicators Project.* www.scotland.gov.uk/Publications/2008/05/30104057/0.

Scottish Government (2010) *The Healthcare Quality Strategy for NHSScotland.* Scottish Government.

Scottish Office (1997) *Designed to Care.* London: The Stationery Office.

Simmons M (2004) 'Facilitation' of practice development: a concept analysis. *Practice Development in Health Care* 3:36–52.

Sirkin H, Keenan P and Jackson A (2005) *The Hard Side of Change Management. Harvard Business Review* 83(10) (Accessed 10 January 2011) http://web.ebscohost.com/ehost/detail?hid=113andsid=58ca46b9-8636-4623-8de3-1c1a1b9c17e7%40sessionmgr104and vid=6andbdata=JnNpdGU9ZWhvc3QtbGl2ZQ%3d%3d#db=buhandAN=18501198.

Stanley D (2008) Congruent leadership: values in action. *Journal of Nursing Management* 16:519–24.

Stanley D (2006) Recognising and defining clinical nurse leaders. *British Journal of Nursing* 15:108–11.

Titchen (2004)In McCormack B, Manley K and Garbett R (eds) *Practice Development in Nursing.* Oxford: Blackwell Publishing, Chapter 5.

Wilkinson J, Rushmer R and Davies H (2004) Clinical governance and the learning organization. *Journal of Nursing Management* 12(2):105–13.

Wong C and Cummings G (2007) The relationship between nursing leadership and patient outcomes: a systematic review. *Journal of Nursing Mangement* 15(5):508–21.

FURTHER RESOURCES

www.fons.org/ – Foundation of Nursing Studies

www.leadershipfoundation.no – Leadership Foundation

McCormack B, Dewar B, Wright J, *et al.* (2006) *A Realist Synthesis of Evidence Relating to Practice Development: Final Report to NHS Education for Scotland and NHS Quality Improvement Scotland.* Quality Improvement Scotland

www.rcn.org.uk/development/researchanddevelopment/kt/pd – RCN Practice Development

www.realworld-group.com/ – Real World Group: Engaging Leadership

Learning and teaching in the community

Virginia Radcliffe

LEARNING OUTCOMES

- Discuss the relationship between teaching, learning strategies and learning styles
- Analyze learning theories and discuss how they can be applied to learning in practice
- Reflect and evaluate on the process and outcomes of learning in practice
- Understand the importance of lifelong learning and continuous professional development to professional practice

INTRODUCTION

This chapter will examine learning through practice, what it is and why it is important, not only for your professional practice but for supporting the learning of others. The chapter will help you to make the best use of clinical learning opportunities, identify individual learning needs and understand the importance of continuing professional development. Learning is not a passive exercise, and participating in the reflective activities is the most effective way to learn from the written materials. Learning is defined by Kolb (1984: 41) as 'the process whereby knowledge is created through the transformation of experience', and combines experience, perception, cognition and behaviour. The way in which we learn varies and is dependent on the skills and attributes we have as well as what is being taught. Knowledge is grasped in different ways, therefore it is important to understand how you learn and how others learn so that teaching methods can be suitably matched.

NMC STANDARDS TO SUPPORT LEARNING AND ASSESSMENT IN PRACTICE: 2008

It is every qualified nurse's responsibility to facilitate students and others to develop their competence (NMC, 2008a). All staff with responsibilities for learning and teaching are under growing pressure to enhance teaching and learning quality and participants' learning experience in a climate of constant change and uncertainty (DH, 2002, 2007). Teaching staff, whether new or with considerable experience, require opportunities to learn and review methods and strategies and to be able to justify the use of particular learning and teaching methods. The *Standards to Support Learning and Assessment in Practice* (NMC, 2008b) provides an education and development framework to support learning and assessment in practice. It defines and describes the knowledge and skills nurses and midwives need to apply in practice when they support and assess students undertaking NMC-approved programmes that lead to registration or a recordable qualification.

The NMC has identified outcomes for mentors, practice teachers and teachers so that there is clear accountability for making decisions that lead to entry on the register. The framework has five underpinning principles for supporting learning and assessment in practice for each of the four developmental stages of a practitioner's career (NMC, 2008a). The four stages are:

1 nurses and midwives
2 mentors
3 practice teachers
4 teachers.

Within the framework are eight domains with identified outcomes for each of the four developmental stages. The overarching domains are:

1 establishing effective working relationships
2 facilitation of learning
3 assessment and accountability
4 evaluation of learning
5 creating an environment for learning
6 context of practice
7 evidence-based practice
8 leadership.

The NMC requires all practitioners who have responsibilities for supporting pre-registration nurses and midwives to hold a mentor's qualification. Practitioners who have responsibilities for supporting Specialist Community Practitioners should hold a practice teacher qualification (NMC, 2008a). If you are undertaking a programme of study, you will have been allocated a mentor or practice teacher. Mentors and practice teachers facilitate learning in practice and are responsible for supervising and assessing in the practice setting (NMC, 2008a).

ACTIVITY 16.1

Reflection point
What do you think is the role of the mentor?

There are many competencies that the mentor must demonstrate, including

- identify the needs of the learner
- provide guidance and support about the available facilities
- use knowledge of the student's stage of learning to select appropriate learning opportunities to meet individual needs

- use a range of learning experiences, involving patients, clients, carers and the professional team, to meet defined learning needs
- act as a resource to facilitate personal and professional development of others
- assess the learner against the defined learning outcomes or needs
- provide constructive feedback to students and assist them in identifying future learning needs and actions
- refer students with particular problems to the appropriate agencies
- be accountable for confirming that students have met, or not met, the NMC competencies in practice.

LIFELONG LEARNING, CONTINUOUS PROFESSIONAL DEVELOPMENT AND PREP

Lifelong learning has its basis in adult learning and is defined as a process of accomplishing personal, social and professional development through formal and informal learning (Wigens, 2006). It is the responsibility of every qualified nurse to keep their knowledge and skills up to date throughout their working life and they must take part in appropriate learning and practice activities that maintain and develop competence and performance (NMC, 2008b). Continuous professional development (CPD) is the way in which healthcare professionals demonstrate that they are up to date and safe and competent practitioners. The way in which you take part in CPD will depend on your opportunities at work, your personal learning style, your profession or speciality and your individual learning needs (Wigens, 2006). CPD activities include work-based learning such as a journal club, reflective practice or clinical audit, professional activities such as conference presentations or mentoring a student, formal learning such as undertaking a course or conducting research, and self-directed learning such as reading a professional journal article or updating your knowledge via the Internet.

The NMC has produced post-registration education and practice (PREP) standards and guidance that are designed to help practitioners to provide a high standard of practice and care. PREP provides an excellent framework for demonstrating CPD, which, although not a guarantee of competence, is a key component of clinical governance (NMC, 2010). A professional portfolio is one way in which you can provide evidence of your competence, demonstrate critical thinking and meet the NMC PREP requirements. An effective portfolio is a visual representation of a practitioner's experience, strengths, abilities and skills (Wigens, 2006). Endacott *et al.* (2004) describe four main forms of portfolio.

1 **The shopping trolley** – this resembles an unstructured resource file with many copies of articles and lecture notes.
2 **The toast rack** – more organized with evidence collated under learning outcomes but again with many photocopied articles.
3 **The spinal column model** – uses learning outcomes or competencies to structure the portfolio, with evidence and reflective accounts to support each one.

4 **The cake mix model** – a reflective commentary to demonstrate what has been learnt with evidence to support the learning.

Ideally, your portfolio should include your curriculum vitae, current job description, copies of relevant certificates and academic awards and a record of your learning activities and be based on models 3 or 4.

ACTIVITY 16.2

Reflection point
How current is your portfolio? What model do you think yours follows? Is it easy to understand and navigate? How would you improve it?

USING EVIDENCE TO DEMONSTRATE LEARNING THROUGH PRACTICE

You may have individual learning needs that have been identified as part of your personal development plan or have specific learning outcomes to achieve while you are in clinical practice. Learning outcomes are what it is intended that the learner will be able to achieve by the end of a period of learning. They can be categorized into three domains of learning: the cognitive domain considers knowledge outcomes and how information is acquired; the psychomotor domain relates to the development of skills and performance outcomes; and the affective domain refers to the formation of beliefs, attitudes and values.

Often the most difficult part of portfolio development is demonstrating how you have achieved the learning outcomes. Creating a learning contract helps the mentor and student share the responsibility for achieving desired outcomes. Learning contracts can help to increase accountability and can provide feedback to the learner regarding their progress towards meeting their agreed goals. A learning contract should include details of how you intend to achieve the learning outcomes, a review of outcomes which identifies what you have learned, with evidence of achievement included, dates of when each outcome has been met and a plan for future changes for the next practice period.

So how do you document your learning? Break the learning outcome down into manageable chunks. Consider what exactly you need to learn, how you will learn it, where you will learn and what help you will need. Consider splitting it up into theory, practice and progress (Table 16.1). You will find that this will become easier with practice.

Table 16.1 Documenting learning

Theory	Practice	Review/progress
Familiarize myself with – give some examples	Observe	What you have learned
Read – give some examples	Attend...	Any barriers to learning

Theory	Practice	Review/progress
Explore – give some examples	Carry out a...	Any further steps to be taken
	Participate in...	Any further deadlines
	Make contact with...	

LEARNING STYLES

Preference for a particular style of learning is not fixed and may change over time or with the type of skills you are trying to learn. There is no best or better style; all have equal value and only represent different ways of gaining knowledge. You may find that you learn better once you know how you learn. Begin by thinking about your beliefs and theories about a particular subject, as individuals learn in different ways and so there are many different learning styles. Knowing your learning style can also help you avoid repeating mistakes by undertaking activities that strengthen other styles.For example, if you tend to 'jump in at the deep end', consider spending time reflecting on experiences before taking action. Consider for a moment how you like to learn and which methods are most successful.

ACTIVITY 16.3

Reflection point

Can you identify an incident where you have learned something without being taught?

For example: you have been asked to teach a patient how to use their new glucometer. How would you ensure that you knew how to use it first? Would you:
• read the instructions booklet?
• ask someone to show you how to use it?
• try to work it out as you go along by trial and error?

A learning style refers to the way in which individuals process information. There are many models that help identify learning styles. In fact, Coffield *et al.* (2004) identified over 70 models of learning styles and categorized 13 of these into major models. These include models based on personality type (Myers and McCaulley, 1998) and flexible learning preference (Kolb, 1984; Honey and Mumford, 1992).

THE MYERS BRIGGS TYPE INDICATOR

The Myers Briggs Type Indicator (MBTI) is based on Jung's theory of the human psyche. This inventory considers normally observed personality traits and categorizes them into four pairs of preferences: attitudes, judging functions, perceiving functions and lifestyle. They are:

Attitudes: Extraversion (**E**) -------------- (**I**) Introversion
Judging: Sensing (**S**) ------------------------- (**N**) Intuition
Perceiving: Thinking (**T**) ---------------------- (**F**) Feeling
Lifestyle: Judgement (**J**) ------------------- (**P**) Perception

The results categorize individuals into one of 16 personality types such as **ISFP** (introversion, sensing, feeling, perception).

ACTIVITY 16.4

> **Reflection point**
> There are many online tools adapted from the MBTI that you could try such as those on www.businessballs.com.
>
> Having used one of the above tools, what are your thoughts on your own identified learning style?

KOLB'S LEARNING STYLES INVENTORY AND EXPERIENTIAL LEARNING THEORY

Kolb (1984) proposed that 'knowledge is created through the transformation of experience' and his theory of experiential learning combines behavioural and cognitive theories. Experiential learning is based on the notion that we bring our own ideas and beliefs to the learning situation and our understanding is not fixed but is reformed through experience. Kolb found that an individual will pass through all types of learning depending on what is being learnt as well as using their past experience, but suggests individuals will have one style in preference to others (Oliver and Endersby, 1994). Learning is seen as a continuous, cyclical process which works on two levels. A four-stage cycle of learning is shown in Fig. 16.1.

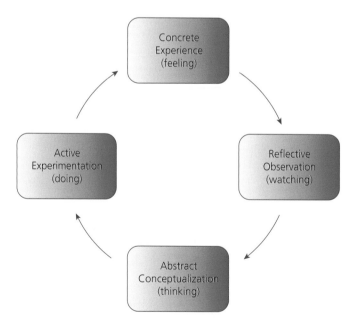

Figure 16.1 Kolb's experiential learning cycle.

- **Concrete Experience (feeling – CE)** – learners are fully involved in new experiences
- **Reflective Observation (watching – RO)** – reviews the experience, makes time and space to reflect

- **Abstract Conceptualization (thinking – AC)** – forms, reforms and processes ideas, takes ownership of and integrates ideas into logical theories
- **Active Experimentation (doing – AE)** – uses new understandings to make decisions, problem solve and test implications.

The second level is a four-type definition of learning styles, each representing the combination of two preferred styles, for which Kolb used the terms:

- Diverging (feeling and watching – CE/RO). Imaginative ability and generation of ideas, values people, enjoys being involved, likes novelty, good at brainstorming, easily bored, open-minded, feelings are emphasized more than thinking, places value on understanding rather than practical application of knowledge.
- Assimilating (watching and thinking – AC/RO). Creates theoretical models and makes sense of disparate observations, likes time to think, values facts and knowledge, is thorough and observant, likes time to reflect on what has been learned so that knowledge can be integrated into past experiences, avoids reaching conclusions, is scientific rather than artistic.
- Converging (doing and thinking – AC/AE). Practical application of ideas, likes knowledge that can be applied, is pragmatic, analytical and systematic, can reason, problem solve and make decisions, likes to know the logic behind the actions and observations, has an emphasis on thinking rather than feeling.
- Accommodating (doing and feeling – CE/AE). Carries out plans and tasks that involve them in new experiences, is intuitive, artistic and a risk taker, likes to see the results and enjoys technical hands-on activities, is receptive to new ideas, is open minded, likes things to happen quickly, learns by trial and error and so likes to experiment.

Kolb (1984) claims that an appreciation of different learning styles helps people to work more effectively in teams, resolve conflicts and communicate more effectively (Wigens, 2006). Understanding which learning style you are will help you to engage in learning and teaching activities. For example, Accommodators will enjoy role play, whereas Assimilators may prefer lectures.

HONEY AND MUMFORD'S LEARNING STYLES (1992)

Honey and Mumford (1992) developed their learning style questionnaire as a variation on the Kolb model and changed the four categories to:

- **Reflector (diverger)** reviews, stands back and observes, is cautious, takes a back seat, collects and analyzes data about experiences and events, is slow to reach conclusions, uses information from past, present and immediate observations to maintain a big picture perspective.
- **Theorist (assimilators)** concludes, thinks through problems in a logical manner, values rationality and objectivity, assimilates disparate facts into coherent theories, is disciplined, aims to fit things into rational order, is keen on basic assumptions, principles, theories, models and systems thinking.

- **Pragmatist (converger)** plans, is keen to put ideas, theories and techniques into practice, searches for new ideas and experiments, acts quickly and confidently on ideas, gets straight to the point, is impatient with endless discussion.
- **Activist (accommodator)** does, immerses themselves fully in new experiences, enjoys the 'here and now', is open minded, enthusiastic and flexible, acts first and considers consequences later, seeks to centre activities around themselves.

ACTIVITY 16.5

Reflection point
Which learning styles do you think will be most successful in clinical practice? Why do you think this is?

Reflectors learn best when they are observing others at work and have the opportunity to review what has happened and think about what they have learned.They are able to produce reports and essays when they do not have a tight deadline to meet. Reflectors learn less well when they are acting as a leader or role-playing in front of others. They do not like to do things when they have not had time to prepare and do not like being thrown in at the deep end or feeling rushed or worried by deadlines.

Theorists learn best when they are put in complex situations where they have to use their skills and knowledge. They like structured situations with a clear purpose where they have the chance to probe and question the ideas behind things. Theorists learn less well when they have to participate in situations which emphasize emotions and feelings. They do not like to do activities that are unstructured, where they do not know the principles or concepts involved or where the briefing is poor.

Pragmatists learn best when there is an obvious link between the topic and the job and are shown techniques with clear advantages such as saving time. They like to be shown a model that they can copy and enjoy role playing so that they have a chance to try out techniques with feedback. Pragmatists learn less well when there is no obvious or immediate benefit they can recognize. They do not like events or learning that are 'all theory' and dislike activities where there are no guidelines on how to do it and do not have an apparent payback to their learning, such as shorter meetings.

Activists learn best when they are involved in new experiences, problems and opportunities. They like being thrown in at the deep end with a difficult task and enjoy business games and team activities. They enjoy chairing meetings and leading discussions. Activists learn less well when they are listening to lectures or long explanations. They dislike reading, writing or thinking on their own, absorbing and understanding data and following precise instructions to the letter.

EDUCATIONAL THEORIES AND CLINICAL PRACTICE

There are many educational theories which can help you understand learning through practice. Some have common themes such as higher education and adult learning. There are a number of theories collectively termed behaviourist, cognitive and humanist and these will be considered in relation to healthcare environments.

There are two main stances to learning. It can be seen as outcome based or process based. Outcome-based learning is seen as where knowledge is taken in and absorbed and kept for future use. Gagné (1985) suggests that learning is systems based, where the key elements are the learner, the stimulus situation, the learner's memory and their response to the situation. Outcome-based learning may include intellectual skills, cognitive strategies and psychomotor skills. Process-based learning, on the other hand, entails a flexible network of ideas, knowledge and feelings, where learning is assimilated to modify understanding. Learning is grounded in experiences where interactions between the learner and the environment lead to the creation of new knowledge (Kolb, 1984).

Learning can be categorized into five levels, from surface to deep learning, where the deeper the learning, the more is understood. Marton and Saljio (1984) suggest five levels where the first three levels are perceived as surface learning and levels four and five are deep:

1 Learning is about increasing knowledge
2 Learning is about memorizing and remembering
3 Learning is about acquiring facts or skills to be used
4 Learning is about making sense and determining the meaning
5 Learning is about understanding reality.

So it is suggested that learning which is deep and process based is the most typically used in healthcare education programmes. Whether learning is meaningful depends on the learner's relationship with the new knowledge and is affected by the experience of others who are learning with them. Learning is usually a shared experience and can be influenced by many factors. Some of the factors that influence learning include age; status in family and society; language; social class; previous experience of learning; health status (physical and mental); shock or bereavement; stress or fatigue; intellectual ability (learning difficulties); disability, e.g. hearing or sight; and self-esteem.

ACTIVITY 16.6

Reflection point
What factors do you think may influence your learning?

As well as the process of learning, there are three main approaches to understanding learning: behaviourist, cognitive and humanist perspectives.

BEHAVIOURIST APPROACH

Behaviourist theories focus upon learning in terms of stimulus, response and reinforcement. These theories are based on forming associations, thus learning that certain events go together. Within **a classical conditioning** model, learning starts with an unconditioned (positive or negative) stimulus as demonstrated by Pavlov and his dogs, which associated food with a ringing bell and eventually salivated when they heard the bell, even if food was not present. **Operant conditioning**, on the other hand, concerns shaping behaviour through a process of positive and negative reinforcement. Skinner (1968) is perhaps the best-known behaviourist to demonstrate operant conditioning using the now famous Skinner's box. In his experiments, rats and other animals such as pigeons were placed in a box where pressing a bar resulted in the reward of food being delivered. After pressing the bar several times accidentally, the animal demonstrated that pressing the bar became intentional behaviour. Further experiments by Skinner showed that behaviour could be shaped by applying specific reinforcements, and he was able to teach animals some quite complex behavioural patterns. Operant conditioning contributes in a major way to learning. Reinforcement is not necessarily given in material rewards. In this theory, reinforcement will lead to a change in behaviour.

Consider how you could incorporate a range of methods of positive reinforcement into your teaching. In your clinical practice, this may be done by praising your student for a job well done or feeling confident with a new clinical skill you have learnt. Words of encouragement and praise, such as 'much better', 'well done', 'you're really getting the hang of it now', are probably the most obvious means of reinforcing correct behaviour. Non-verbal encouragement is equally important. Nods and smiles can be useful, especially while the skill is being practised. You might consider giving marks out of 10. All such rewards are aimed at enhancing self-esteem and self-confidence, at making the learner feel good about their performance of the new skill and more likely to maintain good technique.

But what about the learner who gets it wrong? Negative reinforcement, i.e. punishment in the form of put downs, criticism, sarcasm, decreases the possibility of unwanted behaviour but it fails to give the learner an alternative choice of behaviour. One way of overcoming the negative effects of criticism is to ask the learner how well he/she feels he/she is doing, e.g. you are nearly there, but what did you forget to do? Behaviourist theories of learning have importance and relevance to teaching. Behaviours that result in success or reward are more likely to be repeated than behaviours that do not. Learning should be regularly rewarded and the reward should follow immediately or as soon as possible after the desired behaviour.

COGNITIVE APPROACH

Cognitive psychologists argue that learning is not just explained in terms of stimulus–response association alone. Learning takes place as a result of interaction between new information being acquired and the existing cognitive structures. Thus it is the assimilation of new material with past experience that results in the formation of a new, more detailed cognitive structure. Cognitive learning is sometimes described as learning by problem solving. Learners are not seen as simply absorbing information but making tentative interpretations of experiences where feedback on learning is internal to the individual. Three factors need to be considered in order to achieve meaningful learning:

- the learner must be ready to learn
- material must be presented in a logical way, so that new material builds on old and it can be related to the learner's own cognitive structures

- the learner's own cognitive structures, e.g. memory, must contain specifically relevant ideas so that new information can be integrated with it.

SOCIAL LEARNING APPROACH

This type of learning straddles behaviourist and cognitive approaches. Learning by observation of role models is the basis for this theory. It is suggested that student nurses acquire much of their professional behaviour by a process of identification with skilled practitioners and imitate this behaviour until it becomes part of their own behavioural repertoire. The valuable roles played by preceptors and supervisors cannot be overestimated. They are not, however, without their pitfalls. It is generally recognized that not all practitioners make good preceptors and supervisors, that there is a need for appropriate preparation for the role and staff need support to undertake these roles.

ACTIVITY 16.7

Reflection point
Can you recall a mentor or colleague who was inspiring or a positive influence on your practice? Can you pinpoint why you think this was? What makes a good role model?

HUMANIST APPROACH

The focus of this perspective is on personal growth, the development of self-direction and interpersonal relationships. Learning is not just a behavioural change but changes in values, attitudes and beliefs where the goal is in self-actualization where an individual is able to fully express their talents, capabilities and potential. The humanist approach to learning is based mostly on the work of Carl Rogers (1969). His view is that individuals have an innate ability to learn together with a natural drive to do so. Following this theory, the teacher would take a non-directive approach, acting as a facilitator to the process of learning. The student would be encouraged to be creative, self-reliant and to self-evaluate. Mutual participation and respect of learner and teacher are key elements of this approach, with an emphasis on learning through experience.

Humanism is often linked to adult education, lifelong learning and the concept of andragogy (Knowles, 1985). Andragogy is defined as the 'art and science' of helping adults learn. Knowles (1985) explains how adults prefer to be actively involved, while initially needing support in the early stages of learning. There may need to be time for reorientation to prepare for self-directed study. Andragogy is based on six main assumptions:

1   Adults prefer to learn things that relate to real life
2   Adults are able to use their past experiences as a resource for learning
3   Adults are familiar with problem-solving and task-centred approaches
4   Adults are motivated by learning that leads to job satisfaction and improved quality of life
5   Adults need to know the reasons for learning new skills and knowledge
6   Adults can take responsibility for their own learning

Knowles (1985) suggests that adult learners respond best in a non-threatening learning environment where there is a good relationship between the teacher and learner. He views adult learners as self-directed, preferring a problem-orientated patient-based approach to learning.

ACTIVITY 16.8

Reflection point

Consider at least two ways in which you might apply the principles of adult education in one of the following situations:
- Teaching a daughter about nursing her elderly hemiplegic father at home following a stroke.
- Teaching a first-time mother about weaning.
- Teaching a student nurse on community placement about the roles of the members of the primary health care team.

There are numerous ways in which to incorporate the principles of adult education into teaching.

TEACHING AN ADULT CARER

First, the carer's knowledge and understanding of her father's condition would be assessed. Taking into account the adult as an independent learner, you may find that she has already got books from the library, used the Internet or other sources to help her. If not, you might suggest this, or that she contacts a self-help or voluntary organization for information and support.

You would also want to find out what previous experience she has of caring, such as child-rearing or caring for other dependent adults. By relating the demands of the new caring role with past experience, you may well be able to boost her confidence. For example, by comparing her ability to raise children to independence, including the pleasure and frustrations involved, you may be able to help the carer to understand the importance of encouraging her father to follow the recommended rehabilitation exercises and routines.

By acknowledging her unique situation, you will be able to put the information and teaching you are giving into context. For instance, her readiness to learn may be influenced by her own priorities. If her main concern is how to cope with her father's incontinence then that needs to be the first area of teaching, even if you feel that something else is more important.

TEACHING A FIRST-TIME MOTHER

Again you would want to assess the mum's existing knowledge. As an independent learner, she will probably have asked other people, such as her mother, sister or friends. She may have read information online or books on child-rearing. If not, you will probably want to give her some written material (in appropriate language) so that she can be helped to take an active role in learning and make informed decisions about weaning her baby.

You will probably want to find out what previous experience she has, such as weaning of younger siblings, nephews or nieces. Even if these experiences were not what you would recommend, they can still be used in the learning process. for instance by asking, 'Do you think it was a good thing for your niece to have packet foods and no home cooking?'

Adult learning is task or problem orientated (Knowles, 1985). By identifying the mother's need for information at the right time, you should be able to catch a teachable moment and make weaning more of a task and less of a problem.

TEACHING A STUDENT PRACTITIONER

It is probably appropriate to recognize him/her as an independent learner with a task or problem-solving orientation to learning. Therefore it may be a more effective teaching strategy to arrange for the student to meet the members of the primary healthcare team and ask them questions about their roles than to sit the student down and teach him/her.

Acknowledgement of previous experience and learning such as asking about recent study and experiences in his/her practitioner education and relating these to the task in hand will enhance the learning potential. For instance, you might ask about previous community placements or involvement in discharge planning and build on his/her relevant existing knowledge.

PLANNED TEACHING VERSUS OPPORTUNISTIC TEACHING

Here it is useful to use the analogy of the nursing process. In most situations planning care based on needs and goals is the best approach, with all concerned knowing what is to be expected of each other and of the planned care. However, unexpected situations, such as emergencies, can arise when there is no time to plan and action is required on the spot. The same applies to teaching and the analogy is valid since teaching is often part of the plan of care. On the whole, planning for teaching and recording the plan saves time in the long run since it prevents repetitions, omissions and confusion. It ensures continuity since all concerned are aware of the plans. A teaching plan also provides a framework for evaluation. A teacher/learner interaction that has been planned in advance can be described as formal teaching (Table 16.2).

However, unanticipated situations may occur when it is evident that teaching is appropriate at that very moment, i.e. opportunistic. You may recognize a 'teachable moment' when your student or client is clearly ready to learn. For instance, a client may ask a very pertinent question that it would be inappropriate not to deal with immediately, such as 'My baby always sleeps on his tummy, do you think that this is safe?' Or a student may be present when an ideal opportunity for teaching occurs. For instance, you may be driving through your patch with a student and he/she asks about the demography of the area. Opportunistic teaching, sometimes called informal teaching, takes advantage of the situation as it arises, but can be followed up with further planned teaching as necessary.

Table 16.2 An example of a teaching plan for the parents of a child with diabetes

The practitioner suggested the following:
Learners: Mr and Mrs Smith
Venue: Clinic
Date: 24/3/2012
Time: 10 am
Length of session: 30 minutes
Summary of learning needs: This session relates to the learning needs in relation to coping with illness, i.e. what to do if blood sugars become unstable, how to anticipate problems, when to seek medical advice.
Aim: To help Mr and Mrs Smith to develop an understanding of what to expect and what to do if their daughter becomes ill so that they will feel more confident about her care.
Objectives: By the end of the session Mr and Mrs Smith will be able to:

(i) List three situations in which their daughter's blood sugar is likely to become unstable
(ii) Describe what they should do if the blood sugar is raised
(iii) Discuss two situations in which they should consult the doctor.

Timing
Content
Teaching methods (including visual aids)

10.00
How illness affects diabetes
Explanation, discussion and handout

10.10
How to cope with high blood sugar levels
Discussion, questioning and handout

10.20
Causes for concern and occasions to seek medical advice, home visit or hospital treatment
Scenario, discussion and questioning

10.25
Review and questions
Discussion and questioning

Methods of evaluation and assessment: At the end of the session, she/he would go over the material and check their understanding by questioning. When she/he saw them again, she/he would ask them if they had thought about what was covered in the previous session and whether they had any questions. Self-evaluation and observation of the parents were used as part of the evaluation.

THE TEACHING PLAN

You may be planning for teaching a single session or a programme of learning. In either situation you should address the following questions in the planning:

- Why is teaching needed?
- Who is/are the learner/s?
- What are their learning needs?
- What are the aims and objectives?
- When is the teaching to take place and for how long?
- What is to be learned?
- What is to be taught?
- How are the teaching and learning to be evaluated?

You may wish to use a pre-formatted teaching plan or it may be incorporated into the client's notes or student's records. Whatever the format, the plan should be recorded, not least because you may wish to repeat the teaching on a different occasion. The teaching plan not only helps you to organize yourself and your materials, it also communicates to others involved in the learner's education what you have covered. This helps to prevent overlaps, omissions and confusion.

By planning in advance and writing down the factors needed in a teaching plan, you can consider the appropriateness of each factor and the plan can be modified accordingly. For instance, as you record where the teaching is to take place you can decide whether this venue will provide a suitable environment for learning and, if not, you may explore alternatives. Similarly, by identifying the time and duration of teaching and the teaching methods to be used you can question their appropriateness for the learner/s. You will need to consider such factors as how long can a tired carer concentrate effectively, or what is the best time of day for a group of busy parents?

ADVANTAGES AND DISADVANTAGES OF ONE-TO-ONE TEACHING

One-to-one teaching sessions can be advantageous as a rapport can be established more quickly, the learner gets the undivided attention of the teacher and individual progress can be monitored. However, individual teachings may mean that the learner feels under the spotlight and may miss the support of other learners. The learner may feel that the teaching is going too fast for him or her and may feel embarrassed if they do not learn quickly (Quinn, 2007). Careful consideration of the learner's individual needs will avoid these feelings and the teacher must ensure that the teaching session is pitched at the learner's level and pace.

PATIENT EDUCATION

Patient education is the process by which health professionals inform patients about their clinical condition and how best to manage it. By providing information and health promotion, it is hoped that patients will alter their health behaviours and improve their health status. Important elements of patient education are developing self-management skills and patients need to know when, how and why they need to make a lifestyle change. Each member of the patient's healthcare team needs to be involved in this process.

The value of patient education can be summarized as follows:

- Improved understanding of clinical condition and how to manage it.
- Patients have increased confidence, have less anxiety and feel more in control of their lives.
- Informed consent and increased concordance with treatment options and are willing to share responsibility for treatment.

- Improved patient outcomes – patients more likely to respond well to their treatment plan, have fewer complications, are less likely to suffer acute episodes requiring admission to hospital and have an improved quality of life.
- More effective use of healthcare services – fewer unnecessary phone calls and visits, patients can communicate better with health professionals.

There are many patient education models which provide structure guidance for practitioners on how to support their patients. In particular, the National Institute for Health and Clinical Excellence (NIHCE) guidance on Dose Adjustment for Normal Eating (DAFNE), which is a structured educational programme for people with type 1 diabetes that teaches individuals to adjust their insulin to match carbohydrate intake and lifestyle on a meal-by-meal basis (NIHCE, 2010).

The Expert Patients Programme (EPP) provides courses which are designed to help patients with long-term conditions – to give people the tools, techniques and confidence to manage their condition better on a daily basis (DH, 2001). Expert patients are defined as people living with a long-term health condition who are able to take more control over their health by understanding and managing their conditions, leading to an improved quality of life. Becoming an expert patient is empowering for people with chronic conditions. Expert patient courses normally run for two and a half hours per week for 6 weeks and are usually delivered by people who live with a long-term condition, or by people who have direct experience of living with someone who has a long-term condition.

In these programmes, people learn a variety of relevant skills, which include

- setting goals
- writing an action plan
- problem-solving skills
- fitness and exercise
- healthy eating
- relaxation skills
- communication with family
- working better with healthcare professionals, including communicating better with them
- making better use of medications.

ACTIVITY 16.9

Reflection point
Consider how you might teach one of these skills. What learning and teaching strategies would you choose, and why?

SMALL-GROUP TEACHING

Small-group teaching can be a very useful strategy for teaching patients, clients and their families and for formal and informal carers. Group size is important and it is recommended that the maximum number of participants should not be more than

10 (Quinn, 2007). Groups can be used for a variety of purposes such as discussions of health issues, demonstration of a particular skill or a class on a specific topic. Small-group teaching requires a good understanding of group dynamics and skills in facilitation. This method of teaching allows opportunities for face-to-face interaction with other group members in order to share ideas and feelings (Box 16.1).

Box 16.1 Principles of patient education

Say the important things first as patients are more likely to remember what was said at the beginning of the session.

Stress and repeat the key points. For example, you could say '*the most important thing for you to remember today is…*'

Avoid using jargon and long words when a short one will do.

Use visual aids, leaflets, handouts and written instructions.

Avoid saying too much in one session; three or four key points is all that you can expect someone to remember from one session.

Get feedback from patients to ensure that they understand.

For more information about patient education, see Chapter 12, 'Helping people to learn' in Ewles and Simnett (2003).

CONCLUSION

This chapter has examined learning through practice, what it is and why it is important, not only for your professional practice but for supporting the learning of others. This chapter has explored some of the theories about how people learn. It is clear that there is no one definitive theory, but that they all contribute to our understanding of how people acquire knowledge, skills and attitudes. If teaching is viewed as facilitating learning in others, then some comprehension of the process of learning is essential. The chapter should have helped you to make the best use of clinical learning opportunities, and given you some ideas about planning teaching for patient education, identifying individual learning needs and understanding the importantce of continuing professional development.

REFERENCES

Coffield F, Moseley D, Hall E and Ecclestone K (2004) *Learning Styles and Pedagogy in Post-16 Learning: A Systematic and Critical Review*. London: Learning Skills Research Council.

Department of Health (DH) (2001) *The Expert Patient: A New Approach to Chronic Disease Management for the 21st Century*. London: DH.

DH (2002) *Liberating the Talents*. London: DH.

DH (2007) *Skills for Health*. London: DH.

Endacott R, Gray M, Jasper M, McMullan M, *et al.* (2004) Using portfolios in the assessment of learning and competence: the impact of four models. *Nurse Education in Practice* 4:250–7.

Ewles L and Simnett I (2003) *Promoting Health: A Practical Guide*, 5th edn. London: Bailliere Tindall.

Gagné R (1985) *The Conditions of Learning*, 4th edn. New York: Holt, Rinehart & Winston.

Honey P and Mumford A (1992) *The Manual of Learning Styles*. Maidenhead: Peter Honey Publications.

Hull C, Redfern L and Shuttleworth A (2005) *Profiles and Portfolios*, 2nd edn. London: Palgrave Macmillan.

Knowles M (1985) *Andragogy in Action: Applying the Principles of Adult Education*. San Francisco, CA: Jossey Bass.

Kolb D (1984) *Experiential Learning: Experience as a Source of Learning Development*. Englewood Cliffs, NJ: Prentice Hall.

Marton F and Saljio R (1984) Approaches to learning. In Marton F, Hounsell D and Entwistle N (eds) *The Experience of Learning*. Edinburgh: Scottish Academic Press.

Myers I and McCaulley M (1998) *Manual: A Guide to the Development and Use of the Myers-Briggs Type Indicator*. Palo Alto, CA: Consulting Psychologists Press.

National Institute for Health and Clinical Excellence (NIHCE) (2010) *Final Appraisal Determination: Patient-education Models for Diabetes*. London: The Stationery Office.

Nursing and Midwifery Council (NMC) (2008a) *Standards to Support Learning and Assessment in Practice*. London: NMC.

NMC (2008b) *The Code: Standards of Conduct, Performance and Ethics for Nurses and Midwives*. London: NMC.

NMC (2010) *The PREP Handbook*. London: NMC.

Oliver R and Endersby C (1996) *Teaching and Assessing Nurses*. London: Bailliere Tindall.

Quinn FM and Hughes SJ (2007) *Quinn's Principles and Practice of Nurse Education*, 5th edn. Cheltenham: Nelson Thornes.

Rogers C (1969) *Freedom to Learn: A View of What Education Might Become*. Columbus, OH: Charles Merill.

Skinner BF (1968) *The Technology of Teaching*. Boston, MA: Prentice Hall College.

Wigens L (2006) *Optimising Learning through Practice*. Cheltenham: Nelson Thornes.

FURTHER READING

Gopee N (2011) *Mentoring and Supervision*, 2nd edn. London: Sage Publications.

Quinn F and Hughes S (2007) *Quinn's Principles and Practices of Nurse Education*, 5th edn. Cheltenham: Nelson Thornes.

Race P (2007) *The Lecturer's Toolkit: A Practical Guide to Assessment, Learning and Teaching*, 3rd edn. Abingdon: Routledge.

eHealth

Heather Bain

LEARNING OUTCOMES

- Explore the meaning of eHealth including the associated terminology of telehealth and telecare
- Appraise the suitability of eHealth for use within community nursing practice
- Explore the professional and ethical issues in the use of technology within community nursing
- Discuss the educational needs of the future eHealth community nurse

INTRODUCTION

One of the most significant developments in health and social care in recent years has resulted from the increased use of information and technology (IT), in particular the Internet and the World Wide Web. Considering the changing demographics of society and the fact that advances in technology can save time and money, national strategies are seeing eHealth as an approach to improve healthcare (Scottish Government, 2007; Cruikshank *et al.*, 2010; DHSSPS, 2011). All four UK countries have identified national IT programmes which support the diverging health policies in the UK countries and have developed supporting websites, which are identified in the further reading section. eHealth is about improving health outcomes, the safety of care and providing efficient care; it is not just about technology (NHS Scotland and the Scottish Executive Health Department, 2007). It is therefore clear that eHealth needs to be an integral part of nursing practice and it is important that community nurses have the underpinning knowledge relating to this technology and can use it effectively to meet the healthcare needs of individuals, families and communities. This chapter therefore aims to explore eHealth within community nursing. First, the associated terminology will be examined, then the evidence base to support its use using the management of people with diabetes in their own home as an example. Finally, some professional, ethical and contemporary issues will be considered specific to nursing in the community.

Action point

Before reading this chapter, draw a concept map/mind map/spider diagram outlining what you think eHealth is. Include in your map not only what you think eHealth is, but also its main features and the infrastructure that needs to be in place in order to effectively implement it in community nursing. You may wish to use this concept map to inform Activity 17.4.

THE TERMINOLOGY

eHealth

The term eHealth first appeared in the literature in the 1990s (Booth, 2006) but has since been increasingly and inconsistently used. The widespread use of the term suggests it is a significant concept that is commonly understood despite the lack of a precise definition. Oh *et al.* (2005) undertook a systematic review of definitions and identified 51 unique definitions with no clear consensus. However, they did identify two universal themes, health and technology, and six less mentioned themes of commerce, activities, stakeholders, outcomes, place and perspectives. Therefore, it can be concluded that the various definitions reflect different perspectives, settings and contexts where technology is used to support healthcare needs. The World Health Organization (2011), which was not included within this systematic review, encompasses the two universal themes and defines eHealth as the use of information and communication technologies for health to, for example, treat patients, pursue research, educate students, track diseases and monitor public health.

NHS Scotland and the Scottish Executive Health Department (2007) suggest eHealth is an umbrella term with wide parameters that include

- Internet or intranet to access health information by patients and healthcare professionals
- eLibrary to support access to literature and information
- teleconferencing, videoconferencing and computer-based learning applications to support education and clinical networks
- the use of mobile technology such as mobile phones and portable devices to record, view and communicate information
- email or other messaging devices to support communication
- telehealth to monitor, consult, diagnose or treat remotely
- the electronic health record
- software applications that support the management of health service resources.

Within this definition of eHealth it is recognized that there are many evolving terms encompassed, such as health informatics, nursing informatics, information communication technology, assistive technology, telemedicine, telenursing, telecare, telehealth, electronic patient record, and they are often used interchangeably (Cowie and Bain, 2011). It is not possible to cover them all in depth here; however, it is important that there is an understanding of the broad principles of the key terms, in order that technology can be used appropriately within the community.

Health and nursing informatics

Health informatics is the process of generating, recoding, classifying, storing, retrieving, analyzing and transmitting health information (RCN, 2010). Nursing informatics is similar in that it is the collection of data and use of information to support nursing practice. The term informatics has been used to cover information, technology processes, analytical tools and techniques, governance and the skills required to improve healthcare (DH, 2008). This encompasses the electronic patient record.

Electronic patient record

The electronic patient record is, as it sounds, an electronic copy of a person's nursing or medical record. The aim within the NHS is for a single integrated electronic health record to be available to authorized users, including the service user (RCN, 2010). In the UK the development of the healthcare record is at varying stages, with some GP surgeries having used electronic records for many years; however, the challenge is for the record to cross primary and secondary care boundaries, allowing access to authorized individuals while safeguarding patient confidentiality (Scottish Government, 2008).

Telehealth

Telehealth is the provision of health services at a distance using a range of digital technologies (JIT, 2011; Telecare Services Association, 2011). This can be to promote self-care, for example to enable a patient to monitor their own vital signs such as blood pressure, or from a monitoring perspective, physiological data could be transferred to a remote monitoring centre to allow for health professionals to intervene if measurements fall outside of expected parameters. The RCN (2010) suggests telehealth is an overarching term, as it is seen to be inclusive, focusing on health rather than illness, and it encompasses both telemedicine and telenursing, which can be defined as the practice of medical and nursing care using interactive audiovisual and data communication. The services could involve consultation, patient monitoring, diagnosis, prescriptions or treatment and can be done in real time or delayed through media such as teleconferencing, videoconferencing or the Internet. It should be a targeted approach to enhance service delivery focused around the service user, enabling a more efficient and effective use of clinical resources (Cruickshank *et al.*, 2010; NHS Scotland and the Scottish Executive Health Department, 2007).

CASE STUDY

Mrs A is a 31-year-old lady who has recently been diagnosed with type 1 diabetes. She has been commenced on twice daily insulin and has received education from the diabetic clinic at her local hospital, and has been followed up by her practice nurse. Her blood glucose levels remain unstable.

She is therefore identified as suitable for the telehealth programme until her blood glucose stabilizes. A telehealth monitor is installed in her home and she is shown how to connect her glucometer to the telehealth monitor.

Mrs A then daily carries out a monitoring session using the telehealth monitor. The monitor gathers her blood pressure, heart rate, oxygen levels and weight, and some data from prescribed questions. Finally, she connects her glucometer to the monitor and the readings from the past 24 hours are transmitted.

Her data are then analyzed by a triage nurse at the local community hospital. The triage nurse then contacts her to discuss the readings that are outside of normal limits and provides the relevant education and support. A weekly report is then sent to the diabetic clinic.

Following 8 weeks of this high intervention Mrs A's blood sugars stabilize and she is confident to self-care for her condition.

Telecare is defined as the use of communications technology to provide health and social care direct to the patient (Barlow *et al.*, 2007). Earlier development of telecare also referred to assistive technology and smart homes or smart technology (Sergeant, 2008). Assistive technology is another collective term for devices for personal use to enhance people's functional ability (JIT, 2011). It may include fixed assistive technologies such as stair lifts or portable devices such as bath seats. Therefore, this can include telecare, but is not limited to the kind of technology normally considered within eHealth.

Telecare has now become an umbrella term for all assistive and medical technology that enables people to maintain their independence in their own environment (Doughty *et al.*, 2007), which is more commonly their own home but it can be in any care setting. The Audit Commission (2004) identified three components of telecare: providing information; monitoring the environment; and monitoring the person. JIT (2011) has more recently categorized telecare into three generations.

- First-generation telecare refers to equipment found in most Community Alarm schemes. It involves user activation, for example a cord is pulled which triggers an alarm at a control centre where someone can organize a response of some kind. They have the benefit of providing 24-hour care; however, a major limitation is the reliance on the user to raise the alarm.
- Second-generation telecare is based on first generation but provides a more sophisticated and comprehensive support to managing risk and is less reliant on the user. It involve sensors to collect and transmit information, such as a door opening, movement within the home and bathwater running.
- Third-generation telecare is based on the automatic detection of the second generation, but with the increased availability of broadband, wireless and audiovisual technology it offers the potential for virtual or teleconsultations between the service user and the health professional or support worker. This has the potential to reduce home visits or hospital appointments and provides more opportunities for people unable to leave their own homes.

CASE STUDY

Mrs B is an elderly lady living in sheltered accommodation. She has a medical history of rheumatoid arthritis, angina, deafness and a history of falls.

Following discharge from hospital after a fall she was assessed by a district nurse who arranged for care workers to attend four times a day to meet her personal needs. However, Mrs B became increasingly confused and was getting out of bed and wandering through the sheltered housing complex at night.

Mrs B was then referred for a telecare assessment to identify the risks and to see if there were any interventions that could manage these risks. This resulted in the property being fitted with a wandering client detector (property exit device), flood detectors, a gas sensor and a bed sensor, which will detect if Mrs B has failed to return to bed in the time set. This ensures that if she gets out of bed and falls the warden can intervene accordingly.

Telehealthcare

Considering all the definitions above, it is evident that there are interrelationships between all the terms. Doughty *et al.* (2007) have reviewed the terminology used and acknowledge it will evolve as technology develops, although to avoid confusion the term telehealthcare may be more appropriate as it clearly integrates both telehealth and telecare. However, they suggest this does not necessarily include traditional forms of assistive technology. NHS 24 and the Scottish Centre for Telehealth (2010)also acknowledge this. Although there will be parallel developments between telecare and telehealth, as technology develops there will be the convergence of telecare and telehealth to provide effective high-quality healthcare, particularly around services delivered in the community. The key terms within eHealth are conceptualized in Fig. 17.1.

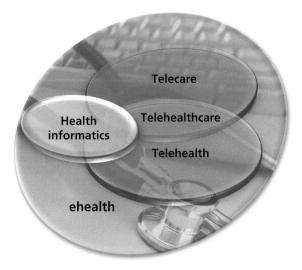

Figure 17.1 Diagram conceptualizing eHealth.

ACTIVITY 17.2

Discussion point

Considering the terminology of eHealth and areas of telehealth and telecare convergence, reflect on how eHealth can support your role as a community nurse.
• What are the challenges?
• What are the opportunities?

Taking into account all the various concepts within eHealth, it is clear that there are many overlaps and all have a potential use within community nursing. The opportunities and challenges are summarized in Table 17.1. There are also many ways that eHealth can be used by a variety of methods, some of which are identified in Table 17.2.

Table 17.1 Summary of opportunities and challenges of eHealth

Strengths	Challenges
Reinforces existing advice	May be expensive to develop
Overcomes challenges of distance	Lack of access to software and hardware
Addresses needs of remote and rural areas	Lack of eHealth in curriculum
Reduces unnecessary outpatient appointments	Technical problems and compatibility
Out-of-hours access	Relies on technical competence of staff and service users
Quicker access to specialist advice	Potential health and safety risk with equipment
Improved safety because of up-to-date recording of information	Maintaining confidentiality
Improved continuity of care	
Portable information	
Improved health outcomes	
Early diagnostic capability	
Evidence-based healthcare accessible to all 24 hourly	

Table 17.2 Examples of how eHealth can be used

Method	Example	Uses
Telephony	Mobile phones: calls and text	Message delivered via text to reinforce health education; phone applications to monitor health status
Videoconferencing	Patient monitoring	Remote advice from specialists
Internet/World Wide Web	Use of search engines and touch-screen internet kiosks	Accessing clinical decision support systems Provide healthcare advice and education
Digital imagery	Digital cameras, webcams, podcasts	Image of wound of housebound patient can be shared with specialist
Gaming	Games consoles	Interactive games can provide education
Email	Communication at a distance	Referral between health professionals

Method	Example	Uses
eHealth record	Patient-held medical record	Care pathways can be shared among professionals
Sensors	Fall detectors, flood detectors, smoke detectors, bed occupancy detectors	Allow high-risk people to stay in their own home
Electronic databases	Caseload management	Audit practice and aid planning

There have been several projects across the UK to ensure that eHealth becomes an integral part of community care provision. However, one of the challenges has been to accurately quantify the benefits, due to the small scale of the projects and the differing methods of evaluation. To further confirm the contribution of eHealth to healthcare, evaluation needs to integrate monitoring, outcomes and personalized feedback (Currell *et al.*, 2000; Verhoeven *et al.*, 2007).

EHEALTH TECHNOLOGY WITHIN COMMUNITY NURSING

Currently the evidence to support the use of eHealth and in particular telehealthcare by community nurses to manage individuals in the community is limited; however, as technology develops and eHealth is integrated within everyday practice the evidence base will be added to. This can provide a dilemma for the practitioner, who until the evidence gap is addressed faces difficult decisions about adopting such concepts into their practice. However, current government policy does support this development and it is clear that eHealth has huge potential, particularly in the management of long-term conditions at all three levels of the Kaiser Permanente triangle: supporting self-care; disease-specific care management; and case management (Cruikshank *et al.,* 2010).

The evidence base

Evidence does exist for the clinical effectiveness of telehealthcare in diabetes, mental health, high-risk pregnancy monitoring, dermatology, heart failure and cardiac disease (Bensink *et al.*, 2006; Barlow *et al.*, 2007). However, the evidence at the highest levels of reliability is variable. Using the management of people with diabetes within their own home as an example, a structured search of literature identified the following relevant systematic reviews and randomized controlled studies: Barlow *et al.* (2007), Boaz *et al.* (2009), Dale *et al.* (2009), Farmer *et al.* (2005), Garcia-Lizana and Sarria-Santamera (2007), Shea *et al.* (2006) and Verhoeven *et al.* (2007).

Garcia-Lizana and Sarria-Santamera (2007) undertook a systematic review focusing on clinical effectiveness, containing 24 randomized controlled trials, of which seven were for interventions specific to diabetes. It found telecare usually has the objective of educating patients and monitoring blood glucose. They found that more complex systems such as web-based medical records and permanent healthcare professional support achieved significant benefits in maintaining appropriate blood glucose levels.

A systematic review by Boaz *et al.* (2009), including 68 randomized controlled trials and 30 observational studies with 80 or more participants, examined the benefits of home telecare for frail elderly people and those with long-term conditions (31% of these studies focused on people with diabetes). This review identified three main functions: vital signs monitoring; safety and security monitoring; and information and support provided by the telephone and the Internet. However, the strength of evidence depends on the type of telecare application. The most effective intervention appeared to be vital signs monitoring and telephone monitoring by nurses for support. However, there was insufficient evidence in many of the other interventions to draw conclusions.

Verhoeven *et al.*'s (2007) systematic review of 39 studies to determine the benefits and deficiencies of teleconsultation and videoconferencing with diabetic clients found most of the reported improvements concerned satisfaction with technology, improved metabolic control and cost reductions. Improvements in quality of life, transparency and better access to care were hardly observed. Teleconsultation programmes involving daily monitoring of clinical data, education and personal feedback proved to be most successful in realizing behavioural change and reducing costs. Similarly a randomized controlled trial that demonstrated the feasibility of using telecommunications for motivation and support of clients provided inconclusive evidence of improved clinical outcomes or reduction in complications (Dale *et al.*, 2009). It also concluded telehealthcare is more valued if delivered by diabetic specialized nurses. However, it was recognized that using telecommunications does not suit all service users.

Another randomized controlled trial compared telehealthcare case management with usual care in older, ethnically diverse medically underserved patients with diabetes mellitus (Shea *et al.*, 2006). The telehealthcare involved in this study consisted of web-enabled computer connection with videoconferencing; remote monitoring of glucose monitoring; Internet access to patient's own clinical data and secure messaging with nurse case managers; and access to an educational website. In the intervention group blood glucose, blood pressure and cholesterol levels improved at 1-year follow-up. However, it must be noted that this was a medically focused study supported by medication changes by physicians.

Farmer *et al.* (2005) performed a systematic review to evaluate evidence for feasibility, acceptability and cost-effectiveness of diabetes telehealthcare applications. No conclusions were made relating to cost-effectiveness and they found no evidence to support the fact that telehealthcare interventions were effective in improving clinical outcomes, but it was seen as feasible and acceptable. Boaz *et al.* (2009) found similar results in their randomized controlled trial of participants with similar demographic and baseline diabetic profiles. No significant deficiencies were found in clinical outcomes, but patients in the telemedicine group reported being clinically symptom free more frequently. The telehealthcare group reported improved quality of life and sense of control with their diabetes.

From this literature it is evident that telehealthcare requires different clinical skills approaches to care, and the following practice recommendations can be made:

- Practitioners must assess the suitability of telehealthcare to manage healthcare needs on an individual basis.

- The use of telecommunications is feasible for the motivation and management of patients with long-term conditions, and can be cost-effective and reliable.
- Telehealthcare is feasible and acceptable for educating patients, monitoring and assessing clinical outcomes.
- Telehealthcare is more meaningful to service users if delivered by specialized nurses and prescribers.
- More complex systems such as web-based medical records and permanent healthcare professional support can achieve significant benefits in improving clinical outcomes.
- Effective management and improved clinical outcomes in the management of long-term conditions involves medicines management.

ACTIVITY 17.3

Action point

Identify an area of practice relevant to your role, access one of the websites from one of the UK countries and then undertake a small literature review to examine the evidence base to support the use of telehealthcare to manage healthcare needs in your chosen area.

Professional and ethical issues

A comprehensive understanding of professional and ethical issues is a fundamental part of community nursing and is discussed more fully in Chapter 3. This section therefore focuses on some of the main issues related to eHealth. Baker *et al.* (2007) explored professional and ethical issues that have emerged with the use of technology and articulated a gap between the potential of eHealth as positively perceived by eHealth leaders and the reality experienced by nurses in clinical practice. However, all respondents clearly identified the global eHealth future. Professional and ethical issues of eHealth can all be directly mapped to the Nursing and Midwifery Council's (NMC, 2008) code of conduct and in particular to the following clauses:

1. You must act as an advocate for those in your care, helping them to access relevant health and social care, information and support.

5. You must respect people's right to confidentiality.

6. You must ensure people are informed about how and why information is shared by those who will be providing their care.

12. You must share with people, in a way they can understand, the information they want or need to know about their health.

13. You must ensure that you gain consent before you begin any treatment or care.

24. You must work cooperatively within teams and respect the skills, expertise and contributions.

35. You must deliver care based on the best available evidence or best practice.

46. You must ensure any entries you make in someone's electronic records are clearly attributable to you.

ACTIVITY 17.4

Reflection point

Reflect on the case examples of telehealth and telecare provided in this chapter, or examples of the use of eHealth available in your area of practice, and consider the following:
* What are the professional and ethical issues?
* How can eHealth support you to manage healthcare needs in the community in a more effective and timely manner?

While undertaking Activity 17.4 many professional and ethical issues will have been identified. You may also have considered the following issues.

Access to information

Assessment of individuals, families, carers and communities as identified in Chapters 1, 7, 8 and 9 is a core skill in community nursing to address healthcare needs. However, often the first assessment of a change in health status is not undertaken by a health professional, but by the individual. The Picker Institute (2006) estimated that a third of the 80% of people actively accessing information about their health first do it through the Internet. Increasingly information is accessed via a search engine on the Internet. Although there are many benefits to this, such as quicker access to information, there is the danger that service users can access incorrect information or it can be of variable quality (BMA, 2010). However, the NHS in the UK provides much credible information to the public via the Internet promoted through media campaigns. For example, NHS Direct online allows users to check their symptoms online and provides advice accordingly. User friendliness is an important consideration as many older people are not familiar with such technology, and therefore alternative methods may be used to access information, such as telephone help services, NHS Direct or NHS 24, for a similar purpose. This technology is changing the balance of power between health professionals and the public. However, it provides nurses with the opportunity to empower and enable people (RCN, 2010), which has always been a key concept within community nursing practice (NMC, 2001, 2004).

Decision-making

When an individual chooses to consult with a community nurse or is referred to a community nurse, eHealth can play a supportive role in the decision-making process of the assessment. Clinical decision support systems can be utilized for this purpose (RCN, 2010). Increasingly, these clinical decision systems are being integrated with electronic patient records or are applications that can be downloaded onto a mobile phone and are therefore a useful tool for the community nurse, who is often working in people's homes. However, as with all expert systems, they should be seen as tools and not as a replacement to clinical judgement. In fact, Courtney *et al.* (2008) suggest that to maintain safe practice, clinical decision systems should be developed to address the differing needs of various practice levels.

Equity and access to services

A major challenge in addressing healthcare needs within the community is the concept that everyone should have equal access to services regardless of where they live, which has been a core concept of the NHS since its inception. This can be considered on two levels: first, access to clinical services and, second, equity of access to eHealth services (Audit Scotland, 2011). However, often there is a sound reason for unequal approaches to addressing healthcare needs. For example, third-generation telecare relies on the availability of broadband; however, in some social housing this is not yet available, or patients may not have the ability to adapt to such technology. This is when the concepts of telehealthcare need to be embedded into care pathways, and, following the assessment of the service user, have suitable exit criteria for its use (Cruikshank *et al.*, 2010) and the use of ethical frameworks by the practitioner needs to accompany this process (Eccles, 2010).

It is clear from considering the above that the professional and ethical issues in the use of eHealth are similar to other areas of nursing practice and many of the skills are transferable. However, the focus can be different and there is a need to develop new approaches and additional knowledge to use eHealth efficiently and effectively to address healthcare needs in the community.

EDUCATING THE FUTURE EHEALTH COMMUNITY NURSE

It is evident that technology will not address healthcare agendas unless practitioners are provided with the education (Booth, 2006) to use it effectively. However, currently nursing education programmes provide little in relation to the necessary knowledge, skills and practice competencies required for nurses to practise in the evolving eHealth world (Scottish Government, 2009). The emphasis in the current curriculum is on computer literacy rather than information literacy and eHealth. Community nurses need to understand the technology and be confident in its use to adequately address healthcare needs (RCN, 2010). It is suggested that particularly undergraduate nursing must take a proactive approach to integrating eHealth within the curriculum, and educators should take a leading role in this (Booth, 2006). The NMC *Standards for Pre-registration Nursing Education* (2010) acknowledge the importance of nurses being competent in the use of technology.

Learning to Manage Health Information (NHS Information Authority, 1999) has been the source of guidance within the UK. The *Learning to Manage Health Information: A Theme for Clinical Education* (NHS Connecting for Health, 2009) provides guidance and suggested learning outcomes for informatics in education.

It is aimed at clinical educators, commissioners, policy-makers and regulatory and professional bodies. It covers seven main themes:

- protection of individuals and organizations
- data, information and knowledge
- communications and information transfer
- health and care records
- the language of health: clinical coding and terminology
- clinical systems and applications
- eHealth: the future direction of clinical care.

Within these themes there are learning outcomes to achieve depending on whether it is a first professional qualification, postgraduate qualification or continuing professional development, or for clinical and management development.

ACTIVITY 17.5

Training need analysis

Access Learning to Manage Health Information: A Theme for Clinical Education (NHS Connecting for Health, 2009). Reflect on your role. Make a self-assessment on your knowledge and skills by completing a tool such as in the table below. Consider any supporting evidence and then identify any areas where you would benefit from further training, education and development.

Outcome: Clinical systems and applications	1	2	3	Evidence
1. Demonstrate understanding of how and why information technology is able to support clinical practice and new ways of working				
2. Demonstrate understanding of the functionality of the clinical systems and applications used in healthcare practice				
3. Demonstrate understanding of the advantages and disadvantages of patient-focused versus speciality, procedure or disease-focused systems				
4. Demonstrate understanding of the key NHS national projects initiatives and developments in the field of healthcare information technology				

1. I require training and development in most or all of this area
2. I require training and development in some aspects of this area
3. I am confident I already do this competently

There will obviously be a period of transition required to address the learning needs of the current workforce, including existing practitioners and educators, as well as undergraduate students in relation to eHealth. The NHS 24 and Scottish Centre for Telehealth (2010) in their strategic framework identify that local training programmes are required to facilitate the use of communication technology for existing staff as well as actively promoting the inclusion of telehealthcare teaching in all core curriculums for pre-registration, doctors, nurses, midwives and allied health professions.

CONCLUSION

This chapter has provided an overview of eHealth considering some of the key terminology. The suitability of its use has been briefly explored within community nursing and some of the associated professional and ethical issues have been highlighted. It is recognized that eHealth is not just about technology, it is about using technology to communicate more effectively to address healthcare needs. Although eHealth is becoming an integral part of government policy, applying the principles in practice can be a challenge and it is therefore essential that healthcare professionals are provided with appropriate education and training to prepare them for the development of eHealth.

REFERENCES

Audit Commission (2004) *Implementing Telecare: Strategic Analysis and Guidelines for Policy Makers, Commissioners and Providers*. London: Audit Commission.

Audit Scotland (2011) *A Review of Telehealth in Scotland, Project Brief*. Edinburgh: Audit Scotland.

Baker B, Clark J, Hunter E, *et al.* (2007) *An Investigation of the Emergent Professional Issues Experienced by Nurses when Working in an eHealth Environment*. Bournemouth: Bournemouth University.

Barlow J, Singh D, Bayer S and Curry R (2007) A systematic review of the benefits of home telecare for frail elderly people and those with long term conditions. *Journal of Telemedicine and Telecare* 13:172–9.

Bensink M, Hailey D and Wotton R (2006) A systematic review of successes in home telehealth: preliminary results. *Journal of Telemedicine and Telecare* 12:8–16.

Boaz M, Hallman K and Wainstain J (2009) An automated telemedicine system improves patient-reported wellbeing. *Diabetes Technology and Therapeutics* 11:181–6.

Booth R (2006) Educating the future eHealth professional nurse. *International Journal of Nursing Education Scholarship* 3:article 13.

British Medical Association (BMA) (2010) *Health Information: Finding Reliable Sources on the Internet*. (Accessed 8 April 2011) www.bma.org.uk/patients_public/finding_reliable_healthcare_information/healthinfonet.jsp.

Courtney K, Alexander G and Demiros G (2008) Information technology from novice to expert: implementation implications. *Journal of Nursing Management* 16:692–9.

Cowie J and Bain H (2011) Development and implementation of policy – communities and health. Scottish perspective. In Porter E and Coles L (eds) *Policy and Strategy for Improving Health and Wellbeing*. Exeter: Learning Matters.

Cruikshank J, Beer G, Winpenny E and Manning J (2010) *Healthcare Without Walls, A Framework for Delivering Telehealth at Scale*. London: 2020health.org.

Currell R, Urqhart C, Wainwright P and Lewis R (2000) Telemedicine versus face to face patient care: effects on professional practice and health care outcomes. *Cochrane Database of Systematic Reviews* Issue 2: CD002098.

Dale J, Caramlau I, Sturt J, *et al.* (2009) Telephone peer-delivered intervention for diabetes motivation and support: The telecare exploratory RCT. *Patient Education & Counselling* 75:91–8.

Department of Health (DH) (2008) *Health Informatics Review.* London: DH.

Department of Health Social Services and Public Safety (DHSSPS) (2011) *Living with Long Term Conditions, A Policy Framework.* (Accessed 14 March 2011) www.dhsspsni.gov.uk/living_with_long_term_conditions_-_consultation_docum.

Doughty K, Monk A, Bayliss C, *et al.* (2007) Telecare, telehealth and assistive technologies – do we know what we are talking about? *Journal of Assistive Technologies* 1:6–10.

Eccles A (2010) Ethical considerations around the implementation of telecare technologies. *Journal of Technology in Human Service*s 28:44–59.

Farmer A, Gibson O, Tarassenko L and Neil A (2005) A systematic review of telemedicines interventions to support blood glucose self-monitoring in diabetes. *Diabetes UK* 22:1372–8.

Garcia-Lizana F and Sarria-Santamera A (2007) New technologies for chronic disease management and control: a systematic review. *Journal of Telemedicine and Telecare* 13:62–8.

Joint Improvement Team (JIT) (2011) *National Telecare Development in Scotland, Glossary of Terms and Definitions.* (Accessed 4 January 2011) www.jitscotland.org.uk/action-areas/telecare-in-scotland.

NHS Connecting for Health (2009) *Learning to Manage Health Information: A Theme for Clinical Education.* London: NHS Connecting for Health.

NHS Information Authority (1999) *Learning to Manage Health Information.* Birmingham: NHS Information Authority.

NHS 24 and Scottish Centre for Telehealth (2010) *Scottish Centre for Telehealth Strategic Framework 2010–2012.* Aberdeen: Scottish Centre for Telehealth.

NHS Scotland and Scottish Executive Health Department (2007) *NHS Scotland eHealth Strategy – The Nursing, Midwifery and Allied Health Professions' Contribution to Realising the Benefits of the National eHealth Programme.* (Accessed 8 April 2011) www.ehealthnurses.org.uk/pdf/NMAHP%20eHealth%20Action%20Plan.pdf.

Nursing and Midwifery Council (NMH) (2001) *Standards for Specialist Education and Practice.* London: NMC.

NMC (2004) *Standards of Proficiency for Specialist Community Public Health Nurses.* London: NMC.

NMC (2008) *The Code: Standards of Conduct, Performance and Ethics for Nurses and Midwives.* London: NMC.

Nursing and Midwifery Council (NMC) (2010) *Standards for Pre-registration Nursing Education.* London: NMC.

Oh H, Rizo C, Enkin M and Jadad A (2005) What is eHealth: A systematic review of published definitions. *Journal of Medical Informatics* 7(1).

Picker Institute (2006) *Assessing the Quality of Information to Support People in Making Decisions about their Health and Healthcare.* (Accessed 8 April 2011) www.pickereurope.org/page.php?id=48.

Royal College of Nursing (RCN) (2010) *Putting Information at the Heart of Nursing Care.* London: Royal College of Nursing.

Scottish Government (2007) *Better Health, Better Care.* Edinburgh: Scottish Government.

Scottish Government (2008) *Better eHealth, Better Care.* Edinburgh: Scottish Government.

Scottish Government (2009) *NMAHP eHealth Education Project: Scoping of and Recommendations for pre-Registration NMAHP Curricula*. Edinburgh: Scottish Government.

Sergeant E (2008) *Aberdeenshire Council Telecare Project*. (Accessed 8 November 2010) www.aberdeenshire.gov.uk/about/departments/AberdeenshireTelecareProjectEvaluationReport.pdf.

Shea S, Weinstock R, Starren J, *et al*. (2006) A randomised trial comparing telemedicine case management with usual care in older, ethnically diverse medically underserved patients with diabetes mellitus. *Journal of the American Medical Information Association* 13:40–51.

Telecare Services Association (2011) *Telehealth and Telemedicine*. (Accessed 4 March 2011) www.telecare.org.uk/information/42290/46200/telehealth_and_telemedicine.

Verhoeven F, van Gemert-Pijnen L, Dijkstra K, *et al*. (2007) The contribution of teleconsultation and videoconferencing to diabetes care: a systematic literature review. *Journal of Medical Internet Research* 9:5.

World Health Organization (2011) *eHealth*. (Accessed 2 March 2011) www.who.int/topics/ehealth/en.

FURTHER READING

Royal College of Nursing (2006) *Use of Text Messaging Services. Guidance for Nurses Working with Children and Young People*. London: RCN.

FURTHER RESOURCES

The eHealth programme in each country can be found by going to the following websites:

www.connectingforhealth.nhs.uk – England

www.wales.nhs.uk/ihc – Wales

www.ehealth.scot.nhs.uk – Scotland

www.dhsspsni.gov.uk – Northern Ireland

Other useful resources are:

www.ehealthnurses.org.uk – Health Nurses Network

www.jitscotland.org.uk/action-areas/telecare-in-scotland – Joint Improvement Team: Telecare in Scotland

www.telecare.org.uk –Telecare Services Association

Development of community nursing in the context of changing times

Anne Smith and Kirsten Jack

LEARNING OUTCOMES

- Identify the key policy drivers that impact on delivering effective healthcare
- Examine the new ways of working that are emerging in response
- Analyze personal skills development that may enable practitioners to contribute more effectively
- Explore the impact of enhanced skills such as non-medical prescribing on the delivery of services

INTRODUCTION

It is important to have a working understanding of health policy in order to contextualize the changes that are occurring in commissioning, managing and delivering community services. The four nations of the UK are responsible for managing their own NHS services. This is achieved in different ways according to the priorities set by each one, but the principles are common to all. There is a common commitment across the four nations to integrate primary and secondary care provision, aiming for a smoother transition for patients between the two, but more importantly trying to reduce hospitalization by anticipating potential problems and providing support services to prevent admission. There is an increasing emphasis on public health and health promotion. It is recognized that with the changing demographics in the population, with life expectancy now extended, services must be reconfigured to respond. A higher percentage of the population is now living with long-term conditions or terminal illnesses, increasing the challenges on health and social care services. The nations face similar issues trying to devise a workable framework on which to base their service delivery. These will be explored further within this chapter.

Since its inception the NHS has been a service free to all, but there has been a conceptual shift away from illness orientation and paternalism over recent years to a more egalitarian approach, with the user taking interest and responsibility for making decisions about their care. The language has changed from that of 'patient', suggesting dependency, to that of 'client', 'consumer' or 'service user', all of which suggest a partnership approach (Hinchliff *et al.*, 2008). The 'Expert Patient' programmes (DH, 2001) were indicative of this shift of emphasis. These programmes were designed to enable people to become more confident in making educated decisions about their condition and their care, rather than relying on professionals.

This chapter will first briefly examine the ways in which healthcare is managed by the devolved governments of the UK. The underlying influence is one of financial austerity, resulting from the economic difficulties currently being experienced across all sectors. Essentially the challenge for staff is to reflect on current practice and consider whether this is ritualistic and routine. Practitioners will be required to adopt effective and efficient approaches in a climate driven by limited financial resources.

KEY POLICY DRIVERS THAT IMPACT ON DELIVERING EFFECTIVE HEALTHCARE

England

The implications of the Department of Health White Paper *Equity and Excellence: Liberating the NHS* (DH, 2010a) will have far-reaching consequences. The paper defined the government's vision that the NHS should become 'the largest and most vibrant social enterprise in the world' (36, 4.21). The need for practitioners to demonstrate innovation and efficiency has never been more necessary. The government is trying to engage front-line staff in developing new ways of working to provide a service that is fit for purpose. There is an emphasis on developing 'social enterprise' as a model of service provision, but many people are sceptical, perhaps due to lack of familiarity with the model, or the inability to work through the demanding bureaucracy surrounding it (Milton, 2010). Following the publication of the White Paper there was widespread discontent, to the extent that the reforms were put on hold and a 'listening exercise' instigated. The NHS Futures Forum was established to examine the substance of the White Paper and collate responses from professionals who expressed concerns about the content of the Bill. In summary the revised Bill 'proposes to create an independent NHS Board, promote patient choice, and to reduce NHS administration costs'.

Key areas

- Establish an independent NHS board to allocate resources and provide commissioning guidance
- Increase GPs' powers to commission services on behalf of their patients
- Strengthen the role of the Care Quality Commission
- Develop Monitor, the body that currently regulates NHS foundation trusts, into an economic regulator to oversee aspects of access and competition in the NHS
- Cut the number of health bodies to help meet the government's commitment to cut NHS administration costs by a third, including abolishing Primary Care Trusts and Strategic Health Authorities (Parliament, 2011).

The White Paper (DH, 2010a) recommended the dissolution of Strategic Health Authorities and Primary Care Trusts (PCTs) and the introduction of Practice

Based Commissioning (PBC) with the GP taking responsibility for 80% of the NHS budget. The original idea of GP 'consortia' has been replaced by Clinical Commissioning Groups (CCGs) and the members of these must be representative of the local stakeholders. The requirements for membership have been revised to be more representative. Crucially the groups must include a nurse member and a specialist doctor. The major implications of the White Paper are concerned with commissioning and service delivery. The consequences surrounding the new proposal about commissioning will be immense, and the plan to combine the management of service provision across the acute and primary care sectors will have implications for all staff. Those individuals and groups with entrepreneurial skills have already seen the potential associated with the reorganization (Duffin, 2011).

The Royal College of Nursing (RCN) and Queens Nursing Institute (QNI) responded promptly to the White Paper, particularly in relation to primary care, as this is where most patient contact occurs and most patient journeys commence. In its position statement (RCN, 2010a) the RCN recognized that practitioners are operating in a rapidly changing landscape. The document stresses the importance of nurses' role in shaping and delivering services. There is concern over the increasing use of skill mix within nursing teams, with healthcare assistants (HCAs) being employed and educated to adopt roles previously undertaken by qualified nurses. However, their role is not regulated and the RCN has identified their vulnerability, with debate around whether they should be permitted to become full members of the RCN. In a toolkit devised by the RCN (2010b) to guide HCA development as part of the Working in Partnership Programme (WIPP), their role is defined as 'someone who works under the guidance of a qualified healthcare professional' (RCN, 2010b, Unit 2: 2). Lepper (2010) cautions that while there is definitely a place for HCAs, until their training is as rigorously monitored as registered nurse education, their roles must be carefully considered within the environments in which they are employed.

Meanwhile the QNI promoted a campaign, 'Right Nurse, Right Skills' (QNI, 2011) which highlighted the necessity to ensure that nurses working in the community are appropriately educated to undertake their roles, as often they are working alone and unsupervised in patients' homes.

Scotland

In Scotland, social care has been free for some time (Scottish Government, 2010a), which is at variance with England. This is a significant variation that also has financial implications as the elderly population increases, because the financial burden of such a policy could well become unsustainable. The devolved governments have some autonomy to operate in different ways and this has an impact on the management of services. Implementation of the NHS Scotland Quality Strategy (Scottish Government, 2010b) aims to ensure public participation, improve access and maintain safety. Already the emphasis has been shifted to consider anticipatory care rather than reactive treatment options. The key themes were influenced by the impact of caring for the ageing population, recommending that a proactive and anticipatory approach was needed. One action resulting from this was closer support and supervision of the most vulnerable, and the creation of personal care plans for the 5% of the population with the most complex needs (Scottish Government, 2010b: 7). Other major strategies have also been developed, for example to assist with caring for patients with dementia or cancer. This is set against the background of the modernization programme which commenced with the introduction of the Modernization Community Nursing Board in December 2009 (RCN, 2010a). The Board's main aim was to provide a more cohesive approach to the delivery of community services across Scotland. The 'Remote and Rural Healthcare Action Plan' (Scottish government, 2008) identified that 79% of the Scottish population live in remote or rural locations and life expectancy in these areas is the third worst in Scotland. The Scottish government commissioned the development of a toolkit to support the work of the Modernization Board. NHS Education for Scotland (NES) is examining the educational requirements of the workforce and a framework is to be developed to ensure that the community workforce offers safe, effective and person-centred care (QNIS, 2010).

Wales

The Welsh Assembly has taken a radical approach by removing the 'internal market' and implementing an integrated organizational structure. The detail concerning how this will be effected was set out in *Setting the Direction* (WAG, 2009). The reorganization took place in 2009, creating seven Local Health Boards (LHBs) responsible for all aspects of healthcare in their area. The purpose of this strategy was to improve the delivery of community-based services in Wales by adopting a more integrated approach between the sectors that offer support in the community. Interestingly, a primary principle of this strategy is to encourage 'citizens' to 'develop confidence in their ability to manage their own health' (p. 6). This reinforces the sentiment stated previously that ultimately the service user is being handed some responsibility as well as being involved in the decisions that affect their care. Like Northern Ireland, another decision taken regarding health care in Wales is that there are no prescription charges (Health in Wales, 2007), with Scotland following in 2011. This decision was taken in Wales in 2007 in an attempt to reduce health inequalities, as it was considered that this policy discriminated against patients who could not afford prescription charges as they were unable to receive their medication. A contributory factor was the variability in exemptions, particularly for those with long-term conditions, some of whom qualified for free prescriptions and others who did not.

Northern Ireland

Health and social care in Northern Ireland is more integrated than in the other countries of the UK. Concern about budget cuts and the potential effect on front-line services and patient care was highlighted in 2010 by the Director of the RCN in Northern Ireland, Janice Smyth. A document published in March 2010, *Healthy Futures*

(DHSSPSNI, 2010), identified a looming crisis in primary care focusing particularly on the needs of children. This provided a strategic overview of the issues affecting vulnerable children and families and demonstrated that early interventions should be considered to channel services to these groups. Health visitors and school nurses were the professionals targeted to make a difference in offering front-line interventions.

Community nursing services have also come under the spotlight and a consultation document was published in June 2011 (DHSSPSNI, 2011). Key messages that emerged from this related to the pivotal role of the district nurse in providing person-centred care in the community. The document advises that care management must include a proactive and anticipatory approach rather than a reactive one. The need to move funding across to community services from the acute sector is highlighted and a model of 'outreach' and 'in reach' suggested (p. 55) which would enable staff to rotate between the sectors. This was further supported by the intention for district nurses to have a presence within the secondary care sector to facilitate discharge planning and thus enable a more seamless approach to patient care. It also identifies that patients with long-term conditions would benefit from a care management approach (p. 52). This had already been piloted with 600 patients and demonstrated positive outcomes. This model mirrors that adopted in England with the introduction of community matrons (DH, 2005). The report suggested that district nurses, if appropriately trained, could fulfil the role of the care manager.

ACTIVITY 18.1

Discussion point
Examine the relevant government policy and/or professional guidelines that relate to your area of work. Consider how changes in your work place have been influenced by the policy decisions made at national or local level.

All four countries recognize the benefits of shifting balance of care from the acute sector to the community. While there are differing opinions on how to develop health services, all the nations are challenged with the same issues associated with the changing demographics of the population. People are living longer, but associated with this is the potential for ill health and compromised quality of life. It is clear that one approach to coping with the increased demand on services is to proactively seek out and support the highest users of services. However, in tandem with this there is the need to actively promote a healthy lifestyle for individuals, families and communities. Community nurses have a key role in delivering this new policy agenda and the new models of care emerging across the UK offer opportunities for community nurses to develop new ways of working (Dickson *et al.*, 2011).

NEW WAYS OF WORKING

It is clear that all nations of the UK are examining how the workforce can be organized to promote efficiency and effectiveness. Employers are being urged to consider deploying resources (including staff) in new ways. Lord Crisp, former Chief Executive of the NHS, has warned that too many resources have previously been ploughed into hospitals and that investing in primary care is the solution to sustaining the future of the NHS (2011). He recognized that this was the best approach to managing the situation where the greatest demand is from an ageing population with long-term conditions.

This approach is coupled with another key element of government health strategy across the four UK countries concerned with increasing the focus on public health. More emphasis is placed on healthy behaviours and this was firmly endorsed by a recent publication in England (DH, 2010b). The Minister for Health defended the White Paper by saying that the intention was to 'nudge' the population into adopting healthy behaviours rather than preaching to them. Anne Milton, Junior Minister for Health, stated that the government was committed to reducing the bureaucracy that often acts as a barrier to realizing innovation (Milton, 2010). Chapter 2 explored these issues. Milton cited the example of the 'family nurses' project that has been piloted following the success of the Sure Start Programmes (DH, 1999). Initially funded by PCTs, their work is largely with teenage mothers, giving support on parenting and on other lifestyle issues such as smoking cessation and healthy eating. Evaluation research of the first 10 projects was very positive (Barnes *et al.*, 2009) and this project is now being introduced in Scotland. Anne Milton suggested that there will be more scope for nurses to establish social enterprises to run such initiatives as this. In line with the public health focus, there are many examples of practitioners developing innovative services. However, funding streams will need to be identified if such ventures are to be supported.

Proactive rather than reactive care was the ideal behind the introduction of the role of the community matron in England (DH, 2005). This was an initiative driven by the Department of Health based on the Evercare model that had provided positive results in the United States. Funding was ring-fenced to support the venture. Community matrons were to adopt a case finding and case management approach to offer holistic care to vulnerable older people in the community with long-term conditions. The key objective was to prevent hospital admissions and therefore to reduce the pressure on hospital beds. Chapman *et al.*'s (2009) research identified that 5 years on, the outcomes of this initiative appeared to have missed the target, but patient satisfaction with the service was high. Community matrons are an expensive commodity and their future is uncertain. Local implementation of their role has varied tremendously and tension has been caused with community nursing teams due to lack of clarity about their roles and caseloads. One example of a successful intervention is with care home residents in Cumbria, where community matrons have reviewed medication and advised care home staff on other general care issues. This demonstrated measurable savings in the drug budget but also achieved other positive outcomes in relation to reduced hospital admissions and GP visits (Sprinks, 2010). In Scotland and Northern Ireland, as indicated earlier, the principles embodied within the community matron role, such as anticipatory care and reduction in hospital admission, have been adopted, although the key player in their introduction has been the district nurse.

Audit and community (or practice) profiling are useful tools with which to examine the uptake and the success of services, as previously discussed in Chapters 1 and 7. In order to provide cost-effective, appropriate care, audit and evaluation are essential (Jack and Holt, 2008). Without such data it is difficult to justify changing services. Front-line practitioners should be proactively involved in this process, contributing to the decision on changes. The QNI (2010) has cautioned that nurses may well end up as merely the 'passengers' as the governmental reforms take place. However, there are opportunities for staff to contribute to the agenda. Burke and Sheldon (2010) describe the benefits of using such information-gathering models as the 'World Café' model. This is an exercise organized at local or national level in which groups of practitioners meet in a relaxed café-style environment in order to network and share ideas about new ways of working and innovative approaches.

This model was utilized to explore the 'Transforming Community Services' (TCS) initiative in England (DH, 2010c), a programme with a variety of work streams examining the Quality Innovation, Productivity and Prevention agenda (QUIPP). This calls for practitioners to be personally equipped with the skills to engage with the vision which aims to transform services in the community in several key areas. There will be an increasing emphasis on public health and illness prevention but equally there is a focus on care of the dying as one of the categories is end-of-life care. This type of consultation enables nurses to be actively involved at a critical time when services are being reshaped.

The whole idea of nurses being at the forefront of service redesign can seem daunting and the concept of new business approaches such as creating a social enterprise is alien to many nurses. Rather than being viewed as passengers (QNI, 2010), the community nursing workforce remains central to the implementation of these far-reaching reforms. It is pertinent to explore social enterprise in more depth to see the relevance of this model to the modern-day NHS.

SOCIAL ENTERPRISE AS AN EMERGING RESPONSE

Social enterprise is not a new term and is closely linked to the concept of social marketing. Social marketing (Lefebvre, 2003) is a concept underpinned by empowerment, with the focus on the service user taking responsibility for their wellbeing. This is an ideal which many community nurses already promote in their current day-to-day practice, for example promoting an egalitarian approach when managing chronic disease such as diabetes. However, Lefebvre (2003) also suggests, that social marketing is 'a problem solving process that may suggest new and innovative ways to attack health and social problems' (2003: 220) and this is where social enterprise may be a useful concept to consider.

An early example of such a model is that of Mary Seacole, who set up a social enterprise aimed at providing healthcare through hotels in the late nineteenth century (Dawes, 2009). Any profits made from the hotel were then used to buy medicines to treat British soldiers. A more recent example is that of university lecturer Barbara Hastings Asatourian, who invented a board game aimed at taking embarrassment out of sexual education. Her social enterprise has grown and she has developed many more products to assist in the delivery of contraception education (Cahalane, 2010).

Social entrepreneurs have a social rather than business focus (Leadbetter, 1997), tending to reinvest profits into the enterprise rather than take it for themselves. Motivation to become a social entrepreneur may be due to what are traditionally described as 'push' or 'pull' factors, for example community nurses may be 'pushed' into entrepreneurial activity due to unemployment, or 'pulled' by the attraction of greater independence (Granger *et al.*, 1995). Indeed independent nurse practitioners can now find themselves in the position of employing salaried general practitioners (Baraniak and Gardner, 2001) in deprived communities, pulled by the opportunities to develop healthcare in these areas.

The ideals of social enterprise may seem attractive to many although internationally only 1% of registered nurses are nurse entrepreneurs (ICN, 2004). Nurses may perceive that they do not have the relevant skills or knowledge to be able to set up a social enterprise. In addition those who have many years of NHS pension contributions may not want to give up the financial security by branching out alone (DH, 2006). Traynor *et al.* (2006) suggest factors such as lack of mentorship and business support for entrepreneurs, the need to combine family and business responsibilities, and lack of self-belief and self-confidence as being prohibitive factors. Indeed, it could be suggested that nurses are not prepared during their undergraduate pre-registration education to even consider this sort of activity as a future option. The move to an all-graduate profession may have some impact on this perception and the new NMC standards (NMC, 2010) acknowledge the need for nurses to adapt to changing needs of service users and communities. However, it may be difficult for nurses to know where to start and the barriers to starting a social enterprise may seem too great. When considering whether there is potential to develop a service the EPOCH model (Entreprenurses, 2008) may be valuable. This model consists of a set of questions with each question feeding into the next one. It encourages the nurse entrepreneur to consider what their strengths are, who would benefit and the potential commissioners (Box 18.1).

Box 18.1 EPOCH model (Entreprenurses, 2008)

1. What are you **E**xcellent at?
2. What **P**eople would benefit?
3. What are the **O**utcomes?
4. Who would **C**ommission it?
5. **H**ow much would the commissioner pay?

The RCN (2007) has published supportive guidance aimed at nurse entrepreneurs who are looking to set up their own enterprise, exploring issues such as becoming self-employed and providing advice on costs and cash flow, for example.

Discussion point
Read the RCN (2007) publication *Nurse Entrepreneurs. Turning Initiative into Independence* in more detail. Then consider this model and apply it using a scenario related to an area of personal interest.

PERSONAL SKILLS DEVELOPMENT AND MANAGING CHANGE

In order to continue to work in an arena that is constantly changing and manage services effectively, it is imperative for practitioners to develop personal skills in managing and coping with change. They must be able to critically reflect on their current roles and have the ability to respond by having the appropriate skills in leadership and management to effect change, whatever their role. The morale of the workforce is dependent on the motivation and enthusiasm that can be generated despite the regular requirement to implement and adjust to change. However, it could be argued that the expectation that practitioners can adjust, frequently not knowing what the system is about, and then provide high-quality outcomes, is unrealistic. There is a personal cost related to instability which may manifest itself either physically or psychologically (Nazarko, 2007). Individuals may feel a sense of loss or feel uncertain about their future in the new system. Transition has to be managed carefully and for change to be successful all parties need to understand and sign up to the vision. Leadership is a crucial aspect of the change process and much has been written about how to develop leadership potential among staff (Taylor, 2010). Clinical leadership is discussed in Chapter 15. Interestingly, while leadership is a quality frequently defined and discussed it is equally important for that leader to be supported by a good follower. As Whitehead *et al.* (2007) suggest, 'followership' is not a passive role but requires the individual to display active participation towards achieving the common goal. The follower is there to support the leader and to provide critical feedback on the progress of the change. The leader is reliant on the advocacy of their colleagues. Although not everyone is able to perform the leadership role, the supporting cast has a vital part to play in ensuring that change is implemented effectively and sustained. Maintaining a balanced approach is conducive to reducing the stress that inevitably accompanies change. It has been suggested that emotional intelligence (Goleman, 1998) is a quality that helps leaders and followers to manage the uncertainties often associated with the change process. If the practitioner has a range of coping strategies within their personal armoury they will be better placed to manage the demands of the constantly fluctuating environment.

There is a wide range of models that can be of assistance when examining the process of change within the organization, which also explore the rationale for change. Theoretical frameworks can be helpful in determining the forces that will impact on the change process. The Department of Health published a document in 2001 (Iles and Sutherland, 2001) called *Managing Change in the NHS* in which it proposed a variety of models that may provide frameworks for underpinning the change process at organizational level. It identified models such as 'PESTELI' and the '5 whys', both of which could be applicable in certain situations. The PESTELI model is defined in Box 18.2.

Box 18.2 PESTELI model

P – determine any political factors influencing the need to change

E – economic constraints impacting on the process

S – social determinants such as the changing demographics of the population or cultural changes

T – technological changes or aspirations can be either a help or hindrance to change and innovation

E – environmental issues including moving work place bases may provoke anxiety

L – legal aspects of any change must be carefully considered.

I – A recent addition to the model has been a consideration of the 'industry'. As the NHS is increasingly becoming a business environment, with Foundation Trusts, GP consortia and other business models emerging for the commissioning and delivery of services, this will influence the change arena.

The '5 whys' model can trace problems back to a root cause to enable a solution to be found. It is best applied to more specific situations rather than the broader application of the previous model. It is important to use the model that is best suited to the change being considered.

DEVELOPING ENHANCED SKILLS TO CONTRIBUTE TO THE NEW AGENDA

Different ways of delivering care are emerging in all areas of the NHS. Some of these changes were generated by the Darzi report (DH, 2008). Lord Darzi reviewed the NHS workforce in England, which then led to the publication of a new NHS constitution with far-reaching consequences (Lilley, 2008). It contained a range of ideas including the move for nursing to become a graduate profession. One initiative that had national interpretation was the introduction of 'Darzi centres', which basically were offering a multitude of services under one roof, a 'one stop shop'. There was a commitment to enabling the general public easy access to care without the need to book a doctor's appointment. 'Darzi centres' were also to stay open for longer hours than surgeries and were intended also to reduce the pressure on A&E departments. The employers mainly relied on nurse practitioners to staff these centres. It was imperative therefore that practitioners were able to operate autonomously for these centres to achieve their targets.

Other services that have developed over recent years are telephone support systems such as NHS Direct and NHS 24. Again the intention was to divert patients from attending A&E unnecessarily. There is an abundance of examples of new and innovative ways of working but in order for these to have an impact it is essential that the workforce is appropriately trained. Within general practice various services such as telephone triage, minor illness clinics and disease-specific clinics are increasingly available, all of which are managed by nurses. Technology is being embraced increasingly to supplement face-to-face care, as discussed in Chapter 17. These services are heavily reliant on having the right nurse with the appropriate skills to manage them.

One aspect of skills development that has become more firmly established in the last few years is non-medical prescribing. This has had a huge influence on the roles adopted by nurses. As independent prescribers were legally able to prescribe from virtually the whole British National Formulary (BNF) their roles also extended to take over certain roles previously only undertaken by doctors (Brookes and Smith, 2007). The NMC issued the Standards for Prescribing (2006) but the devolved governments in the UK have been responsible for the development of prescribing within their own country and the governance issues surrounding it. Services have been transformed through this extension of the nurse's role, with the evolution of services such as Walk-In Centres and Out of Hours rapid access centres. The NMC has also expanded the use of the Community Nurses Formulary (NMC, 2009), previously only available for specialist practitioners to prescribe from, to enable appropriately qualified community staff nurses to prescribe from this formulary. Historically non-medical prescribing has been an important factor in expanding the nurse's role and has been the trigger for the introduction of a variety of services, and it continues to evolve.

CONCLUSION

The NHS and primary care are in the midst of radical change. Professional nursing organizations are campaigning throughout the UK nations to ensure that standards are not compromised by the new agenda. Community nurses must ensure that they are involved in the decisions about how services will be developed. It is crucial that practitioners prepare to assert themselves as key members of the primary care team, demonstrating the range of skills that they bring to contribute to the emerging landscape.

REFERENCES

Baraniak C and Gardner L (2001) Nurse-led general practice for nurses, doctors and patients. In Lewis R, Gillam S and Jenkins C (eds) *Personal Medical Service Pilots.* London: King's Fund, pp. 75–87.

Barnes J, Ball M, Meadows P, *et al.* (2009) Nurse-family partnership programme second year pilot sites implementation in England. The infancy period. *Primary Care Nursing* 19:6–8.

British Medical Association and Royal Pharmaceutical Association (2009) *The Nurse Prescribers' Formulary for Community Practitioners.* London: BMJ Group and RPS Publishing.

Brookes D and Smith A (eds) (2007) *Non-medical Prescribing in Healthcare Practice. A Toolkit for Students and Practitioners.* Basingstoke: Palgrave.

Burke C and Sheldon K (2010) Encouraging workplace innovation using the 'world cafe' model. *Nursing Management* 17:14–19.

Cahalane C (2010) *The CIC Profile: Contraception Education.* (Accessed 27 October 2010) www.socialenterpriselive.com.

Chapman L, Smith A, Williams V and Oliver D (2009) Community Matrons: primary care professionals' views and experiences. *Journal of Advanced Nursing* 65:1617–25.

Cooper C (2010) Remote control. *Nursing Standard* 25:18–19.

Cross Government Obesity Unit (2008) *Healthy Weight Healthy Lives. A Cross Government Strategy for England.* London: HMSO.

Dawes D (2009) How nurses can use social enterprise to improve services in health care. *Nursing Times* 105:22–5.

Department of Health (DH) (1999) *Health Service Circular 199/002:LAC 99(1) Sure Start.* (Accessed 1 December 2010) www.dh.gov.uk/prod_consum_dh/groups/dh_ digitalassets/@dh/@en/documents/digitalasset/dh_4012568.pdf.

Department of Health (2001) *The Expert Patient: A New Approach to Chronic Disease Management in the 21st Century.* London: HMSO.

DH (2003) *General Medical Services Contract.* (Accessed 1 November 2010) http:// webarchive.nationalarchives.gov.uk/+/www.dh.gov.uk/en/Managingyourorganisation/ Workforce/Paypensionsandbenefits/GPcontracts/index.htm.

DH (2005) *Supporting People with Long Term Conditions.* London: Department of Health.

DH (2006) *Our Health Our Care Our Say: A New Direction for Community Health Services.* London: HMSO.

DH (2008) *High Quality Care for All: NHS Next Stage Review Final Report.* London: HMSO.

DH (2010a) *Equity and Excellence: Liberating the NHS.* London: HMSO. (Accessed 1 November 2010) www.dh.gov.uk/prod_consum_dh/groups/dh_digitalassets/@dh/@ en/@ps/documents/digitalasset/dh_117794.pdf.

DH (2010b) *Healthy Lives, Healthy People. Our Strategy for Public Health in England.* London: HMSO. (Accessed 1 December 2010) www.dh.gov.uk/prod_consum_dh/ groups/dh_digitalassets/@dh/@en/@ps/documents/digitalasset/dh_122252.pdf.

DH (2010c) *Transforming Community Services.* (Accessed 1 November 2010) www.dh.gov. uk/en/Healthcare/TCS/Abouttheprogramme/DH_121964.

Department of Health, Social Services and Public Safety (DHSSPSNI) (2010) *Healthy Futures 2010–2015: The Contribution of Health Visitors and School Nurses in Northern Ireland.* Belfast: DHSSPSNI. (Accessed 20 February 2010) www.dhsspsni.gov.uk/ healthy_futures_2010–2015.pdf.

DHSSPSNI (2011) *A District Nursing Service for Today and Tomorrow. Consultation Document. Supporting People at Home.* Belfast: DHSSPSNI.

Dickson C, Gough H and Bain H (2011) Meeting the policy agenda, part 1: the role of the modern district nurse. *British Journal of Community Nursing* 16:495–500.

Duffin C (2011) Wider representation on new consortia puts nurses in the spotlight. *Primary Health Care* 21:6–7.

Entreprenurses CIC (2008) *How the EPOCH Business Model Will Increase Your Turnover or Your Money Back.* (Accessed 8 November 2010) www.entreprenurses.net.

Foresight (2007) *Tackling Obesities: Future Choices.* London: Government Office for Science.

Goleman D (1998) *Working with Emotional Intelligence.* New York: Bantam Books.

Granger B, Stanworth J and Stanworth C (1995) Self employment career dynamic: the case of the 'Unemployment Push' in United Kingdom book publishing. *Work, Employment and Society* 9:499–516.

Health in Wales (2007) *Free Prescriptions for Wales Approved.* (Accessed 1 November 2010) www.wales.nhs.uk/news/6081.

Hinchliff S, Norman S and Schrober J (2008) *Nursing Practice in Health Care*, 5th edn. London: Hodder Education.

Iles V and Sutherland K (2001) *Managing Change in the NHS: Organisational Change: A Review for Healthcare Managers, Professionals and Researchers.* London: National Co-ordinating Centre for NHS Delivery and Organisation R and D.

International Council of Nurses (2004) *Guidelines on the Nurse Entre/intrapreneur Providing Nursing Service.* Geneva: ICN.

Jack K and Holt M (2008) Community profiling as part of a health needs assessment. *Nursing Standard* 22:51–6.

Leadbetter C (1997) *The Rise of the Social Entrepreneur.* London: Demos.

Lefebvre C (2003) Social marketing and health promotion. In Bunton R and Macdonald G (eds) *Health Promotion. Disciplines, Diversity and Developments,* 2nd edn. London: Routledge.

Lepper J (2010) The role and regulation of health care assistants. *Independent Nurse* 17 May:32–3.

Lewin K (1958) *Field Theory in Social Science.* New York: Harper and Row.

Lilley R (2008) Social enterprise will be your future employer. *Primary Health Care* 18:12–13.

Milton A (2010) Nurses can adapt to new models of care. *Nursing Standard* 24:12–14.

Nazarko L (2007) Primary Care reconfiguration: managing the transition. *Primary Health Care* 17:14–16.

NHS Education for Scotland (NES). Edinburgh. (Accessed 1 November 2010) www.nes.scot.nhs.uk/disciplines/nursing-and-midwifery.

Nursing and Midwifery Council (NMC) (2006) *Standards of Proficiency for Nurse and Midwife Prescribers.* London: NMC.

NMC (2009) *Standards of Education for Prescribing from the Nurse Prescribers Formulary for Community Practitioners for Nurses Without a Specialist Practitioner Qualification – Introducing code V150.* London: NMC.

NMC (2010) *Standards for Pre-registration Nursing Education.* London: NMC.

Queen's Nursing Institute (QNI) (2010) *Position Statement March 2010. Nursing People in their Own Homes – Key Issues for the Future of Care.* London: QNI.

Queen's Nursing Institute (QNI) (2011) *Nursing People at Home: the Issues, the Stories, the Actions.* London: QNI.

Queen's Nursing Institute Scotland (QNIS) (2010) *News – Framework for Community Nursing.* Edinburgh: QNIS. (Accessed 29 November 2010) www.qnis.org.uk/index.php?option=com_content&view=article&id=51&Itemid=128.

Royal College of Nursing (RCN) (2007) *Nurse Entrepreneurs. Turning Initiative into Independence.* London: RCN.

RCN (2010a) *Pillars of the Community. The RCN's UK Position on the Development of the Registered Nursing Workforce in the Community.* London: RCN. (Accessed 27 August 2010) www.rcn.org.uk/__data/assets/pdf_file/0007/335473/003843.pdf.

RCN (2010b) *WIPP Healthcare Assistants Toolkit Unit 2. The Employment of Health Care Assistants in General Practice.* London: RCN. (Accessed 17 February 2011) www.rcn.org. uk/__data/assets/pdf_file/0007/159442/unit2.pdf.

Scottish Government (2008) *Delivering for Remote and Rural Healthcare.* Edinburgh: Scottish Government. (Accessed 1 December 2010) www.scotland.gov.uk/Resource/ Doc/222201/0059769.pdf.

Scottish Government (2010a) *Free Personal and Nursing Care in Scotland.* Edinburgh: Scottish Government. (Accessed 1 November 2010) www.scotland.gov.uk/Topics/ Health/care/17655.

Scottish Government (2010b) *The Healthcare Quality Strategy for NHS Scotland.* Edinburgh: Scottish Government. (Accessed 1 December 2010) www.scotland.gov.uk/Resource/ Doc/311667/0098354.pdf.

Smyth J (2010) *RCN Warns of Threat to Frontline Services in Northern Ireland.* London: RCN. (Accessed 17 December 2010) www.rcn.org.uk/newsevents/news/article/ northern_ireland/rcn_warns_of_threat_to_frontline_services_in_northern_ireland.

Sprinks J (2010) Nurse Prescribers boost patient well being and satisfaction levels. *Nursing Standard* 25:8.

Taylor R (2010) Leadership theories and the development of nurses in Primary Care. *Primary Care Nursing* 19:40–5.

Traynor M, Davis K, Drennan V, *et al.* (2007) *The Contribution of Nurse, Midwife and Health Visitor Entrepreneurs to Patient Choice: A Scoping Exercise.* London: NCCSDO.

UK Parliament (2011) *Health and Social Care Bill 2010.* (Accessed 9 September 2011) http:// services.parliament.uk/bills/2010–11/healthandsocialcare.html.

Welsh Assembly Government (WAG) (2009) *'Setting the Direction'. Primary and Community Services Strategic Delivery Programme.* Cardiff: Welsh Assembly Government. (Accessed 27 August 2010). www.wales.nhs.uk/sitesplus/867/opendoc/157 072?uuid=4E4F17BD–1143–E756–5C1BCD843D069AE5.

Whitehead D, Weiss S and Tappen R (2007) *Essentials of Nursing Leadership and Management,* 4th edn. Philadelphia, PA: F.A. Davis Co.

FURTHER READING

Dickson C, Gough H and Bain H (2011) Meeting the policy agenda, part 1: the role of the modern district nurse. *British Journal of Community Nursing* 16:495–500.

Iles V and Cranfield S (2004) *Managing Change in the NHS: Developing Change Management Skills.* London: SDO.

Iles V and Sutherland K (2001) *Managing Change in the NHS: Organisational Change: A Review for Healthcare Managers, Professionals and Researchers.* London: National Co-ordinating Centre for NHS Delivery and Organisation R and D.

Royal College of Nursing (RCN) (2006) *Policy Briefing 04/2006 Nurse Led Social Enterprise.* London: RCN.

RCN (2010) *Pillars of the Community. The RCN's UK Position on the Development of the Registered Nursing Workforce in the Community.* London: RCN.

INDEX

Page numbers in *italics* refer to boxes, figures and tables.